# PSYCHOLOGICAL THEORIES OF DRINKING AND ALCOHOLISM

THE GUILFORD ALCOHOL STUDIES SERIES
HOWARD T. BLANE AND DONALD W. GOODWIN, EDITORS

# PSYCHOLOGICAL THEORIES OF DRINKING AND ALCOHOLISM

Edited by
**HOWARD T. BLANE AND KENNETH E. LEONARD**
*State University of New York at Buffalo*

The Guilford Press
NEW YORK    LONDON

PRINTED IN THE UNITED STATES OF AMERICA

**Library of Congress Cataloging-in-Publication Data**

Psychological theories of drinking and alcoholism.

Includes bibliographies and indexes.
1. Alcoholism—Psychological aspects. 2. Drinking of
alcoholic beverages—Psychological aspects. I. Blane,
Howard T., 1926–    . II. Leonard, Kenneth E.
[DNLM: 1. Alcohol Drinking. 2. Alcoholism—psychology.
WM 274 P9744]
HV5045.P74    1987        616.86′001′9        86–18472
ISBN 0–89862–166–6

# Contents

# II
## RECENT THEORETICAL MODELS

# 10

## Opponent Process Theory                                         346

THOMAS E. SHIPLEY, JR.

# 11

## Conclusion                                                      388

KENNETH E. LEONARD AND HOWARD T. BLANE

# Contributors

DAVID B. ABRAMS, PhD, Division of Behavioral Medicine, The Miriam Hospital, Brown University, Providence, Rhode Island.

STEVEN BERGLAS, PhD, Department of Psychiatry, Harvard Medical School/ McLean Hospital, Boston, Massachusetts.

HOWARD T. BLANE, PhD, Research Institute on Alcoholism and Department of Psychology, State University of New York at Buffalo, Buffalo, New York.

SANDRA A. BROWN, PhD, Veterans Administration Medical Center and Department of Psychiatry, [University of California, San Diego, San Diego, California.

HOWARD CAPPELL, PhD, Addiction Research Foundation and University of Toronto, Toronto, Ontario, Canada.

BRUCE A. CHRISTIANSEN, PhD, Mt. Sinai Medical Center, Milwaukee, Wisconsin.

W. MILES COX, PhD, Veterans Administration Medical Center and Department of Psychiatry, Indiana University School of Medicine, Indianapolis, Indiana.

MARK S. GOLDMAN, PhD, Department of Psychology, University of South Florida, Tampa, Florida.

JANET GREELEY, MA, Addiction Research Foundation and University of Toronto, Toronto, Ontario, Canada.

JAY G. HULL, PhD, Department of Psychology, Dartmouth College, Hanover, New Hampshire.

KENNETH E. LEONARD, PhD, Research Institute on Alcoholism and Department of Psychology, State University of New York at Buffalo, Buffalo, New York.

RAYMOND S. NIAURA, MS, Division of Behavioral Medicine, The Miriam Hospital, Brown University, Providence, Rhode Island.

STANLEY W. SADAVA, PhD, Department of Psychology, Brock University, St. Catharines, Ontario, Canada.

KENNETH J. SHER, PhD, Department of Psychology, University of Missouri, Columbia, Missouri.

THOMAS E. SHIPLEY, Jr., PhD, Department of Psychology, Temple University, Philadelphia, Pennsylvania.

# 1 Introduction

HOWARD T. BLANE

KENNETH E. LEONARD

This volume on psychological theories of drinking and alcoholism is a testament to the growing maturity of thinking and research about the initiation and maintenance of drinking, the principles that govern transitions between one drinking status and another, and the interrelations among individual, situational, and sociocultural variables. This volume also recognizes and responds to needs to summarize and systematize the large body of psychological research and theory that has accumulated during the past 40 years and to provide a common forum for theoretical models that have been recently proposed. The impetus for embarking on this project grew out of conversations between the editors concerning the lack of suitable texts for undergraduate and graduate courses on alcoholism. There are, to be sure, any number of excellent reviews on specific topics of interest to psychologists buried away in the ubiquitous all-purpose volume, but there is virtually no single source the psychologically minded reader can turn to that provides comprehensive coverage in depth within a historical context. This seems all the more deplorable considering recent developments in the field that suggest that the psychological study of alcohol is fast becoming an area of specialization in its own right. These developments include the proliferation of research in the past 10–15 years, the increased sophistication in methods and conceptualizations, and the formalization of a growing "invisible college" of colleagues. There is little doubt that the force behind these developments was the creation of a Federal presence, including monies, in the alcohol area, represented by the establishment in 1970 of the National Institute on Alcohol Abuse and Alcoholism. Historically, however, psychological research on alcohol began much earlier.

HOWARD T. BLANE and KENNETH E. LEONARD. Research Institute on Alcoholism and Department of Psychology, State University of New York at Buffalo, Buffalo, New York.

1

While studies of the acute effects of alcohol on psychomotor and cognitive functions occurred as early as the mid-1800s, modern psychological research on alcohol dates from about 1940, when the Yale Center of Studies on Alcohol was established along with the *Quarterly Journal of Studies on Alcohol*.[1] Much of the early research was atheoretical and guided implicitly by the Zeitgeist, dominated on the one hand by psychoanalysis and its offshoots, and by Hullian learning theory on the other. The notion of tension reduction, while formalized by learning theorists, initially appealed to adherents of both schools of thought. Subsequently, however, two divergent traditions emerged: personality studies deriving from a psychodynamic orientation, and laboratory studies focusing upon tension reduction. From the 1960s, social learning and interactional approaches added to earlier traditions without supplanting them. These four broad approaches to understanding drinking still play vital roles in alcoholism research and theory, and form significant aspects of the nexus out of which contemporary models have developed. That is to say, one cannot fully appreciate these newer models without knowing the conceptual–empirical background from which they emerged.

The impact of the availability of federal funds on psychological research on alcohol only began to be felt in the mid-1970s, and has been increasing significantly since that time. This impact has meant greater integration between mainstream psychology and the alcohol field, manifest in several ways: There are more psychologists in alcohol research and, due to competition for funding, its quality, as measured by publication in American Psychological Association and other refereed journals and presentations at major professional meetings, has increased. More students are exposed to knowledgeable mentors, and recent PhDs with a background in alcohol research are increasingly sought after. The number of universities with major research programs in alcohol studies is growing and there is a sense that no solid graduate program in psychology should be without an alcohol studies component. There has always been an "invisible college" of colleagues working in the alcohol field. This "college," so necessary to intellectual vigor, has grown among psychologists to the point that it was recently formalized as the Society of Psychologists in Addictive Behaviors, a group of a few hundred psychologists, many of whom are engaged in alcohol-related work. The formation of the society is a step preliminary to achieving status as a division of the American Psychological Association.

More important than these organizational and professional indicators of growth and stability, however, are the substantive effects on theory and research. The increased integration of psychological alcohol research with its

---

[1] The Center moved from Yale University to Rutgers University in 1961; the *Quarterly Journal of Studies on Alcohol* is now the *Journal of Studies on Alcohol*.

parent discipline has led to several salutary developments: important conceptual developments in alcohol theory occur concurrently with theoretical developments in psychology; methodological refinements in psychology are quickly reflected in alcohol research; and there is greater reciprocity concerning conceptual–empirical advances in psychology and in alcohol studies.

Until recently, alcohol theory and research were highly dependent upon theoretical developments within psychology, with relatively little theorizing emanating from within the field itself. Thus, we saw studies of alcoholics around field dependence, locus of control, self-concept, and so on, which tended to be little more than mechanical extensions of a technqiue or a conceptual framework rather than tests of hypotheses generated specifically to explain alcoholism. Currently, however, investigators draw upon the accumulated knowledge of both the alcohol field and developments in psychology in developing hypotheses about aspects of drinking. Similarly, the level of methodological sophistication was much less than the state-of-the-art in psychology generally. As recently as 1978, Nathan and Lansky documented methodological weaknesses in the field, including attention to definitional–diagnostic issues, inadequate sampling, noncomparable or nonexistent control groups, faulty designs, inappropriate or "shotgun" measures, poor analytic strategies and techniques, and so on. While it would be an error to say that these lacks are no longer with us (in alcohol research or in psychological research generally), there have been singular advances in the quality and sophistication of alcohol research. Alcoholism treatment outcome research, for example, is now comparable in quality and vigor to outcome research generally, and increasingly follows a clinical trials model (e.g., see Sanchez-Craig, Annis, Bornet, & Mac Donald, 1984).

Perhaps the clearest evidence demonstrating the influence of integration can be found in the cross-fertilization between alcohol studies and mainstream psychology. Neuropsychology, for instance, has contributed much to the understanding of alcohol's acute and chronic effects on cognitive functioning, memory, and higher-order abstraction, in particular. These understandings, in turn, have contributed to furthering explanation of memory functioning in general (Butters & Cermak, 1980). Another example may be found in the increasingly sophisticated conceptualizations and methodologies being developed in alcoholic family interaction research. This research, initially proceeding from the state-of-the-art in family research generally, is now making important methodological and theoretical contributions to our knowledge of the stability, reliability, and substance of sequential interactions over time (Jacob, in press). These examples, which are not isolated, show that the psychological study of alcohol benefits from and contributes to psychology in ways that simply did not exist before.

These considerations suggest the need for a work that on the one hand provides a systematic frame of reference for comprehending early theoretical efforts and their contributions to current thinking and research, and on the other accords systematic treatment to recently postulated theoretical models. In regard to the presentation of early theories, we could have proceeded by devoting a chapter to specific early models. One might, for example, devote a chapter to psychoanalytic theory, which has had and continues to have an influence on conceptualizations about alcohol. Despite this influence, no research tradition has built up around psychoanalytic ideas nor is their current impact strong. Or one might devote special attention to dependency or power models, both of which find their roots in psychodynamic conceptions of human experience. Similarly, one might concentrate upon a host of models and hypotheses that have been proposed and studied over the years: the first drink experience, field dependence, locus of control. Rather than follow these paths, we chose to adopt broader categories of approach that would subsume and integrate these often isolated and scattered efforts by enlisting authors with grasp and mastery of the content, issues, methods, development, and current status of an area. The areas we chose were tension reduction, personality, interactionism, and social learning. Each area has a unique focus and has made important contributions to the field. Chapters on each of these areas provide both a historical context within which newer models may be appreciated and an assessment of the current status of the area within the alcohol studies field.

## Traditional Approaches

### Tension Reduction Theory

The original formulation of the tension reduction hypothesis, based on behavioral learning principles, held that drinking alcohol was not some unique manifestation but simply one "response among many in the (behavioral) repertoire of an organism: The existence of a tension state energized the response and the relief of tension provided by alcohol reinforced the drinking response" (Cappell & Herman, 1972, pp. 33–34). Later formulations distinguished between two hypotheses; namely, alcohol reduces tension, and individuals drink alcohol for its tension-reducing properties. Howard Cappell and Janet Greeley, after considering the origins of tension reduction theory (TRT), trace developments in conceptualizations and empirical research with regard to tension reduction since the early 1970s, providing a critical assessment of TRT's current status. They first examine evidence for the proposition that alcohol reduces tension, drawing upon animal and human studies on experimental conflict, response to physically noxious stimuli, response to social stressors, expectancies, and affect. They then evaluate recent work on self-administration of alcohol designed to investigate TRT's second proposition that organisims drink in order to reduce tension. Their conclusions place TRT within the context of current thinking about alcohol: TRT is not tenable as a single factor explanation (alcohol does many things besides reducing tension), is valid within a relatively circumscribed portion of the dose–response curve, and makes its greatest contribution as a crucial component of more complex models such as that represented, for example, by stress response dampening.

### Personality Theory

Less a coherent body of theory than a point of view concerning drinking and alcoholism, the notion of the importance of personality factors and how these factors are organized in distinguishing alcoholics from nonalcoholics, heavy drinkers from light drinkers, drinkers from nondrinkers, and, more recently, among alcoholics themselves, has had a long and empirically productive history in attempts to understand drinking and alcoholism psychologically. In Chapter 3 of this volume, W. Miles Cox delineates early approaches to personality and alcohol, including psychoanalytic, dependency, and tension reduction formulations, and subsequent models, including power theory and femininity theory (the only female-specific formulation to date). He organizes the wide array of personality factors that have been pursued in the search for the elusive personality of the alcoholic into a meaningful set of categories: nonconformity and impulsivity, negative affect and self-esteem, cognitive–perceptual styles, and motivational determinants. The importance of personality for understanding drinking and alcoholism is recognized now more than ever before, but emphasis has shifted from unifactorial, global explanations to the reconceptualization of personality constructs as contributory to multilevel causal schemes as, for example, in the work of Jessor (1983) and his colleagues, or as mediating complex causal chains as in the work of Huba and Bentler (in press).

### Social Learning Theory

Bandura's (1969) early formulation about alcohol use and abuse from a social learning theory (SLT) standpoint assumed that all drinking, from incidental social use through abuse and alcoholism, is governed by similar principles of learning, cognition, and reinforcement. In Chapter 5, David Abrams and Raymond Niaura examine the details of this formulation against the background of a consideration of the assumptions of SLT generally and then provide an integrated analysis of the more sophisticated and refined set of principles that has emerged from theoretical–empirical developments since 1969. These principles, arranged developmentally, offer an understanding of psychosocial and cultural predisposing influences on drinking as well as the interactive role of predisposing individual differences that may be biological and/or psychological and genetic and/or acquired. These influences are critical for understanding experimentation in adolescence and subsequent use, which varies according to positive and negative reinforcing effects mediated by expectations and situational demands. Abuse is likely to occur under conditions that overwhelm effective coping ability and reduce one's perception of efficacy. Continued use of alcohol results in acquired tolerance which may act as another mediator of additional consumption, heightening the risk for developing physical and/or psychological dependence. The consequences of abusive drinking episodes in themselves can exacerbate further drinking (reciprocal determinism), while recovery depends upon the individual's ability to acquire general coping skills and self-control skills required to manage drinking. The central thesis of the SLT of alcohol use and abuse put forward by Abrams and Niaura is that alcohol abuse is a method of coping with the demands of everyday life. As such, it is related to both tension reduction theory and to stress response dampening, and its progeny also include expectancy theory.

### Interactional Theory

Interactional theories conceive of behavior as a function of codetermination and reciprocal effects among person, environment, and behavior. In Chapter 4 of this volume, Stanley W. Sadava argues that as methodologically sound information about alcohol use and abuse has expanded almost exponentially in the past decade, the need for comprehensive explanatory and ordering schemes has become more evident. An interactionist approach is both useful and necessary in understanding the reality of an interrelated system. While there is no single, widely used interactionist theory of alcohol use, several investigators, coincident with renewed interest in interactionism during the 1970s, developed models relevant to drinking as jointly determined by aspects of the person and the social environment. These include Richard Jessor's problem behavior theory, George Huba and Peter Bentler's domain model, and Robert Zucker's developmental model. Sadava identifies several general principles that characterize these theories: Personality is a multivariate system in which variables may be grouped in domains; environment consists of characteristics that are relatively consistent across time and situations; variables are either proximal or distal to the behavior of interest. Furthermore, the models are more or less developmental in approach, employing longitudinal designs and multivariate analyses. These interactional conceptualizations of drinking provide rich and complex models and have especially contributed to our understanding of the initiation of drinking and the transitions from one drinking status to another.

## Recent Theoretical Models

The choice of recently developed models was dictated by two criteria: (1) the exposition of a systematic conceptual model aimed at the explication of important aspects of the initiation and maintenance of drinking behavior that eventuates in alcohol problems, and (2) a beginning body of empirical support for the model. The five models selected include expectancy, stress response dampening, self-awareness, self-handicapping, and opponent process theory. There is always a certain amount of arbitrariness in choices of this sort and other editors may well have come up with a different list. Our review of the recent psychological literature, however, suggests that the models cited provide comprehensive coverage of contemporary theoretical activity in the field. This is not to say that we have attempted to provide a purview of all research activity relevant to psychologists and in which psychologists are usually involved. To include work on such areas as treatment and prevention outcome research, neuropsychological studies, family interaction research, studies of high-risk populations, and measurement and classification research would be simply beyond the scope of this volume. In enlisting the authors for each of the newer models, we attempted whenever possible to obtain the person most closely identified with the original statement of the model or, in lieu of that, the person known as a spokesperson for the model.

### Expectancy Theory

The importance of cognitive factors in the initiation and maintenance of drinking behaviors is central to expectancy theory. The construct "expectancy," the history of which is thoughtfully delineated by Mark Goldman, Sandra Brown, and Bruce Christiansen in Chapter 6 of this volume, "refers to the anticipation of a systematic relationship between events or objects" in a specific situation. The authors, drawing upon their own research as well as that of other investigators, examine how expectancy theory answers four basic questions: initiation of alcohol use, maintenance of drinking, acceleration of drinking in some individuals, and continuing use of alcohol even when its consequences have become physically and behaviorally destructive. They evaluate expectancy theory in light of other models, concluding that while the theory is insufficiently formalized at this point in time, it has nonetheless resulted in the discovery of important new information relative to the nonpharmacologic effects of expectancies in blanced-placebo designs, as well as to prediction strategies by means of expectancy assessment instruments.

## Stress Response Dampening

Quite closely aligned with the tension reduction hypothesis, stress response dampening (SRD) focuses on alcohol's effects on the individual when stressed. The stressed individual reacts physiologically in several different systems. In Chapter 7 of this volume, Kenneth Sher argues that alcohol dampens this physiologic response, subjectively alleviating stress and thereby reinforcing drinking in other similar stress situations. Viewing SRD theory as an essentially psychopharmacologic approach to alcohol, he examines the psychophysiologic effects of alcohol, its relation to other drugs, and the possible direct and indirect pharamacologic mechanisms involved. Sher also assesses the importance of nonpharmacologic cognitive effects (i.e, expectancies) and the role of individual differences in sensitivity to SRD. While acknowledging the importance of the tension reduction hypothesis to the development of SRD theory, he distinguishes the latter as being more molecular and relying on fewer hypothetical constructs; he considers the SRD model as a "psychobiological minitheory" that may be viewed within the larger context of cognitive–social learning theory.

## Self-Awareness

Like the stress-response dampening model, the self-awareness model attempts to understand some of the causes and effects of alcohol use in terms of alcohol's pharmacologic action. Unlike SRD, the self-awareness model posits that this action affects cognitive processes, specifically the self-aware state, rather than the physiologic stress response. The model, as explicated in Chapter 8 of the current volume by its progenitor, Jay Hull, contains four basic propositions: (1) alcohol decreases self-awareness (2) by inhibiting cognitive processes related to encoding information according to its self-relevance. By reducing self-awareness, (3) drinking has affective and behavioral consequences opposite to those associated with increased self-awareness, thus decreasing appropriate behaviors (i.e., behavioral disinhibition) and self-evaluation based on past performance. (4) Alcohol decreases negative evaluation of the self following failure and this is sufficient to induce and sustain drinking. Hull provides conceptual and empirical evidence for each assumption, relying on several studies conducted by his colleagues and himself, designed specifically to test aspects of the model. Like some of the other, more recent models (such as stress-response dampening and self-handicapping), the self-awareness model is molecular, attempting to explain some causes and effects of drinking. Hull argues that drinking to avoid negative self-evaluation is orthogonal with respect to other alcohol consumption motives such as expectancy and tension reduction, and thus has a unique though circumscribed explanatory value.

### Self-Handicapping

This nonpharmacologic model, with origins in the theories of attribution and impression management, addresses a major gap in our knowledge, that is, the explanation of alcohol abuse among successful individuals. In Chapter 9, Steven Berglas, the originator of the model, asserts that self-handicapping involves the use of a tactic that enables these individuals to protect a positive competence image by controlling the attributions drawn from their behavior. Consuming alcohol prior to evaluation of performance is one such tactic. If failure occurs under the influence of alcohol, the individual's own competence is not assailed since poor performance is charged to alcohol; with success, the individual's image of competence is enhanced since he or she performed well under handicapping conditions. Citing evidence from research conducted by himself and others, Berglas explores the implications of this formulation, showing that self-handicappers' successful performance histories are marred by subjective ambiguity as to whether success was due to their personal abilities or to factors external to themselves (noncontingent reinforcement). The consequent threat of performance anxiety, often accompanied by an exaggerated competency image, sets the stage for the use of alcohol to self-handicap. As with the stress-response dampening and self-awareness models, self-handicapping may be thought of as a model that attempts to understand the causes and effects of one type of abusive drinking in a specifically pre-disposed individual.

### Opponent Process Theory

Opponent process theory is a general theory of acquired motivation developed in the early 1970s and applied to a variety of motivational phenomena, including addictive behaviors. As applied to alcohol abuse, the theory, which is basically a classical conditioning approach, holds that the intake of alcohol has a direct effect on physiologic processes, an effect that is counteracted by a homeostatic rebound mechanism which has physiologic effects opposite to that of alcohol. As described by Thomas Shipley in Chapter 10, the formulation differs from other homeostatic theories in that the rebound mechanism overcorrects, leading to a "failure of equilibrium." According to the theory, this rebound mechanism becomes stronger with repetition, diminishing the immediate effect of alcohol such that the individual requires more alcohol than before to achieve the same effect (i.e, tolerance). Furthermore, this homeostatic process is experienced as a decidedly negative state (i.e, withdrawal) and can be linked to external cues related to drinking. Addiction to alcohol occurs when the person begins to drink to alleviate this conditioned homeostatic process. Shipley critically examines evidence for the basic propositions of the theory and considers recent alternative explanations of addiction. Furthermore, he carefully integrates implications of opponent process theory with clinical aspects of alcoholism, including relapse, recovery, and treatment strategies.

The volume is designed to be useful in several ways to several audiences. First, it fills a major gap in instruction for undergraduate and graduate psychology courses. As noted, there is no single comprehensive source for psychological theory and research concerning alcohol. The present volume is intended to fill this gap by presenting current models within a historical context of theory and research. As such, it may be used as a primary text for courses specifically on alcohol studies or as a secondary reading for courses that deal with other addictive behaviors. It may also be used as a reading in general social science, behavioral science, and psychiatry courses on alcohol studies. Second, the volume is designed for those investigators in psychology, psychiatry, and related fields who are not involved in the alcohol field but who wish to learn more about the psychological aspects of alcohol behavior or who are planning to conduct research in the area. For these readers, the book provides an up-to-date, comprehensive, and sophisticated introduction to psychological thinking about alcohol as well as a consideration of major current methodological strategies, thereby providing a solid platform from which more specialized interests may be pursued. Third, for the alcohol investigator in psychology and the biomedical or social sciences, the book offers an in-depth survey of important recent developments in the specialty of alcohol psychology that will help the reader to stay abreast of new knowledge, to prepare for cross-disciplinary research, to provide new theoretical insights, or simply to broaden one's knowledge in the field.

## References

Bandura, A. (1969). *Principles of behavior modification*. New York: Holt, Rinehart & Winston.

Butters, N., & Cermak, L. S. (1980). *Alcoholic Korsakoff's syndrome: An information-processing approach to amnesia*. New York: Academic Press.

Cappell, H., & Herman, C. P. (1972). Alcohol and tension reduction: A review. *Quarterly Journal of Studies on Alcohol, 33*, 33–64.

Huba, G. J., & Bentler, P. M. (in press). *Antecedents and consequences of adolescent drug use. A psychosocial study of development using a causal modeling approach*. New York: Plenum Press.

Jacob, T. (in press). Alcoholism: A family interaction perspective. In C. Rivers (Ed.), *Nebraska Symposium on Motivation*. Lincoln, Nebraska: University of Nebraska Press.

Jessor, R. (1983). The stability of change: Psychosocial development from adolescence to young adulthood. In D. Magnusson & V. Allen (Eds.), *Human development: An interactionist perspective* (pp. 321–341). New York: Academic Press.

Nathan, P. E., & Lansky, D. (1978). Common methodological problems in research on the addictions. *Journal of Consulting and Clinical Psychology, 46*, 713–726.

Sanchez-Craig, M., Annis, H. M., Bornet, A. R., & MacDonald, K. R. (1984). Random assignment to abstinence and controlled drinking: Evaluation of a cognitive–behavioral program for problem drinkers. *Journal of Consulting and Clinical Psychology, 52*, 390–403.

# I TRADITIONAL APPROACHES

# 2 Alcohol and Tension Reduction: An Update on Research and Theory

HOWARD CAPPELL

JANET GREELEY

## Origins of the Tension Reduction Theory

Like all psychological theories relating to alcohol and drug use, the tension reduction theory (TRT) is predicated on prior developments in basic research. Tension reduction theory is a direct outgrowth of the application of drive reduction theory to an understanding of how alcohol is reinforcing. Although drive reduction theory applies equally to appetitive and aversive motivational states, where alcohol is concerned, aversive states have been the primary focus of attention. An aversive state such as anxiety "is conceived of as a drive, with anxiety reduction playing the role of reinforcer," asserts a vintage textbook on learning (Kimble, 1961). This approach to learning, associated with such names as Hull, Mowrer, and Spence, took root in the 1940s and dominated motivational research for many years thereafter.

Motivational theory addresses itself not only to the energy that drives behavior, but also to the acquisition and performance of behavior that an organism can use to regulate its drives. Hungry organisms learn how to acquire food, and thirsty ones to find water. What can the tense and anxious rat or human do to relieve its aversive state? Clearly there are a number of possibilities, among which drinking alcohol is perhaps one. That this might be so became the center of psychological theories of both normal and pathological drinking, and until the appearance of Cappell and Herman's critical review in 1972 the merit of tension reduction theories went unquestioned.

HOWARD CAPPELL and JANET GREELEY. Addiction Research Foundation and University of Toronto, Toronto, Ontario, Canada.

In 1944, the Yale Summer School of Alcohol Studies was the scene of a series of lectures by eminent scholars from a variety of scientific and other disciplines concerned with accounting for alcohol consumption and its attendant problems. Twenty-nine of these were published as a volume entitled *Alcohol, Science, and Society* (Yale Studies on Alcohol, 1945). Although none of the lectures espousing the TRT referred to experimental data, they anticipated the questions that would occupy the attention of researchers as appropriate methodologies became available. Jellinek's lecture, the second in the series (Jellinek, 1945), presented an elaborate treatise that addressed itself to everything from the behavior of the individual alcoholic to the behavior of the state, all of which stemmed, in his view, from the need to manage various sources of tension. The model he proposed was a general one (see Figure 2.1) of a "social problem of which the use of alcohol is only a part." According to Jellinek, "When society becomes more complex . . . social–economic restrictions and frustration grow by leaps and bounds . . . tension increases in intensity and frequency. . . . Individual releases are sought. Since there is a substance which can give the desired relief, harassed man will want to take recourse to it" (p. 19). Jellinek certainly did not want to imply that *all* alcohol consumption was motivated by the desire for relief from tension. "It would be sheer nonsense to hold such an opinion. I would say that in modern society the beverages are used more frequently as condiments, as refreshments, as a compliance with custom and for prestige purposes than for conscious or unconscious sedation and relief. The emphasis on relief from tension is only to show the particular function of alcohol through which it

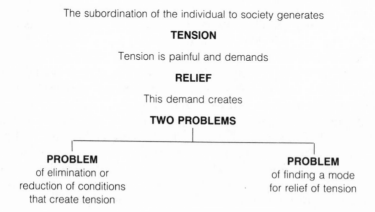

FIGURE 2.1. Jellinek's schematic representation of the origin and consequences of tension. Adapted from Jellinek (1945).

attained such social value as is attributed to it" (pp. 19–20). When it came to pathologic drinking, however, the commitment to the tension reduction model was firmer. "While all drinking is far from being only a seeking of relief from tension, addiction—compulsive drinking—does definitely serve that purpose" (p. 20).

In Lecture 13, Donald Horton (1945) affirmed this conclusion from studies of primitive societies. "In the state of intoxication, and in what it means to men, apparently lies the answer to the positive value of alcohol. By positive value I mean that this is the thing for which the alcoholic beverage is treasured, honored, preserved as a custom throughout the ages. The best possible explanation that I can offer you, based on a review of the use of alcohol in a good many primitive societies, is that the value is primarily in its anxiety-reducing function" (p. 158). Prescient in his anticipation of modern therapists' emphasis on problem-solving and coping skills as the stuff of successful behavioral adaptation, Horton, obviously not given to waffling, asserted simply that "alcohol solves the problem of anxiety-reduction" (p. 162). Selden Bacon (1945) next stated to the students of the summer school: "as you are all aware, alcohol is a depressant. Alcohol allows, through its depressing function, a relaxation of tension, of inhibition, of anxiety, of guilt" (p. 190).

The year 1945 also witnessed the publication of an influential laboratory study in which the credibility of the TRT was enhanced by the experimental method. Masserman's classic study of "experimental neurosis" and its relief by alcohol in cats became widely cited (Masserman, Jacques, & Nicholson, 1945). The creation of an approach–avoidance conflict in cats was thought to provide a reasonable model of human neurosis, a condition for which humankind had through time used alcohol because it could "mitigate the anticipated stresses of impending experiences, or as a hypnotic which blunts and disorganizes neurotic anxieties" (Masserman & Yum, 1946). Other examples based on the experimental study of behavior soon followed. Ullman (1952) explained addictive drinking as an overlearned response to the need for tension reduction that obviated the occurrence of "more appropriate" coping responses. This appraisal has no shortage of supporters today. However, it remained for Conger (1956) to write the theoretical review that became an essential reference for many years afterward. He summarized TRT as follows: "From observation, we know that many people who have once made the response of drinking alcohol continue to do so, and that some of them do to excess. Through experience, the drinking response becomes learned. While this point seems clear, it is by no means as readily apparent that the drinking response is learned *because* it leads to a reduction in drive. But if we are to be consistent in applying a drive-reduction hypothesis, we must maintain that in those cases where the drinking response is learned, it is learned because it is rewarding" (p. 296).

Following a brief review of the support for TRT available in literary, psychoanalytic, and scientific sources, Conger set out to outline a firm experimental basis for it in laboratory data. His experimental test employed the approach–avoidance conflict procedure that had been developed by a pioneer in this area, Neal Miller (1944). Conflict was created by training rats to traverse an alley to a goal box where they were both reinforced with food and punished with electric shock. An intraperitoneal injection of a moderate dose of alcohol could ameliorate this conflict, thus providing crucial support for an important element of the TRT. Moreover, Conger concluded that the resolution of conflict by alcohol was attributable to "a reduction in the avoidance response motivated by fear."

The TRT formulated by Conger was the guiding force for empirical research as the laboratory experiment came to dominate the development of behavioral theory. In 1972, Cappell and Herman reviewed the literature that had accumulated to that time, and an updated version followed (Cappell, 1975). The later review specified that the two main elements of the TRT were the hypotheses that (1) alcohol reduces tension [the original tension reduction hypothesis, (TRH) considered by Cappell and Herman], and (2) organisms drink alcohol for its tension-reducing properties. The bodies of literature pertaining to both hypotheses were examined thoroughly, and it was concluded that plausibility notwithstanding, the TRT had a generally poor record of empirical support. Cappell's review also concluded that approaches other than those predicated on the TRT should be given increased attention as accounts for alcohol consumption.

The development of the TRT subsequent to the mid-1970s will be the subject of the balance of this chapter. It will become evident that the TRT has not been abandoned or supplanted by a novel approach, and indeed, the more limited TRH has attracted a spirited defense (Hodgson, Stockwell, & Rankin, 1979). Although many studies begin with an acknowledgment of the flaws of the TRH, this awareness of imperfection has led not to its rejection, but instead to more careful experiments and more circumscribed theorizing.

## Tension Reduction Theory in Perspective

Cappell and Herman (1972) used the word "tension" to refer generically to a variety of states that could plausibly be considered as aversive sources of motivation, such as fear, anxiety, conflict, and frustration. In the modern lexicon, the word "stress" has supervened, but the change has been primarily semantic. At a recent symposium on alcohol and stress (Pohorecky & Brick, 1983), it was agreed that no universally accepted definition of general concepts like tension and stress is imminent. Thus, while methods for manipulating and measuring stress or tension have improved vastly, it remains necessary to be somewhat vague about their precise connotation. However, it seems fair to say that tension is something that can interfere with performance or well-being, and therefore must be coped with in the service of hedonic balance, perhaps by drinking. There are of course other theories intended to account for variation in alcohol consumption that propose a specific mechanism of reinforcement (e.g., see Hull, 1981), and even one that considers "significant regularities between behavior and its consequences without positing underlying organismic states of any kind" (Vuchinich & Tucker, 1983). Since the birth rate of new theories of drinking behavior appears to exceed the death rate of old ones, the behavior to be explained remains static even as the contenders to explain it continue to multiply.

Until a general integrative theory of alcohol consumption emerges, the only standard for assessing the merit of the TRT as against competing theories is to judge how much it can in some absolute sense survive a reasonable process of scrutiny. Although the appraisal can be based on the results of scientific effort, the final judgment will contain a large subjective component. Previous reviews (Cappell & Herman, 1972; Cappell, 1975) were not optimistic that the TRT deserved to survive. What follows is a consideration of whether new research warrants any revision in this verdict.

**The Evidence**

The basic hypotheses comprising the TRT remain unchanged, and investigators have continued to ask whether alcohol reduces tension and whether tension promotes alcohol consumption. However, behavioral and biological research has improved significantly in both theoretical and methodological sophistication within the last decade. There has been a welcome increase in the number of studies with human subjects, greater attention to individual differences, and a considerable improvement in the technology of behavioral measurement. Our review of these developments will be organized according to the two main hypotheses of the TRT. Within each of these sections, we will attempt to organize studies by type to the extent possible. Only reports considered to make an important contribution to the evaluation of the theory will be considered in any depth.

*Evidence on Whether Alcohol Reduces Tension*
*(the Tension Reduction Hypothesis)*

The research considered in this section reflects a relatively uniform strategy. Beginning with a behavioral or physiologic model, investigators can proceed to a relatively straightforward test of whether alcohol ameliorates tension. The experiments reviewed have varied in methodological rigor (e.g., some may involve more than one dose of alcohol and others not), but generally the studies have been well conceived and to the point.

## Experimental Conflict

The earliest test of the TRH involved an experimental model of approach–avoidance conflict in animals. In this model, conflicting motives and responses are activated, but the strength of the conflict is measured by a single response. Typically, an animal is trained to respond (e.g., run down an alley) for food reward, and once this response is established, punishment of the approach response with shock is introduced. The strength of conflict is reflected in the suppression of responding to obtain food. A tension-reducing agent should be able to restore a suppressed response by weakening the avoidance component created by punishment.

Cappell and Herman (1972) concluded that the conflict paradigm was the only one to provide consistent support for the TRH, but they offered no hypothesis as to why this might be so. More recently, Hodgson et al. (1979) provided their own appraisal of the literature on conflict and some other behaviors based on aversive motivation. Their explicit objective was to reconsider some of the animal studies covered by Cappell and Herman (1972) in order to affirm, rather than doubt, the TRH. Where Cappell and Herman concluded that certain studies failed to support the TRH, Hodgson et al. concluded that the same studies were not really germane and therefore did not provide a fair test of the TRH. In their view, behavioral tests incorporating passive avoidance (i.e., the animal avoids aversive stimulation by inhibiting rather than executing a response) provide the best test of the TRH because they represent the purest example of a behavior truly motivated by fear. Indeed, it does appear that behavioral tests involving passive avoidance do provide the best support for the TRH, and in this, the conclusions of Cappell and Herman and Hodgson et al. were really no different when the same data were being considered. The more important implication of the critique by Hodgson et al. is that Cappell and Herman may have been overinclusive in considering some studies of aversively motivated behavior as being relevant to the TRH when they were not. If it is true that the general success of the TRH in studies of conflict is attributable to the special validity of the passive avoidance component as a model of anxiety or fear, Hodgson et al. may have provided a reconciliation for contradictions that would now be more apparent than real. However, it should be kept in mind that the critique by Hodgson et al. addressed only a limited portion of the range of evidence that Cappell and Herman considered, and cannot therefore be taken as a general appraisal of the TRH.

There have been a limited number of new studies on conflict in animals that on balance, are consistent with the TRH. In one of these (Mansfield, Eaton, Cunningham, & Brown, 1977) there were two unusual features. First, the conflict was between two avoidance tendencies rather than between approach and avoidance. The second unusual feature was in the method of administering alcohol. This was done by restricting fluid intake to 15 min/day; thus on test days, the rats would ingest a reasonably high dosage of ethanol (ranging from 1.0 to 3.6 g/kg) prior to the conflict test. Notwithstanding this unorthodox procedure and the variability in self-administered doses it produced, the result was that alcohol ameloriated an avoidance–avoidance conflict. This finding has proved to be replicable (Mansfield, 1979).

The procedure that has become standard for assessing anxiolytic activity of drugs in animals is a variant on runway studies of approach–avoidance conflict. The newer procedure involves the acquisition of operant responding for food reward, which is subsequently punished with electric shock. Such punishment suppresses responding, and excellent quantification of behavior is possible. The technique is used routinely and effectively to screen minor tranquilizers for anxiolytic activity, and is known to be reliable and sensitive. Effective anxiolytics clearly restore responding suppressed by punishment. In one study, the technique was even adopted for use with goldfish by Geller, Croy, and Ryback (1974) who found that alcohol did not attenuate conflict. In the same study, however, phenobarbital was effective, and the authors therefore concluded that only phenobarital was an anxiolytic in this test. These results are somewhat difficult to evaluate because of the absence of a general experimental context for comparison (i.e., there are not many experiments in which drugs are administered to fish via their living environment, and not much is known of concentration–behavior relationships), but the discrepancy in results with two putative anxiety-reducers cannot be ignored. In experiments with squirrel monkeys (Glowa & Barrett, 1976), and mice and rats (Vogel et al., 1980), however, alcohol was shown to restore responding suppressed by punishment.

The interpretation of this antipunishment phenomenon is not always made in the context of the TRH, and indeed it is possible to question the necessity for a motivational interpretation of such findings. For example, Glowa and Barrett (1976) found that alcohol increased low rates of responding both when they were a reflection of punishment-induced suppression and when they occurred in the absence of punishment. Alcohol's effect was said to be an example of rate dependency (i.e., an effect of alcohol on low rates of responding, however engendered), which is an interpretation of many drug effects favored by behavioral pharmacologists who reject motivational concepts.

There has been some additional work using a variety of nonconflict animal models of tension, such as avoidance and escape behavior, since this work was last reviewed by Cappell (1975). From an overview of these studies (Bammer & Chesher, 1982; Cunningham, 1979; Cunningham & Brown, 1983; Dickerson & Ferraro, 1976; DiGuisto & Bond, 1977; Skurdal, Eckardt, & Brown, 1975) no clear picture emerges as far as the TRH is concerned, and results pro and con continue to be obtained. The problem in obtaining consistent results in this literature appears to be largely methodological, and experimenters typically spend much of their discussion in identifying methodological points that might account for discrepant or unexpected findings.

Some new and important work with human subjects has appeared recently. Lindman's work (1980)[1] deserves to be considered first because it is an exemplary collection of thorough and ingenious studies. In the first experiment of the series, subjects were asked to traverse a floor and then withdraw a plastic ball from a container filled with a solution of electrolyte. As soon as they made contact with the solution, they were administered an unpleasant electric shock. Conflict was measured as the amount of time it took for a subject to cross the floor and touch the surface of the solution. The validity of this index showed up in the fact that subjects approached more slowly when the shock probability was moderate or certain (50% or 100%) than when it was zero. In a dose of 0.9 g/kg, alcohol decreased the reluctance to approach significantly. In a follow-up experiment, the same behavioral test was augmented by the inclusion of an electrodermal measure of tension. Although the results with approach behavior were replicated, and there was evidence that the amplitude of changes in skin conductance was a valid measure of tension, alcohol had no effect on the psychophysiologic index. Thus Lindman concluded that "behavioral fear" was relieved by alcohol although autonomic arousal was not.

Lindman thought it important to determine the effect of alcohol on a "naturally occurring fear." To this end, he included a task in which female subjects were asked to transfer a mouse from one jar to another, with the time taken to effect this transfer as the measure of fear. Specific training in behavioral coping as well as the effect of alcohol (0.9 g/kg) were compared in their ability to reduce fear in this situation. Both manipulations independently reduced the time taken to transfer a mouse, that is, reduced fear. In a subsequent methodological study, it was shown that the effect of alcohol was pharmacologic and not based simply on the *expectation* that alcohol would reduce fear.

There has been another study (Rimm, Briddell, Zimmerman, & Caddy, 1981) that appears superficially similar to the work of Lindman except in the

---

[1] It might be questioned whether this experiment and the one by Rimm *et al.* (1981) are appropriately considered in a section on conflict, since the approach component seems to be missing. It must be assumed that the motivation to approach is created by the experimenter's request to do so.

result. In this case the question was whether alcohol (0.5 g/kg) would affect subjects' willingness to approach and handle a 4-foot boa constrictor. Alcohol was without effect on approach behavior, but it did reduce self-reported fear of the snake. If there is no reason to assume that fear of snakes is more difficult to overcome than fear of mice, perhaps the best reconciliation of the discrepancy with Lindman is that he used nearly double the dose. The issue of dose will emerge as an important one throughout the review.

Cognitive dissonance is a tension state that is not precisely the same as conflict, but it is not inappropriate to consider an excellent study on this phenomenon (Steele, Southwick, & Critchlow, 1981) in this section. A dissonant state can be created in individuals by inducing them to argue in favor of a position that is contrary to their own current attitudes about a subject. For example, Steele *et al.* induced subjects who were *opposed* to an increase in tuition fees to write an essay *favoring* an increase. When this is done by free choice, subjects should experience dissonance, which can be reduced by changing attitudes to become more consistent (in this case, by becoming more favorable to a tuition increase). Indeed this is what happened among control subjects. However, subjects who drank alcohol before measurement of attitude change displayed a reduced amount of attitude change. Therefore, it appeared that alcohol was able to reduce the psychological tension associated with dissonance and hence the need to change attitudes. Steele *et al.* included three separate studies to eliminate various alternative interpretations, and were able to conclude firmly that the phenomenon was genuine. What they could not determine was whether the effect of alcohol was mediated pharmacologically or cognitively. In the latter category would be included behavior caused by expectations or beliefs about the effects of alcohol, which are discussed later. If the effect was mediated pharmacologically, it did not require a large dose, since the maximum was 2 ounces of vodka (roughly 0.3 g/kg in a person weighing 70 kg) in one of the experiments in which a positive result was obtained.

In summary then, experiments on conflict behavior have continued to provide relatively consistent support for the TRH in both humans and a variety of animal species. However, at least some of this support is subject to alternative interpretation based on constructs having nothing to do with motivational states.

## Response to Physically Noxious Stimuli

There have been a number of studies in which behavioral and physiologic responses to unavoidable "physically" noxious stimuli (such as electric shock) have been studied. These are distinguished from studies of "social" stressors which are considered separately. It is recognized that this distinction could be arbitrary in that these different sources of tension may be superficially distinct but functionally similar. Since there has been one reconciliation of discrepant findings based on this distinction (Higgins & Marlatt, 1975), separate sections are perhaps justified theoretically. In any event, the distinction is used here as an organizational device and nothing more.

A good way to begin is by considering a study by Levenson, Sher, Grossman, Newman, and Newlin (1980), since many of the general issues pertinent to the methodology of research on the TRH were explicitly raised by the authors. In this study of male college students, various psychophysiologic indices of stress and a self-report measure of anxiety were repeatedly recorded during a baseline prestress period, a "countdown" period of anticipation of the stressor, and following application of the stressor. Electric shock and the requirement to make a videotaped self-disclosing speech that subjects were told would be rated by observers were the stressors. Subjects consumed 1.0 g/kg of alcohol, which produced a mean blood alcohol concentration (BAC) of 900 mg/liter[2] or a placebo over a 45-min period; the stress procedures began after allowance for the alcohol to be absorbed. Also included was a manipulation of beverage expectancy (see below) that will not be considered here. The study produced a rich yield of data which can only be briefly summarized here. Results were largely similar with both types of stressor.

During the prestress period, alcohol had mixed effects. The physiologic data suggested that alcohol had both "stimulant" and "relaxant" effects. Alcohol reduced self-reported anxiety. Both anticipation (during countdown) and delivery of the stressors affected the physiologic and self-report measures in a predictable way that showed the manipulations to be effective. However, compared to placebo, alcohol dampened the responses to the stressors, giving rise to the coining of the phrase "stress-response dampening" (SRD). A number of mechanisms (direct physiologic damping, disruption of attention to the stressor) were suggested as mediators of SRD. But for present purposes, it is more important that Levenson et al. extracted several important general principles from their study to be kept in mind as others are considered:

1. *Stress-response dampening can be expected only if a bona fide stressor is used.* That is, the stress-induction procedure must be validated.
2. *Stress-response dampening should be most pronounced during anticipation and immediately following onset of the stressor.* That is, a stress-dampening agent should be most effective when the stressor is most salient.

---

[2] The other common ways to express this concentration are 90 mg%, 90 mg/100 ml, or 0.09.

3. *Stress-response dampening should be more evident at high doses of alcohol.* This conclusion was drawn from a comparison to studies by others in which no SRD was found at half the dose used by Levenson *et al.*

One of the studies (Lindman, 1980) appears to meet the requirements set out by Levenson *et al.* in that it employed a high enough dose (0.9 g/kg), a validated index of tension, and measurement at the time of application of the stressor. However, the psychophysiologic measure yielded negative results compared to a behavioral approach measure. Lindman concluded that the two types of measures might be parallel but independent, and therefore need not respond identically to alcohol.

One possibility that needs to be considered when noxious stimuli are applied is that alcohol may have analgesic properties that in turn reduce the stressfulness of such stimulation. Cutter, Maloof, Kurtz, and Jones (1976) tested the response to the pain produced by immersion of the hand and forearm in ice-cold water. The subjects were 29 hospitalized alcoholics and 50 "presumably nonproblem drinking" control subjects and the dose was approximately 0.5 g/kg. Alcohol alleviated pain in the alcoholic group but not among nonalcoholics. In a later study (Brown & Cutter, 1977), a more elaborate design was used that included placebo and two doses of alcohol (0.32 g/kg and 0.63 g/kg), and two different types of pain stimulation. The subjects were college students who were experienced drinkers and provided detailed information about their customary drinking habits. In this case there were interactions between customary drinking habits and the effect of alcohol on pain. Whereas subjects who could be characterized as "problem" drinkers experienced maximal pain reduction at the high dose, "moderate" drinkers experienced maximal pain relief at the low dose and were somewhat sensitized to pain at the high dose. Brown and Cutter made a connection between problematic drinking (i.e., drinking in a bar, alone or with barmates, relatively high dose and frequency) and drinking to escape from "negative feelings"; they suggested that the superior analgesia experienced by problem drinkers at the high experimental dose was related to a general capacity to achieve relief from aversive stimulation at high doses in this population. It was suggested that this was a learned capacity in that problem drinkers acquire a *belief* in the efficacy of alcohol through past experience in using it successfully to ameliorate negative feelings; this transfers to experimentally induced analgesia. The link which makes work on analgesia relevant to the TRH is the assumption that "pain relief by analgesic drugs involves a reduction in the emotional reaction component" (Brown & Cutter, 1977). Thus, it appears that this work on analgesia supports the TRH, and suggests that individual differences are important. The individual difference dimension can be described and related to problem drinking, and a learning mechanism relating alcohol's general relief-giving properties to experimental analgesia among problem drinkers and alcoholics can be suggested. Why it is that this mechanism evolves in some individuals and not others remains obscure. It is also unclear whether the expectation that alcohol will be efficacious in providing relief is related to an innate sensitivity to this source of reinforcement, or is an outgrowth of heavy drinking that develops independently of such a hypothetical sensitivity.

A follow-up of earlier work (Levenson *et al.*, 1980) by Sher and Levenson (1982) further implicates individual differences in the alcohol–stress relationship. Using a reanalysis of data from their earlier work along with an additional experiment, Sher and Levenson studied the relationship between "risk for alcoholism" and the effects of alcohol on the response to their speech stressor. Risk for alcoholism was defined on the basis of existing personality inventories. It is important to note that "risk" was appraised independently of manifest differences in alcoholic behavior; that is, subjects with an alcoholic parent were excluded, and there were no differences found in self-reported quantity and frequency of drinking behavior. Regardless of risk for alcoholism, the effects of alcohol in the prestress period were as in the earlier study— for all subjects there was a mixed arousing and relaxant effect. However, differences emerged when a cardiovascular measure of SRD was used. Alcohol (1.0 g/kg, which produced a peak BAC of 700 mg/liter) exerted the SRD effect for high-risk subjects exclusively. Sher and Levenson went on to suggest that this distinctive response to alcohol provides a unique opportunity for tension reduction as a basis for reinforcement in high risk subjects. Moreover, they suggested that since this difference in SRD antedates any difference in actual drinking behavior, it is probably biologically based. These results parallel those of Brown and Cutter (1977) with analgesia. However, Sher and Levenson clearly require that problem drinking is a *result* of exaggerated sensitivity to the tension-reducing effect of alcohol, whereas Brown and Cutter cannot so clearly direct the causal arrow from their data.

It is an obvious step from Sher and Levenson's interpretation to the suggestion that there is a genetic basis for the differences in biological sensitivity to SRD. They discussed this possibility, and Schuckit, Engstrom, Alpert, and Duby (1981) have reported data relevant to it. Schuckit *et al.* also included risk for alcoholism as a variable, but their criterion of high risk was that their subjects (males aged 21 to 25) have a first-degree relative who could be classified as an alcoholic. The effect of alcohol (peak BAC of approximately 900 mg/liter) on muscle tension (electromyogram; EMG) in this group was compared to matched control subjects with no evidence of alcoholism in first-degree relatives. There was no differential effect of alchol when EMG scores were collected during an "active" period when subjects were filling out a questionnaire; however, muscle tension declined compared to baseline in the high-risk group but not in controls. There were a number of methodological flaws in the study admitted by its authors (e.g., no placebo, only a single measure of tension), but the data again suggest that the TRH may depend on individual differences for its confirmation. It is also worth mentioning that no noxious stimulus was applied in this study, which would make it a relatively weak test of the TRH when the results of Levenson, Sher, and associates are considered.

There is one study in which alcohol (in doses that produced peak BACs of 440 mg/liter and 680 mg/liter) produced *increases* in tension in subjects (the population was not well described, except to note that they were male undergraduates) exposed to a shock stressor (Dengerink & Fagan, 1978). This was true with a self-report measure of anxiety as well as heart rate and skin conductance. The authors' interpretation was that alcohol increased anxiety in a situation that was already anxiety-provoking. This is of course no more than a description of the outcome, with no explanation as to *why* the TRH was contradicted. The result is clearly at odds with what is expected from the work described earlier. There was also no effect of alcohol on subjects' tolerance for shock, which is superficially at odds with Brown and Cutter (1977). It is perhaps not anomalous that no analgesic effect was found, since Brown and Cutter's data would lead to the expectation of a negative result except in a population of alcoholics and problem drinkers. According to Sher and Levenson (1982), an SRD effect might not be expected except in a population including subjects at risk for alcoholism. Even if Dengerink and Fagan had a preponderance of subjects not at risk for alcoholism, the expectation would simply be a negative result rather than an *increase* in tension. The high dose used by Dengerink and Fagan (0.9 g/kg) was also nearly the same as that used by Sher and Levenson (1.0 g/kg). This apparent discrepancy was not addressed by Levenson *et al.* (1980), despite the fact that they cited Dengerink and Fagan in passing.

One study of the effect of alcohol on the response to noxious stimulation in humans (Polivy, Schueneman, & Carlson, 1976) introduced yet another consideration into the literature. Female subjects were told that they would be given a "painful but not dangerous" electric shock in the context of a reaction time task. Prior to the task, they were administered alcohol (0.48 g/kg) or placebo. Within the beverage manipulation, "expectancy" was manipulated as half were told that the drink was alcohol and half were told it was vitamin C. When self-report was measured, the effect of actually being given alcohol was to reduce anxiety; however, the mere instruction that one received alcohol had the paradoxical effect of *increasing* anxiety. The interpretation of this was based on the argument that the *belief* that they had consumed alcohol was anxiety-provoking in subjects who were inexperienced with alcohol and were in an unfamiliar (and perhaps threatening) setting. This would be aggravated by failing to experience the expected effect of alcohol in the placebo condition. However, the *pharmacologic effect* of alcohol was sufficiently powerful to offset the anxiety produced by the threat of shock. Thus according to these results, the pharmacologic effect of alcohol was quite powerful and consistent with the TRH, even though cognition in the absence of pharmacologic action had the opposite consequence.

A final study in this category (Sutker, Allain, Brantley, & Randall, 1982) attempted simultaneously to examine the effects of sex of subject, expectancy, and beverage on psychophysiologic and self-report measures of tension created by fear of electric shock. The alcohol dose was 0.63 g/kg. The data were complex (a theme we will hear of again) and generally failed to illuminate understanding of alcohol's effect on tension. Most of the statistically significant findings were interactions that occurred in no theoretically meaningful pattern.

The recent animal literature on stress induced by noxious stimuli is quite instructive, and it is possible to find some parallels with humans. A complete critical review of this literature would exceed the scope of this chapter. However, there are some strong trends that are worth considering in a selective review. Although there is biochemical evidence that alcohol can act as a stressor (Ellis, 1966; Van Thiel, 1983), there is a growing body of research to show that it can also block biochemical responses to acutely applied stressors. Pohorecky, Rassi, Weiss, and Michalak (1980) reported findings to this effect in rats. Their measures of stress were blood levels of corticosterone and nonesterified fatty acids (NEFA), both of which increase with stress. In a 2 × 2 factorial design, rats were administered foot-shock or confined to the shock chamber with the grid not activated. Within each group, the rats were pretreated with ethanol (0.5 g/kg) or saline. With both biochemical parameters, this modest dose of alcohol substantially blocked the stress responses that were seen in shocked saline controls. In nonshocked animals, however, alcohol produced a small nonsignificant elevation in these indices of stress. Pohorecky *et al.* came to the obvious conclusion that this outcome supports the TRH. This pattern of results was confirmed in a later study (Brick & Pohorecky, 1982) and extended to another form of stress in rats, physical restraint. Like the human research considered earlier, this work confirms that tests of the TRH using a nonstressed organism may be inappropriate.

Other evidence from animal research bears directly on the importance of individual differences in the ethanol and stress relationship (DeTurck & Vogel, 1982). In their work, plasma and brain catecholamine (CA) levels were used to measure stress. Stress was induced in rats by immobilizing them for 30 min. Alcohol (0.5 g/kg) or saline was administered 15 min before the stressor. Immobilization was a potent stressor, causing large rises in plasma norepinephrine and epinephrine. Alcohol caused a significant attenuation of this effect of stress, although it had no effect in nonstressed controls. However, there were noteworthy individual variations in sensitivity, as not all rats were protected equally by alcohol. The results for brain CA were complex, since there were three different biochemical measurements and eight brain sites sampled. Generally, alcohol had no effect on CA concentrations in unstressed animals, but when it did, the effects were comparable to those of immobilization stress. However, in the case of stressed rats, alcohol counteracted many of the chemical changes induced by the stressor.

This is yet another example of the importance of considering the state of the organism when alcohol is administered; alcohol may increase tension in the resting organism and decrease it in one under stress. DeTurck and Vogel adopted this interpretation, but did not consider that the changes in arousal produced by alcohol in the resting organism might be correlates of some affectively positive consequence of alcohol rather than stress (see McCollam, Burish, Maisto, & Sobell, 1980). Interpretation of such data must be speculative and subject to alternatives until there is a better characterization of the relationship between brain chemistry and behavior.

Vogel and DeTurck (1983) recently reported some additional data on individual differences. They bred rats to be "low" or "high responders" to immobilization stress. Alcohol (0.5 g/kg) had little effect on the biochemical responses of low responders, but attenuated the stress response in high responders. Thus there are now animal data to suggest a differential ability to "benefit" from the stress-reducing effect of alcohol (see Brown & Cutter, 1977). This differential sensitivity may take two forms: an exceptional sensitivity to alcohol among those who respond similarly to stress (Sher & Levenson, 1982), or an exceptional response to stress that provides more latitude to achieve a reduction from alcohol (Vogel & DeTurck, 1983).

Research discussed earlier (Vogel et al., 1980) raises an important caveat in the interpretation of biochemical findings. In this study, alcohol, at a dose that had a clear antipunishment or anticonflict effect, did not alter the level of corticosterone in blood as measured following the conflict test. In contrast, the tranquilizer chlordiazepoxide had anticonflict activity as well as blocking the stress response measured biochemically. Clearly, behavioral and physiologic responses can be dissociated where alcohol is concerned. Although other variables might be considered, it is possible that the dosage threshold for achieving tension-reducing effects is different for different response systems. In the experiment by Vogel et al. (1980), the dose of alcohol was 1.5 g/kg, whereas in the studies reporting positive results with biochemical measures the dose has typically been 0.5 g/kg. However, even though reconciliations among discrepant results are possible in principle, the existence of this type of dissociation in outcomes means that the behavioral implications of biochemical results can be equivocal.

Further support for the suggestion that dose is a critical variable is to be found in several investigations. Kakihana (1976) described alcohol as a stressor, and at doses of 1.6 and 2.0 g/kg in mice, plasma corticosterone was elevated compared to saline-treated controls. There was also evidence of genetically transmitted differences in the stress response, as mice bred for susceptibility to the hypnotic effect of alcohol displayed the elevated corticosterone response, whereas insensitive mice did not. There was no test of whether alcohol at these doses would have had a different effect in mice subjected to noxious stimulation. Nonetheless, considering these data along with the positive findings (e.g., Brick & Pohorecky, 1982; DeTurck & Vogel, 1982) and the negative ones (Vogel et al., 1980), the easiest conclusion to draw is that the protection afforded by alcohol against the biochemical consequences of stress is a low-dose phenomenon. Gliner, Horvath, and Browe (1978) studied the effect of tail-shock, alcohol (1.6 g/kg), and interactions between these two manipulations on heart rate and circulatory changes in rats. Shock alone produced a characteristic pattern of cardiovascular effects which was described as an anxiety pattern. Alcohol alone also produced a characteristic pattern of cardiovascular effects; it was different than that produced by shock, but most importantly, there were no alterations in the anxiety pattern when alcohol and shock were given together. For example, heart rate was elevated by shock alone but unaffected by alcohol alone. Alcohol did not attenuate the elevation in heart rate produced by shock. If doses lower than 1.6 g/kg had been included, it would have been possible to comment with some confidence on the possibility that tension reduction is a low-dose phenomenon for some physiologic parameters; as it is, we are left to speculate that the negative results in this study were related to the relatively high dose.

The complexity introduced by multiple measurements of tension in animals has its counterpart in work with humans (Steffen, Nathan, & Taylor, 1974). They examined the relationships among BAC, EMG data, and a self-report measure of "subjective distress." In this study, four alcoholics had free access to whiskey over a 12-day period. The frequency of measurement of the dependent variables was very high, occurring at 2-hour intervals when the subjects were awake. Correlational data indicated that BAC and EMG were negatively associated, which is consistent with the TRH. However, BAC and subjective distress were positively correlated, which is contrary to the TRH. No pattern emerged when EMG and subjective distress were correlated. Recognizing this paradox in the context of the TRH, the authors concluded that the relationships among intoxication level, physiologic situation, and subjective appraisal "are more complex than previously believed."

A few other studies suggest that alcohol can have the effect of a stressor in both humans and rodents. Klepping, Guilland, Didier, Klepping, and Malval (1976) studied the effect of an intravenous infusion of alcohol (peak BAC 950 mg/liter) in 23 hospitalized alcoholics who had been free of alcohol and other drugs for at least 3 days prior to testing. Levels of urinary catecholamines were significantly increased by the procedure. This led Klepping *et al.* to conclude that alcohol should not be considered as "une drogue tranquillisante, mais tout au contraire, comme un stimulant." Unfortunately, needed control subjects were lacking. Moreover, this study was not intended to determine whether alcohol could block the biochemical response to a noxious stressor. Finally, forced consumption of an ethanol-containing diet (Tabakoff, Jaffe, & Ritzmann, 1978) has been found to produce elevations in plasma corticosterone in mice, but again the purpose of this study was not to determine whether alcohol would afford some protection against the effect of noxious stimulation.

To summarize, there is some suggestion that alcohol can attenuate the effects of noxious stimulation in both humans and animals. Most of the confirmatory evidence involves psychophysiologic or biochemical indices. It has been argued that the dose must not be too low to achieve a positive result (Sher *et al.*, 1980) but equally it appears from animal studies that a stress-dampening effect may disappear when the dose becomes too high. It is possible that alcohol's effect on the action of a noxious stimulus will be different than its effect on an otherwise unstressed organism. In the former case, alcohol has often appeared to reduce stress, and in the latter to increase it, at least where biochemical studies are concerned. As far as the TRH is concerned, the data are on balance supportive as long as a few qualifications are made. Among the more interesting qualifiers are individual differences of several kinds.

## Response to Social Stressors

A priori, there is no reason to assume that the effects of alcohol on responses to physically noxious stimuli and what might be called "social stressors" should differ. There is even some arbitrariness in assigning noxious stimuli to these two categories. For example, should fear aroused by mice, snakes, and electrical shock be distinguished from the fear of social evaluation? Empirically, the issue has not been resolved. Levenson *et al.* (1980) found comparable results whether shock or self-disclosure were the tension-inducing manipulations. However, there may be some justification for a psychological distinction between the two. Higgins and Marlatt (1975) postulated that social anxiety could be psychically distinct, in that people expect it will be particularly amenable to alcotherapy, whereas "fear of shock is not a meaningful source of tension as it relates to alcohol consumption." It will have to remain a matter of opinion whether a separate section on this subject represents an artificial taxonomic measure or something of theoretical importance. Much of this literature has also been concerned with "expectancy effects," and they will be considered as necessary. Another important issue that will become evident has to do with the research strategy. In particular, it may be that studies in this group are unwieldy in their complexity.

One of the earliest studies to employ stressful social interaction as the tension manipulation was reported by Wilson and Abrams (1977). The factorial design involved an orthogonal manipulation of the actual beverage administered and subjects' expectations about whether they were given alcohol (0.5 g/kg) or a placebo tonic beverage. The subjects were males whose task was to make "as favorable an impression as possible" on a female confederate. There were psychophysiologic, self-report, and observational measures of tension level. Regardless of the actual beverage consumed, subjects told to expect that they were consuming alcohol had a smaller heart rate acceleration in response to the social interaction than those told to expect tonic. A nonsignificant effect in a similar direction was obtained for one of the several self-report measures of anxiety. There was no effect of any independent variable on verbal behavior recorded during the interaction. Wilson and Abrams concluded that their data were consistent with the TRH, but that it was a nonpharmacologic mechanism that produced the effect. They contrasted this result to that of Polivy et al. (1976), who found that the expectancy that alcohol was consumed *increased* anxiety. Their interpretation was that the most likely reason for this discrepancy was that Polivy et al. manipulated anxiety using shock whereas they used a "clinically relevant" anxiety manipulation. Why they did not focus on the difference in the sex of the subjects (Polivy et al. used females) or on the measurement used (the findings of Polivy et al. were based on self-report, whereas the only significant findings of Wilson and Abrams were for heart rate) remains obscure. Nor did they comment on the relevance of the fact that fully one-third of their subjects reported that for them, no reduction of anxiety by alcohol was expected. However, as we shall see, unaddressed contradictions abound in this literature.

A sequel to the previous study, involving female subjects, was published in 1979 by Abrams and Wilson. The design was a similar 2 × 2 factorial design in which the actual beverage content (alcohol or placebo) and the expected beverage content (subject told alcohol or told placebo) were orthogonally manipulated. The social situation involved a brief interaction with a male confederate. Physiologic, self-report, and observer ratings of anxiety were obtained. There was independent confirmation that the majority of the subjects entered the study with the expectation that alcohol reduces tension in people in general, and for them in particular. However, the experimental data were to the contrary. The belief that alcohol was consumed resulted in elevated physiologic arousal; the actual beverage consumed did not affect the outcome. Although a self-report measure indicated that the social interaction did produce anxiety, none of the independent variables affected this set of measurements. The complex analysis of observer ratings suggested that subjects who believed they had been given alcohol were more uncomfortable in the interaction than those who believed they had been given only tonic water. This is basically the opposite of what was found with men. Thus, despite similar advance beliefs about the effects of alcohol on anxiety in both sexes, the tension of females was increased in the experimental situation. Abrams and Wilson speculated that this might have resulted from a learned habit in women to be apprehensive in some situations involving alcohol, leading to the activation of concerns related to propriety and sexuality. Whether or not they were right, what is important is that a circumstance under which contradiction of the TRH might be expected appears to have been identified.

Another elaborate investigation involving social anxiety was reported by Keane and Lisman (1980). They used males, but added the variation of including subjects described as "clinically shy." There was also a novel variant in the expectancy domain. Instead of manipulating whether they were given correct or false information about their actual beverage, the experimenters told their subjects either that alcohol would facilitate or hinder performance in the social interaction they were to have with a female. Shortly prior to the interaction, subjects received alcohol (0.4 g/kg) or placebo. Observational, psychophysiologic, and self-report measures of tension were obtained. The observational data involved ratings of verbal behavior from audiotapes. Socially anxious males behaved comparably to the females studied by Abrams and Wilson (1979). Alcohol impaired actual performance in the social interaction as reflected in verbal behavior; this was suggestive of augmented social anxiety in the situation. Alcohol had no effects on self-reported fear, but did lead to more "irrational self-statements." The latter finding was taken to reflect increased emotionality. There were no beverage-induced effects on the physiologic measures. The effects of the instructions are of tangential interest here. However, it is worth noting that the positive findings discussed here were main effects of alcohol and not expectancies or instructions. Consequently, they must be interpreted as having a pharmacologic basis.

In a second experiment, Keane and Lisman (1980) used nonshy males and varied the dose (0.26 g/kg and 0.60 g/kg). The instructional manipulation was retained as were the procedures and measurements of tension. There were few differences in actual performance in the interaction, but those that occurred suggested an impairment even in these subjects. In this experiment, one of the psychophysiologic variables showed a difference, as heart rate during the social interaction was increased in the group that received the highest dose. Not surprisingly, the general conclusion by Keane and Lisman was that alcohol failed to reduce tension anxiety. This was conservative in view of the fact that the evidence was that alcohol actually *increased* tension anxiety. Keane and Lisman did not discuss their results in the context of the diverse finings in this line of research.

A potentially valuable insight into the relationship between alcohol, performance, and anxiety is to be had in a study not concerned with performance in a social behavior (Logue, Gentry, Linnoila, & Erwin, 1978). Male and female subjects were asked to perform a test of driving skills after ingesting placebo or alcohol (0.5 g/kg, 0.8 g/kg, or 1.2 g/kg). Self-ratings of anxiety were obtained before and after performance testing. There was a dose-related increase in anxiety in both sexes. The typical effect of alcohol on this type of performance is a dose-related impairment. This raises the possibility that what is anxiogenic about alcohol in performance situations is that, objectively, performance is adversely affected. This could be true whether the task involves social or psychomotor performance. The common mechanism would be that intoxication increases the likelihood of undesirable outcomes. Of course, this does nothing to reconcile the contradictory outcomes that have occurred when socially stressful interactions have been studied, but it does give a rationale for why anxiety might increase in such a situation. Perhaps, for example, this is why women (see Abrams & Wilson, 1979; Polivy *et al.*, 1976) and shy males (Keane & Lisman, 1980) appear likely to become more anxious in potentially threatening situations after drinking.[3]

A few studies have explored the importance of prior drinking history and tolerance using social interaction as the means for inducing tension. Wilson, Abrams, and Lipscomb (1980) used a social interaction situation to study the effects of dose and drinking habits on a variety of measurements of anxiety. The subjects were males who interacted with a female confederate. The doses were placebo, 0.5 g/kg and 1.0 g/kg, administered to subjects classified by a drinking habit inventory as light or heavy drinkers. When heart rate was the measurement, the data suggested that the highest dose of alcohol afforded some protection against anxiety. This was not corroborated by self-report of anxiety. Ratings of anxiety were made by male and female judges

---

[3] It may well be that females have a generalized tendency to become tense in laboratory investigations of alcohol. Myrsten, Hollstedt, and Holmberg (1975) compared the effects of alcohol (0.72 g/kg) on males and females in a situation in which psychomotor performance was measured. Subjects were tested in groups of three individuals of the same sex. Female subjects were less happy, more depressed, more irritated, and less relaxed than males as measured by self-report. They also excreted more adrenaline and noradrenaline in their urine and had higher heart rates than males. Since the subjects in this study were Swedish, comparisons to American women should proceed with caution. However, the consistency in the general direction of sex differences is difficult to overlook where alcohol and tension are concerned.

who viewed videotapes of the interactions. There were complex interactions between sex of observer and dose. Although these were discussed, it is probably best to ignore unpredicted interactions yielded by a five-way analysis of variance. Drinking history had no reported effects.

The interesting conclusion from this study was that the "findings underscore the importance of including multiple measures of anxiety in studies of the tension-reduction hypothesis." Implicit in this was criticism of studies using only a single measure. This research can only be praised for care in its design, use of multiple doses, and other virtues. At the same time, just one of two physiological measurements of tension (the other was skin conductance) yielded an intelligible result related to the TRH and to an extent its significance ($p < .025$) relied on an enormous number of degrees of freedom in the analysis, as the $F$ value was not large. Perhaps it would make more sense to have fewer, more consistent and sensitive measurements, instead of relying on dozens of opportunities (each general type of measurement is represented by a large number of variants) to extract a statistically significant result. Wilson *et al.* saw these discrepancies as "intriguing," but from a theoretical point of view they are distressing. Their final conclusion was that "it is no longer useful to ask whether alcohol reduces tension, but rather to investigate under what conditions, at which dose and on which measures it reduces tension." Were Keane and Lisman to have authored this statement, it might have been the same, with the exception of substituting the word "increases" for "reduces."

The same group of investigators (Lipscomb, Nathan, Wilson, & Abrams, 1980) hypothesized that effects of alcohol on tension would be subject to tolerance. Evidence consistent with this was obtained in a study using the experimental strategy of other studies by this group. Subjects were classified as high or low in tolerance based on the effect of alcohol on body sway. Both low (0.5 g/kg) and high (1.0 g/kg) doses were used. Psychophysiologic, self-report, and observer ratings of anxiety were obtained. Among these there were significant findings only with the psychophysiologic measurements of heart rate and skin conductance. For subjects high in tolerance, there was a large heart rate increase during the social interaction at the low dose, but this was very much reduced when the dose was doubled. For subjects low in tolerance, the heart rate increase was small at both the low and high doses. An analogous pattern was seen in skin conductance. Thus for one type of index of tension, it appeared not only that alcohol reduced tension, but that this phenomenon was subject to tolerance. Furthermore, the data suggest that there is a threshold effect in low-tolerance subjects, since the total benefit was achieved at the low dose and could not be increased by increasing the dose. It is unfortunate that there was no placebo condition included in view of this threshold effect, since in its absence we cannot determine whether low-tolerance subjects are exquisitely sensitive to alcohol in this situation, or simply *insensitive* to the manipulation of social anxiety. This study is also subject to the problem that the hypothesis was confirmed with only one of three classes of anxiety measurement, with no truly satisfactory explanation of why beyond the essentially circular arguments that "anxiety is a multidimensional construct," and that "physiologic data are at least more reliable indices of anxiety than self-report or observer ratings."

There are other studies that could be considered in greater detail here, but they would not add to the patchwork of conclusions already established. These include more results that are simply negative with respect to the TRH (Bradlyn, Strickler, & Maxwell, 1981), or results that are a combination of negative, positive, and contradictory findings, involving complex interactions with sex, dose, and so on (Eddy, 1979). The extent to which these complex, multifactorial, multimeasure designs (including for good measure the manipulation of beliefs and expectation) provide a challenge to theoretical interpretation is evident in still other studies following this strategy (Wilson, Perold, & Abrams, 1981; Woolfolk, Abrams, Abrams, & Wilson, 1979). A major problem with the strategy is that the complexity of the construction of studies can become detrimental to the value of theoretical clarity, although the intent is clearly opposite. Discussion sections too often consist of retrospective rationalizations of bits of outcome in the midst of numerous outcome *opportunities,* only a fraction of which pan out and receive interpretation. Negative results, however abundant, receive scant attention. The conclusion *must* be that the phenomenon is very complex, but it is always difficult to be satisfied with this necessary conclusion, since there is a different complexity with each study. Complexity by itself is not a deadly problem, but it can be a premorbid symptom for a theoretical enterprise if no two studies produce the same complex picture of reality. Perhaps in time a happy medium will be reached where the TRH is concerned. For the moment, however, studies of social anxiety have done little to clarify the TRH.

## Alcohol and Expectancies

In dealing with the literature on expectancy and alcohol effects, it is important to bear in mind that there are two quite distinct subcategories to be considered. In *experiments,* "expectancy" refers to the deception of subjects about whether they are being administered alcohol or a placebo. Subjects' beliefs about the *effects* of alcohol (e.g., on anxiety) are another matter entirely. For example, in the experiment by Wilson and Abrams (1977), although all subjects appeared to be successfully deceived about beverage content, only two-thirds believed that alcohol would have any effect on their tension level. Clearly, it is only by asking subjects to describe their cognitions about alcohol's *effects* that the possible impact of the deception can be understood. Although this has been done on occasion, experimenters have usually talked confidently about the importance of cognitions without taking into account that a manipulation of information about the *beverage* is an "unclean" manipulation of the important cognitions about *effects*.

The other kind of literature in this category is more straightforward. Subjects have been administered questionnaires soliciting their beliefs about the effects of alcohol. There is nothing fundamentally new about this approach (see Keehn, Bloomfield, & Hug, 1970). The methodology in this research, however, reflects the most current procedures used in the analysis of large sets of questionnaire data. There has been a spate of publications of this type in the past few years, beginning with the work of Brown, Goldman, Inn, and Anderson (1980). A large, heterogenous group of subjects, ranging from college students to patients in an alcohol treatment program, was used to develop items for an Alcohol Expectancy Questionnaire (AEQ). The questionnaire was designed to tap alcohol reinforcement expectancies. A refined version of the AEQ was subsequently administered to a group of college students described as "social drinkers" along with questionnaires concerning demographic characteristics and drinking patterns. In a factor analysis of the AEQ, tension-reduction was only one of six factors that emerged. The other five (e.g., expect alcohol to enhance sexual performance and experience) could be described more as positive reinforcement expectancies than negative reinforcement by tension reduction. The relative importance of these potential sources of reinforcement could not be assessed. Brown *et al.* (1980) even suggested that tension-reduction theories of alcohol use might have derived from theorists' own expectancies about alcohol's effects. Whether or not this is so, the existence of an expectancy of reinforcement by tension reduction provides a strong circumstantial case that alcohol *has* such an effect, although of course the *basis* for the expectancy (e.g., is it strictly pharmacologic?) is another matter.

In a related kind of research, Farber, Khavari, and Douglass (1980) reported the results of a factor analysis of self-reported reasons for drinking. They identified two major categories of reasons. One was positive reinforcement, which they equated with "social drinking." An example of an item loading on this factor was "I drink to be sociable." The other category was negative reinforcement, which was equated with "escape drinking." An item loading on this factor was "I need a drink to help me relax." Interestingly, subjects reporting the highest levels of alcohol consumption were also those who had the highest scores on escape drinking.

More recently, research into expectancies using questionnaire methods has been addressed to questions beyond describing these expectancies. In one such study (Southwick, Steele, Marlatt, & Lindell, 1981) an attempt was made to use this kind of data to comment on conflicting experimental results. A distinction was suggested between tension as represented in physiologic arousal on the one hand, and negative affect on the other. Southwick *et al.* reported that their informants (college students) expected alcohol to alleviate tension in the sense of negative affect, but to have the opposite effect on arousal. Although this finding was related in the general context of contradictory research findings, no studies to which the distinction might be relevant were considered. Some experimenters have relied heavily on alcohol-dampened physiologic arousal to support the TRH (see Levenson *et al.*, 1980; Limpscomb *et al.*, 1980). Thus it is not obvious how these data on expectancies help to resolve or explain any conflict in the literature concerning the TRH—certainly one would not expect Levenson *et al.* or Lipscomb *et al.* to embrace any suggestion that reduced physiologic arousal is not a result of alcohol consumption or an appropriate index of tension reduction. Clearly, more consideration needs to be given to the existing empirical literature on "real" alcohol consumption before engaging in speculation based on this type of questionnaire data. There is much yet to be discovered about the relationship between these questionnaire responses and the effects of consumed alcohol.

One way to achieve this is by including variables that have appeared to be important in the laboratory experiment. For example, Rohsenow (1983) found that female undergraduates expected less relaxation from "a few drinks" than did their male counterparts. This seems to correspond with the results on sex differences that have been obtained in the laboratory. In addition, the heavier drinkers in their sample expected to achieve more relaxation from a few drinks than did light drinkers; this seems to fit with Farber *et al.*'s (1980) relationship between heavy drinking and "escape drinking."

Finally, it appears that expectancies concerning the effects of alcohol, including those related to tension are acquired at a young age and without the necessity of personal experience with drinking (Christiansen & Goldman, 1983; Christiansen, Goldman, & Inn, 1982).

The suggestion that what a person expects from a certain experience will color that experience is an ancient notion, and certainly not new to alcohol research (see MacAndrew & Edgerton, 1969). The literature on expectancies concerning alcohol is still immature if promising in some respects. To an extent, the "balanced placebo design" that characterizes the experimental research has been applied reflexively without adequate analysis of the theoretical justification for manipulating expectancy. Moreover, there is yet to emerge a standard approach to the concept of expectancy; some investigators have been simply content to deceive subjects about what drink they get, whereas others have tried to determine what their subjects actually expect alcohol will do to them. No consistent effects of expectancy manipulations with regard to the TRH have emerged in experiments, although the questionnaire research suggests that there is a stable set of beliefs about alcohol's effects in North America. It will be interesting to see the direction that expectancy research takes.

## Alcohol and Affect

One class of experiments not discussed previously deals not with the effects of alcohol on tension states specifically, but on mood generally. It is not our intention to review this literature thoroughly, since this has been done repeatedly by others (Freed, 1978; Pihl & Smith, 1983; Russell & Mehrabian, 1975; Tucker, Vuchinich, & Sobell, 1982). However, a few observations must be made. The nature of the data collected in studies of mood tends to be similar across experiments; subjects are administered alcohol, and at various points in the procedure they self-rate mood on a standardized scale such as the Profile of Mood States (POMS). There appears to be excellent consistency in this literature. Generally, at low doses the effect of alcohol is mood enhancement; subjects will report that they are euphoric, happy, and relaxed. At higher dose levels, however, it is likely that subjects will report increases in anxiety and depression (see Russell & Mehrabian, 1975). This has been found within the context of a single extended drinking session in nonalcoholic subjects (Williams, 1966) and in studies of continuous daily drinking by hospitalized alcoholic subjects (e.g., Mendelson, LaDou, & Solomon, 1964; Nathan, Titler, Lowenstein, Solomon, & Rossi, 1970). Such data have been taken to contradict the TRH (e.g., see Cappell, 1975), and certainly it would seem that they are embarrassing for an unamended version of it. For the purposes of the present discussion, this consistent finding is all that is of importance; readers interested in the details of this literature and the theoretical issues it raises are referred to the articles cited above.

A recent descriptive study of drinking in alcoholics (Stockwell, Hodgson, & Rankin, 1982) is an explicit attempt to defend the TRH against the implications of studies demonstrating deterioration in affect during chronic drinking. Another interesting approach to the "paradox" of people continuing to use alcohol despite suffering what appear to be aversive consequences, has been taken by Mello (1981).

## Tension and Alcohol Self-Administration

All of the work reviewed to this point can at most establish whether *in principle,* tension reduction could be a basis for reinforcement by alcohol. Logically, it would be an error to draw a firm conclusion about the motivation for a behavior from one of its effects. The volume of research on tension and alcohol self-administration over the past 10 years has not been great, but there have been a reasonable number of studies involving human subjects to offset the decline in work with animals. The following section will review experimental studies in humans in which tension manipulation was the independent variable and drinking was the dependent variable. Although some additional data on animals have accumulated, they will be touched upon only briefly. As far as research with animals is concerned, there has been insufficient progress in this literature in the last decade to warrant review. It is not that there has been a failure to show that some stress manipulations may produce elevations in alcohol consumption in rats (e.g., Kinney & Schmidt, 1979; Mills, Bean, & Hutcheson, 1977), but that there has yet to emerge even a rudimentary understanding of the conditions under which various stress manipulations will or will not affect alcohol consumption in animals. Interested readers can find a more thorough appraisal of the recent literature in an article by Pohorecky (1981). Correlational studies examining relationships between self-reports of drinking and some assessment of tension level also will not be included. Although correlational studies can be useful, there is always the problem of assessing the direction of causality.

The research that most studies in this area use as a reference point was conducted by Higgins and Marlatt (1973). The subjects were 20 male alcoholics who were nonabstinent at the time of the study, and 20 "social drinkers." The subjects were given the explanation that the experimenters were interested in "the effect of touch on the taste of alcohol." The "touch" stimulus in this case was electric shock, which subjects were told would be either weak (low threat) or strong (high threat). After concluding the threat manipulation, the experimenters invited the subjects to rate a variety of alcoholic beverages on various dimensions of taste. Of course, they were really interested in the amount of alcohol consumed. There was no effect of the threat manipulation on alcohol consumption in either population of drinkers. Higgins and Marlatt appeared to consider this a failure for the TRT, but it could be argued that they tended to gloss over the evidence that the threat manipulation was relatively ineffective.

A follow-up study was published (Higgins & Marlatt, 1975) in which a social anxiety manipulation was used because unlike fear of shock, this would be a "meaningful source of tension as it relates to alcohol consumption." There were several independent variable manipulations applied to these male undergraduates, but only one exerted an effect on alcohol consumption as measured in the taste-rating task. Subjects who were led to believe that they would be taking part in an evaluative personal interaction with a female drank more than those who thought that they would only be asked to rate some pictures of females for attractiveness. One interpretation of this was that the former subjects drank more to reduce tension.

The relative success of this experiment raised the problem of why such an outcome should selectively apply to fear of evaluation and not fear of shock. Because a nonparsimonious distinction would have been required to explain the discrepancy in results (the fact that the shock manipulation was relatively ineffective was not considered), the authors offered the alternative that high-fear subjects drank more as a "self-control procedure" rather than solely to reduce tension. How this differs in substance from a tension-reduction argument (i.e., people may attempt to establish control because lack of it creates tension) was not made clear, nor was it clear how drinking would produce a feeling of being in control. Nor was there any consideration of why subjects would not seek this form of control in the face of impending shock. There is an interesting test of the self-control interpretation suggested in the experiments in which females more than males appeared to have a strong need not to lose control to alcohol. Such a comparison would test the prediction that females in an anxiety-provoking social situation would drink *less* than males for fear of *losing* control rather than *more* in the hope of asserting it.

Higgins and Marlatt (1973) had both alcoholics and social drinkers in their study, and found that the expectation of electric shock did not affect drinking in either group. Another group of investigators (Miller, Hersen, Eisler, & Hilsman, 1974) had a more positive result using a social stressor which, from its description, could be characterized as a 15-min harassment of subjects over their shortcomings. Prior to this manipulation and after it, subjects were permitted to perform a simple operant response that resulted in the delivery of bourbon and water. There was also a no-stress control condition. The only significant result was an interaction, as alcoholics increased their responding from no-stress to stress conditions, whereas social drinkers *decreased* their responding when stressed. A pulse rate measure validated the effectiveness of the stress manipulation. Since it was equally effective for both drinker populations, the difference was interpreted to indicate that alcoholics learn to drink to cope with stress, whereas nonalcoholics possess a larger repertoire of alternative coping behaviors.

A study bearing more directly on alternative coping mechanisms was conducted by Marlatt, Kosturn, and Lang (1975). In this experiment, male and female subjects were harassed, not unlike those in the study by Miller *et al.* (1974). But Marlatt *et al.* described theirs as a manipulation of anger rather than of stress. Some of the "provoked" subjects were given an opportunity to retaliate against an insulting confederate (by administering shocks) and others were not. Control subjects who were not provoked at all were also included. Subsequently, alcohol consumption was measured using the taste-test deception. The primary finding was that subjects who were insulted but allowed to retaliate drank less wine than those who were insulted without benefit of retaliation. There was no difference in BAC among groups, which was measured at a modest 200 mg/liter. Two accounts of these data were considered. One was that subjects who are made angry become tense. The tension can be reduced through the catharsis of retaliation; failing this, subjects may drink instead. This alternative was less favored than the argument that subjects given the opportunity to retaliate drew from this a sense of control over the source of the insult, and with this coping mechanism at hand required less to drink. While the study does not necessarily affirm the TRT, it is consistent with it. Unfortunately there were several problems. First, nowhere did the investigators report whether there were different levels of anger or tension among conditions; the only data were on ratings of personal attributes of the confederate. Second, there were no differences in drinking between the subjects who were insulted and could retaliate, and those who were not insulted at all. This raises some obvious questions about the manipulation. In summary, conclusions should be taken from this study with caution.

Holroyd (1978) studied the effects of manipulated social anxiety on beer drinking with a result that appears contradictory to the TRT. Subjects also were selected to be high or low in social anxiety. The anxiety manipulation involved giving them either a negative or positive evaluation of their social skills. Following this, subjects were invited to an "informal get-together" in which beer was available. Subjects in the conditions of the 2 × 2 design drank virtually identical amounts of beer; those with high social anxiety who were also given a negative evaluation drank less. This was seen as discrepant with the outcome expected from the work of Marlatt and his colleagues, and at odds with the TRT. One possible explanation was that the group that drank less did so because the subjects became socially withdrawn; in this view, they avoided drinking since it involved social interaction. This is not very satisfying since the subjects did not in fact avoid drinking—they only drank somewhat less. Moreover, the study lacked control subjects who were given no evaluative feedback (see the analogous control condition present in the study of Marlatt et al., 1975).

Subjects have been exposed to a variety of other tension-inducing manipulations. Gabel, Noel, Keane, and Lisman (1980) argued for the importance of comparing the effects of aversive motivation with qualitatively different sources of arousal. For their purposes the comparison involved sexual arousal. In a within-subject design, male undergraduates on separate occasions viewed slides of mutilated accident victims, sexual activity, or neutral scenes. Physiologic recordings were obtained during the slide presentations, which were followed by a taste test version of a drinking opportunity for half the subjects, and an operant response that produced alcohol for the remainder. The effectiveness of the arousal manipulations was ambiguous; although both sexual and mutilation scenes produced increased skin conductance on exposure of the first slide, only the mutilation scene remained arousing compared to the neutral condition by the final slide. No differences in heart rate were found. As for drinking, there was more consumed in the sexual arousal condition than the others, but only in the taste-test. The biggest effects were for type of alcoholic beverage and type of drinking task. Again these results were interpreted as contrary to the TRT, although limitations of the data are obvious.

Alcohol consumption to reduce tension may represent an instrumental adaptive strategy that is applied selectively as needed, according to Tucker, Vuchinich, Sobell, and Maisto (1980). In a complicated experiment, they attempted to create a situation in which male subjects (heavy social drinkers) could balance any desire to reduce tension with the desire to avoid deleterious effects on performance in the tension-arousing task. The results were too complicated to review here in detail, but they did not support the hypothesis that subjects drank according to some instrumental plan. However, subjects in the high-stress (greater task difficulty) condition drank more in a taste-rating task than their less stressed counterparts.

Two studies have attempted to determine the effects of experimentally manipulated depression. Pihl and Yankovsky (1979) manipulated mood by deceiving subjects into believing that they had done either well or poorly in a test of intelligence. The manipulation was effective, in that self-rated anxiety and depression were elevated when subjects were informed that they had done poorly. The results were opposite to what might be predicted from the TRT—when negative affect was induced, subjects drank *less* in a taste-test procedure than control subjects in whom affect was slightly elevated or unchanged. Pihl and Yankovsky concluded that negative reinforcement through tension reduction is at best a limited source of motivation for drinking.

Also pursuing the relationship between depressive affect and drinking, Noel and Lisman (1980) conducted several studies. The first was a survey that revealed that among female but not male undergraduates, respondents rated as moderately clinically depressed according to the Beck Depression Inventory reported greater alcohol consumption than those who were not depressed. Two subsequent studies were experimental. They involved use of a "learned helplessness" manipulation to elicit depression. Only female subjects were used. There was some question as to the overall success of the manipulation with regard to the concept of learned helplessness, but it appeared to be successful in inducing depressive affect. It also produced an elevation in beer consumption compared to a control group in the now familiar taste-rating procedure. A useful additional control was that although ginger ale was also available, only beer consumption was affected. In all, however, trivial amounts of beer were consumed by both the depressed (5.7 ounces) and nondepressed (3.6 ounces) groups. The results were essentially replicated in a second experiment. Noel and Lisman observed that an "impersonal" source of stress could lead to an increase in alcohol consumption, which is somewhat at odds with the position advanced by Marlatt and his associates. The data of Tucker *et al.* (1980) reinforce such a view, but these positive results stand in contrast to those of Pihl and Yankofsky (1979).

In a study considered earlier, Steele *et al.* (1981) reported that alcohol reduced the tension induced by cognitive dissonance. Another important element of this research was to test whether the presence of dissonance would lead to increased alcohol consumption in the taste-rating procedure. However, despite the fact that alcohol reduced the effects of dissonance, dissonance did not lead to increased alcohol consumption. A variety of possible reasons for the discordant results were presented, and notwithstanding that dissonance did not affect drinking, it was suggested that teaching methods of coping with dissoannce would be a useful addition to treatment for alcoholism prevention.

The major advance in research on self-administration has been the addition of experimental work involving human subjects. Methodologically, this has been aided by the taste-test procedure, which may be a relatively nonreactive way of assessing motivation to obtain the postingestional effects of alcohol. However, it seems clear that there is no strong trend in this research yet. Tension need not lead to increased drinking, and has even had an opposite effect. There has also been a tendency at times to go farther in conclusions than the data warrant.

## Current Evaluation of the Tension Reduction Theory

### Overview of the Findings

In earlier reviews on this subject (Cappell, 1975; Cappell & Herman, 1972), it was not difficult to come to the conclusion that there was a huge gap between the apparent faith in the TRT and the quality of the evidence to support it. Although there is still no reason to accept a simpleminded version of the TRT, the major change evident in the literature is that there is now agreement on this point. Indeed, there have been numerous observations of how complex are the relationships determining alcohol's credentials as an anxiolytic agent. Yet within this brew of new findings, there are some new leads that may help to formulate a more supportable theory. This seems especially so for the TRH, since the literature on self-administration has not really yielded much of conclusive theoretical importance.

Studies employing *conflict procedures* in both humans and animals have continued to provide relatively consistent support for the TRH, although it is still difficult to pinpoint what it is about the nature of conflict that makes this so. Certainly there appears to be something about conflict that makes it especially amenable to resolution by an anxiolytic intervention. After all, conflict procedures have emerged as the techniques of choice by drug manufacturers for evaluating anxiolytic agents. Thus, even if the anxiolytic action of a drug is only one in a wide spectrum, these techniques may be particularly effective in detecting it. The direct comparison of alcohol to tranquilizers using the same procedure (Vogel *et al.*, 1980) provides especially important support for the TRH, and is a comparison to which we shall return.

Work described in the section on alcohol and the *response to noxious stimuli* has also provided a rich yield in understanding. The work by Levenson, Sher, and their associates was especially impressive. In particular, the suggestion that there are biological differences that might make some individuals particularly responsive to the tension reducing effects of alcohol is worthy of note and of further research. This theme was echoed in the findings of Cutter and his associates in humans and in recent animal research as well (Vogel & DeTurck, 1983). Nothing could do more to help clarify the status of the TRH than to isolate individual difference factors that can determine whether alcohol is likely to have a tension reducing effect.

The animal literature on responses to noxious stimulation has also been interesting. It suggested that alcohol may effectively block biochemical responses to stress, but most effectively when the dose is not very high. High doses of alcohol seem also to create rather than ameliorate tension states in humans.

In the best of all possible worlds, the literature on the effects of alcohol in *socially stressful situations* in humans would have produced some of the best data with which to appraise the TRH. However, this was not so. With the exception of pointing to potentially important sex differences, this literature is a mass of contradiction and inconsistency. An hypothesis may be confirmed by one response index and not another, and contradicted by yet a third. Although the complex factorial designs that dominate this literature made sense on an a priori basis, it seems that generally the designs and procedures of many of these studies were so complicated as to make consistently interpretable results difficult to obtain. Hence the main conclusion from much of this research was that the phenomenon under study is extremely complex. Perhaps it would be best to retreat to simpler designs in preference to the complicated and numerous alternative explanations that seem endemic to this literature.

The concept of *expectancies* holds out the promise of accounting for some puzzling results. If diverse beliefs in alcohol's effects cause variations in behavior despite ostensibly identical pharmacological stimulation, this might explain why alcohol can reduce tension for one person but not for another.

Unfortunately, the incorporation of expectancy manipulations into research designs has too often been done automatically and without adequate forethought, and it is not always clear enough exactly what is being affected by expectancy manipulations in experiments. The questionnaire approach has certainly helped to describe beliefs about alcohol's effects, but this literature has yet to advance much beyond description. In principle, however, if the belief that alcohol reduces tension is acquired very early in life and is very resistant to change, this could go a long way toward explaining apparently paradoxical results.

*Self-administration studies* in humans have often been ingenious in tests of the TRT. Although there have been some results supportive of the theory, no powerful conclusion can be drawn, and occasionally there have been conclusions that were only weakly supported by the data. However, perhaps not too much is to be expected from such studies in view of the fact that tension reduction is only one of a myriad of potential reinforcers for drinking. This is another area that would benefit from greater concentration on individual differences. Interesting alternative formulations are now available (e.g., Hull, 1981; Vuchinich & Tucker, 1983), and these can be expected to supplement TRT in the near future.

### Limitations of the Tension Reduction Theory

Many of the limitations of the TRT have now been recognized and accepted by the scientists working to support or cast doubt on the theory. The most important limitation is that historically there was too much emphasis on a single-factor theory, and this has been reflected in attempts to devise new theoretical approaches (Hull, 1981; Vuchinich & Tucker, 1983). When the literature on self-report of expectations of reinforcement from alcohol (e.g., see Brown *et al.*, 1980) is considered, it becomes obvious that tension reduction is only one of many motives for alcohol consumption. We can agree with Hodgson *et al.* (1979) that alcohol *can* reduce tension, but it can do other things as well. The issue for research is to determine the conditions in which what *can* happen actually *will* happen. When faced with alternative techniques for coping with tension, what determines that drinking will be chosen? Even if drinking is efficacious for some, other adaptations are nonetheless available.

Another limitation of the theory may stem from a consideration of the pharmacologic actions of alcohol itself. Here it is important to bear in mind that such success as the TRH has enjoyed has involved modest doses of alcohol. High doses appear to generate increases in tension. This pattern of findings should serve to remind that alcohol is a drug with a variety of actions, only one of which may be anxiolytic or tension-reducing. To appreciate the importance of this, it is necessary to turn to some fundamental principles of drug action. Drug effects can be grouped into two main categories. The first category contains the *intended* (therapeutic) *effect,* and the other contains *side effects.* For the present argument, the "therapeutic effect" is tension reduction, and anything else is a side effect. The net effect of any given administration of a drug will be some composite of the therapeutic and side effects associated with a particular dose. In the case of alcohol, the important question is whether there are side effects that can obscure the therapeutic effect. The answer appears to be affirmative, especially at higher doses. If this answer is accepted, then it must be concluded that if alcohol is an anxiolytic, its *potency* as an anxiolytic is not great, and that this is probably due to the fact that as dose increases, the potency of side effects that interfere with tension reduction increases.

This point is easiest to illustrate in a comparison with that group of drugs, the benzodiazepines, that were developed with a view to maximizing anxiolytic potency within their total spectrum of drug actions. Alcohol and benzodiazepines have been shown to differ in a number of respects relevant to present considerations. In particular, they appear to differ in their ability to produce aversive side effects. One paradigm that can be used to make a general assessment of the aversive properties of drugs is conditioned taste aversion. Animals will learn to avoid novel-tasting solutions that are followed by administration of a variety of psychoactive drugs, as if they have been poisoned (Cappell & LeBlanc, 1977). Using this paradigm, it has been shown (Cappell, LeBlanc, & Endrenyi, 1973) that alcohol is a more potent agent than chlordiazepoxide (CDP), which is one of the benzodiazepines; thus, alcohol is in some general way more aversive to rats than is CDP. It has also been shown that whereas CDP *accelerated* the extinction of a conditioned taste aversion, alcohol *retarded* it (Cappell, LeBlanc, & Endrenyi, 1972). That is, CDP was effective in ameliorating a conditioned aversive response which was actually aggravated by alcohol.

Earlier it was noted (see Vogel *et al.*, 1980) that both alcohol and CDP were effective in restoring behavior that was suppressed by shock in both rats and mice. However, there were important differences, at least where rats were concerned. The minimum effective dose (MED) of alcohol to restore punished responding was 0.5 g/kg. Although the effect was still obtained at doses of 1.0 g/kg, 1.5 g/kg, and 2.0 g/kg, no additional "benefit" was observed as the dose was increased. However, at a dose of 3.0 g/kg (six times the MED) punished behavior was even more suppressed than in a saline control condition. For CDP, the MED was 4 mg/kg. At 8 mg/kg the antipunishment effect was stronger still. At a dose of 27 mg/kg (seven times the MED) the antipunishment effect was lessened but it was still slightly greater than the one observed at the MED. Higher doses were not tested. In a variant of the antipunishment test (Breese, Frye, Vogel, Koepke, & Mueller, 1983), it was reported that ethanol in a dose range of 0.25 to 1.0 g/kg was ineffective, whereas CDP was effective in restoring behavior suppressed by punishment at doses of 3.0 mg/kg and 10.0 mg/kg.

What is the point of this comparison? First, the evidence should be summarized:

1. Both alcohol and CDP can be effective in a test that is sensitive to the anxiolytic activity of drugs.
2. As dose increases, the anxiolytic action of alcohol is lost or obscured at a smaller proportional increment.
3. In some tests, CDP is effective when alcohol is not.
4. In some tests, alcohol appears to be a more potent aversive agent than CDP, and can even exacerbate an aversive effect that CDP ameliorates.

Of course, CDP was *specifically developed* to have relatively potent anxiolytic effects compared to its side effects. Such anxiolytic effects that alcohol possesses are as nature has determined. In a comparison, it appears clear that the designed anxiolytic simply has a *greater tension reducing potency* than alcohol. The reason for this appears to be that as one moves up from the MED for an anxiolytic effect, interfering effects will emerge more quickly in the case of alcohol than CDP. In pharmacologic jargon, the "margin of safety" for "therapeutic" (tension reducing) effects versus "toxic" (those that degrade or even reverse the tension-reduction) side effects is less for alcohol than for CDP.

The comparison between alcohol and CDP has been presented in simplified terms, but it is our belief that the analysis will stand empirical scrutiny even if variations and exceptions could be found. The simple conclusion is that even if alcohol is a tension reducing agent, it is a relatively ineffective one, primarily because it has other actions which negate its ability to reduce tension, especially at higher doses. If this line of reasoning is accepted, it is not difficult to understand why the TRT has been so resistant to wide confirmation, or why such effort needs to be invested to achieve a positive result. Of course, the broader implication of this pharmacologic analysis is that a generalized TRT will *never* receive support no matter how much research is done, and that only efforts to delineate the conditions under which alcohol's tension reducing effect is relatively strong and uncontaminated will save what is valid in the theory. Further research not governed by this assumption seems bound to founder, and the example provided by Sher and Levenson (1982) is to be commended as one to follow.

## Implications for Prevention and Treatment

The implications of the TRT for treatment are obvious- if drinking may emerge or has emerged as a pathologic response to tension, therapies directed at alternatives for reducing tension would be indicated. A good example of this rationale is to be found in studies of the relationship between phobic anxiety and alcoholism. Smail, Stockwell, Canter, and Hodgson (1984) reported a remarkable rate of phobias in a sample of alcoholic inpatients in England. Fully 53% of the sample of 60 individuals (40 males and 20 females) were diagnosed as having agoraphobia, a social phobia, or both. There was a positive association between severity of the phobic condition and severity of alcohol dependence. Smail *et al.* reported that, "A majority of alcoholics had suffered mild or severe phobic anxiety when last drinking and this group all attributed tension reducing properties to alcohol", and that "alcohol had helped them to cope with feared situations." The converse relationship also appeared to exist, as 12 of 18 patients with a primary diagnosis of phobia (rather than alcoholism) reported that they self-medicated with alcohol to relieve their phobic condition.

In a related study (Stockwell, Smail, Hodgson, & Canter, 1984), 24 of the patients from the Smail *et al.* (1984) sample who were diagnosed as both alcoholic and phobic were interviewed concerning the relationship between their phobic experiences and their drinking. It was interesting that although such patients had earlier attributed tension-reducing properties to alcohol and found that drinking was an effective coping mechanism, when interviewed "a significant majority of the sample who confessed to experiencing fears believed that a heavy drinking bout worsened their fears."

Like many other students of the relationship between anxiety and drinking, Stockwell *et al.* concluded that they were dealing with a "complex interaction of learning and psychobiological processes." Because of this complexity, they suggested that behavioral interventions meant to deal with anxiety should not be initiated without a good analysis of the functional relationship between drinking and anxiety in each clinical case.

These data on phobias and alcoholism are interesting and will probably lead to yet more interesting findings (see also Bowen, Cipywnyk, D'Arcy, & Keegan, 1984). Yet the suggestion of a functional relationship between some form of affective disorder and drinking is not new or unique to phobias. For example, very similar issues arise in a consideration of the relationship between depression and alcoholism (Goodwin, 1983). Indeed, it may be necessary to consider relationships among phobic disorders, depression, and alcoholism at once (Leckman, Weissman, Merikangas, Pauls, & Prusoff, 1983).

A further review of this literature will not be attempted. It appears that it is in a considerable state of flux, and it remains to be seen what it will yield. There is a recent review of the literature on the efficacy of behavioral anti-anxiety treatments for alcoholism (Klajner, Hartman, & Sobell, 1984). Its conclusion was that a convincing clinical trial of such treatments has yet to be done.

The implications of some of the new findings for prevention are interesting and of considerable potential importance. Primary among these is the emerging evidence that there are individual differences in the efficacy of alcohol to achieve the reduction of tension (e.g., see Sher & Levenson, 1982). Of paramount importance is that these can be determined in advance of the emergence of abusive drinking, which is of course essential to genuine prevention. Not only do such differences appear to exist, but they have been related to the risk for developing problems in the self-management of alcohol consumption or its consequences. If the TRT has a contribution to make to the amelioration of alcohol problems, the most promising research direction to pursue appears now to be evident.

## References

Abrams, D. B., & Wilson, G. T. (1979). Effects of alcohol on social anxiety in women: Cognitive versus physiological processes. *Journal of Abnormal Psychology, 88*, 161–173.

Bacon, S. D. (1945). Alcohol and complex society. In Yale Studies on Alcohol, *Alcohol, science and society* (pp. 179–200). Westport, CT: Greenwood Press.

Bammer, G., & Chesher, G. B. (1982). An analysis of some effects of alcohol on performance in a passive avoidance task. *Psychopharmacology, 77*, 66–73.

Bowen, R. C., Cipywnyk, D., D'Arcy, C., & Keegan, D. (1984). Alcoholism, anxiety disorders, and agoraphobia. *Alcoholism: Clinical and Experimental Research, 8*, 48–50.

Bradlyn, A. S., Strickler, D. P., & Maxwell, W. A. (1981). Alcohol, expectancy and stress: Methodological concerns with the expectancy design. *Addictive Behaviors, 6*, 1–8.

Breese, G. R., Frye, G. D., Vogel, R. A., Koepke, K. M., & Mueller, R. A. (1983). Comparisons of behavioral and biochemical effects of ethanol and chlordiazepoxide. In L. A. Pohorecky & J. Brick (Eds.), *Stress and alcohol use* (pp. 261–278). New York: Elsevier.

Brick, J., & Pohorecky, L. A. (1982). Ethanol–stress interaction: Biochemical findings. *Psychopharmacology, 77*, 81–84.

Brown, R. A., & Cutter, H. S. G. (1977). Alcohol, customary drinking behavior, and pain. *Journal of Abnormal Psychology, 86*, 179–188.

Brown, S. A., Goldman, M. S., Inn, A., & Anderson, L. R. (1980). Expectations of reinforcement from alcohol: Their domain and relation to drinking pattern. *Journal of Consulting and Clinical Psychology, 48*, 419–426.

Cappell, H. (1975). An evaluation of tension models of alcohol consumption. In R. J. Gibbins, Y. Israel, H. Kalant, R. E. Popham, W. Schmidt, & R. G. Smart (Eds.), *Research advances in alcohol and drug problems* (Vol. 2, pp. 177–210). New York: John Wiley & Sons.

Cappell, H., & Herman, C. P. (1972). Alcohol and tension reduction: A review. *Journal of Studies on Alcohol, 33*, 33–64.

Cappell, H., & LeBlanc, A. E. (1977). Gustatory avoidance conditioning by drugs of abuse: Relationships to general issues in research on drug dependence. In N. W. Milgram,

L. Krames, & T. M Alloway (Eds.), *Food aversion learning* (pp. 133–167). New York: Plenum Press.

Cappell, H., LeBlanc, A. E., & Endrenyi, L. (1972). Effects of chlordiazepoxide and ethanol on the extinction of a conditioned taste aversion. *Physiology and Behavior, 9,* 167–169.

Cappell, H., LeBlanc, A. E., & Endrenyi, L. (1973). Aversive conditioning by psychoactive drugs: Effects of morphine, alcohol and chlordiazepoxide. *Psychopharmacologia, 29,* 239–246.

Christiansen, B. A., & Goldman, M. S. (1983). Alcohol-related expectancies versus demographic/background variables in the prediction of adolescent drinking. *Journal of Consulting and Clinical Psychology, 51,* 249–257.

Christiansen, B. A., Goldman, M. S., & Inn, A. (1982). Development of alcohol-related expectancies in adolescents: Separating pharmacological from social-learning influences. *Journal of Consulting and Clinical Psychology, 50,* 336–344.

Conger, J. J. (1956). Alcoholism: Theory, problem and challenge. II. Reinforcement theory and the dynamics of alcoholism. *Quarterly Journal of Studies on Alcohol, 13,* 296–305.

Cunningham, C. L. (1979). Alcohol as a cue for extinction: State dependency produced by conditioned inhibition. *Animal Learning and Behavior, 7,* 45–52.

Cunningham, C. L., & Brown, J. S. (1983). Escape from fear under alcohol: Fear inhibits alcohol-enhanced responding. *Physiological Psychology, 11,* 81–86.

Cutter, H. S. G., Maloof, B., Kurtz, N. R., & Jones, W. C. (1976). "Feeling no pain": Differential responses to pain by alcoholics and nonalcoholics before and after drinking. *Journal of Studies on Alcohol, 37,* 273–277.

Dengerink, H. A, & Fagan, N. J. (1978). Effects of alcohol on emotional responses to stress. *Journal of Studies in Alcohol, 39,* 525–539.

DeTurck, K. H., & Vogel, W. H. (1982). Effects of acute ethanol on plasma and brain catecholamine levels in stressed and unstressed rats: Evidence for an ethanol–stress interaction. *Journal of Pharmacology and Experimental Therapeutics, 223,* 348–354.

Dickerson, L. L., & Ferraro, D. P. (1976). Effects of alcohol on specific and environmental fear. *Psychological Reports, 39,* 1335–1342.

DiGuisto, E. L., & Bond, N. (1977). Enhancement of pseudoconditioning and retardation of escape by low doses of ethanol. *Pharmacology, Biochemistry and Behavior, 6,* 175–177.

Eddy, C. C. (1979). The effects of alcohol on anxiety in problem- and nonproblem-drinking women. *Alcoholism: Clinical and Experimental Research, 3,* 107–114.

Ellis, F. W. (1966). Effect of ethanol on plasma corticosterone levels. *Journal of Pharmacology and Experimental Therapeutics, 153,* 121–127.

Farber, P. D., Khavari, K. A., & Douglass, F. M., IV (1980). A factor analytic study of reasons for drinking: Empirical validation of positive and negative reinforcement dimensions. *Journal of Consulting and Clinical Psychology, 48,* 780–781.

Freed, E. X. (1978). Alcohol and mood: An updated review. *International Journal of the Addictions, 13,* 173–200.

Gabel, P. C., Noel, N. E., Keane, T. M., & Lisman, S. A. (1980). Effects of sexual versus fear arousal on alcohol consumption in college males. *Behaviour Research and Therapy, 18,* 519–526.

Geller, I., Croy, D. J., & Ryback, R. S. (1974). Effects of ethanol and sodium pentobarbital on conflict behavior of goldfish. *Pharmacology, Biochemistry and Behavior, 2,* 545–548.

Gliner, J. A., Horvath, S. M., & Browe, A. C. (1978). Circulatory changes to alcohol, anxiety and their interactions. *Proceedings of the Society for Experimental Biology and Medicine, 158,* 604–608.

Glowa, J. R., & Barrett, J. E. (1976). Effects of alcohol on punished and unpunished responding of squirrel monkeys. *Pharmacology, Biochemistry and Behavior, 4,* 169–174.

Goodwin, D. W. (1983). The management of depression in alcoholism. *Journal of Psychiatric Treatment and Evaluation, 5,* 445–450.

Higgins, R. L., & Marlatt, G. A. (1973). Effects of anxiety arousal on the consumption of alcohol by alcoholics and social drinkers. *Journal of Consulting and Clinical Psychology, 41,* 426–433.

Higgins, R. L., & Marlatt, G. A. (1975). Fear of interpersonal evaluation as a determinant of alcohol consumption in male social drinkers. *Journal of Abnormal Psychology, 84,* 644–651.

Hodgson, R. J., Stockwell, T. R., & Rankin, H. J. (1979). Can alcohol reduce tension? *Behaviour Research and Therapy, 17,* 459–466.

Holroyd, K. A. (1978). Effects of social anxiety and social evaluation on beer consumption and social interaction. *Journal of Studies on Alcohol, 39,* 737–744.

Horton, D. (1945). The functions of alcohol in primitive societies. In Yale Studies on Alcohol, *Alcohol, science and society* (pp. 153–178). Westport, CT: Greenwood Press.

Hull, J. G. (1981). A self-awareness model of the causes and effects of alcohol consumption. *Journal of Abnormal Psychology, 90,* 586–600.

Jellinek, E. M. (1945). The problem of alcohol. In Yale Studies on Alcohol, *Alcohol, science and society* (pp. 13–30). Westport, CT: Greenwood Press.

Kakihana, R. (1976). Adrenocortical function in mice selectively bred for different sensitivity to ethanol. *Life Sciences, 18,* 1131–1138.

Keane, T. M., & Lisman, S. A. (1980). Alcohol and social anxiety in males: Behavioral, cognitive, and physiological effects. *Journal of Abnormal Psychology, 89,* 213–223.

Keehn, J. D., Bloomfield, F. F., & Hug, M. A. (1970). Use of the reinforcement survey schedule with alcoholics. *Quarterly Jorunal of Studies on Alcohol, 31,* 633–658.

Kimble, G. A. (1961). *Hilgard and Marquis' conditioning and learning.* New York: Appleton-Century-Crofts.

Kinney, L., & Schmidt, H., Jr. (1979). Effect of cued and uncued inescapable shock on voluntary alcohol consumption in rats. *Pharmacology, Biochemistry and Behavior, 11,* 601–604.

Klajner, F., Hartman, L. M., & Sobell, M. B. (1984). Treatment of substance abuse by relaxation training: A review of its rationale, efficacy and mechanisms. *Addictive Behaviors, 9,* 41–55.

Klepping, J., Guilland, J.-C., Didier, J.-P., Klepping, C., & Malval, M. (1976). Alcool: Facteur de stress ou tranquillisant? *Revue de l'alcoolisme, 22,* 5–14.

Leckman, J. F., Weissman, M. M., Merikangas, K. R., Pauls, D. L., & Prusoff, B. A. (1983). Panic disorder and major depression: Increased risk of depression, alcoholism, panic, and phobic disorders in families of depressed probands with panic disorder. *Archives of General Psychiatry, 40,* 1055–1060.

Levenson, R. W, Sher, K. J., Grossman, L. M., Newman, J., & Newlin, D. B. (1980). Alcohol and stress response dampening: Pharmacological effects, expectancy, and tension reduction. *Journal of Abnormal Psychology, 89,* 528–538.

Lindman, R. (Ed.). (1980) *Anxiety and alcohol: Limitations of tension reduction theory in non-alcoholics* (Monograph Suppl. 1). Abo, Finland: Abo Akademi, Department of Psychology.

Lipscomb, T. R., Nathan, P. E., Wilson, G. T., & Abrams, D. B. (1980). Effects of tolerance on the anxiety-reducing function of alcohol. *Archives of General Psychiatry, 37,* 577–582.

Logue, P. E., Gentry, W. D., Linnoila, M., & Erwin, C. W. (1978). Effect of alcohol consumption on state anxiety changes in male and female nonalcoholics. *American Journal of Psychiatry, 135,* 1079–1081.

MacAndrew, C., & Edgerton, R. B. (1969). *Drunken comportment: A social explanation.* Chicago: Aldine.

Mansfield, J. G. (1979). Dose-related effects of ethanol on avoidance–avoidance conflict behavior in the rat. *Psychopharmacology, 66,* 67–71.

Mansfield, J. G., Eaton, N. K., Cunningham, C. L., & Brown, J. S. (1977). Ethanol and avoidance–avoidance conflict in the rat. *Physiological Psychology, 5,* 197–203.

Marlatt, G. A., Kosturn, C. F., & Lang, A. R. (1975). Provocation to anger and opportunity for retaliation as determinants of alcohol consumption in social drinkers. *Journal of Abnormal Psychology, 84,* 652–659.

Masserman, J. H., Jacques, M. G., & Nicholson, M. R. (1945). Alcohol as a preventive of experimental neuroses. *Quarterly Journal of Studies on Alcohol, 6,* 281–299.

Masserman, J. H., & Yum, K. S. (1946). The influence of alcohol on experimental neuroses in cats. *Psychosomatic Medicine, 8,* 36–52.

McCollam, J. B., Burish, T. G., Maisto, S. A., & Sobell, M. B. (1980). Alcohol's effects on physiological arousal and self-reported affect and sensations. *Journal of Abnormal Psychology, 89,* 224–233.

Mello, N. K. (1981). The role of aversive consequences in the control of alcohol and drug self-administration. In R. E. Meyer, B. C. Glueck, J. E. O'Brien, & T. F. Babor (Eds.), *Evaluation of the alcoholic: Implications for research, theory and treatment* (MD20014, pp. 207–228). Bethesda, MD: Department of Health, Education and Welfare.

Mendelson, J. H., LaDou, L., & Solomon, P. (1964). Experimentally induced chronic intoxication and withdrawal in alcoholics, Part 3, Psychiatric findings. *Quarterly Journal of Studies on Alcohol* (Suppl. 2), pp. 40–52.

Miller, N. E. (1944). Experimental studies of conflict. In J. McV. Hunt (Ed.), *Personality and the behavior disorders* (pp. 431–465). New York: Ronald Press.

Miller, P. M., Hersen, M., Eisler, R. M., & Hilsman, G. (1974). Effects of social stress on operant drinking of alcoholics and social drinkers. *Behaviour Research and Therapy, 12,* 67–72.

Mills, K. C., Bean, J. W., & Hutcheson, J. S. (1977). Shock induced ethanol consumption in rats. *Pharmacology, Biochemistry and Behavior, 6,* 107–115.

Myrsten, A. L., Hollstedt, C., & Holmberg, L. (1975). Alcohol-induced changes in mood and activation in males and females as related to catecholamine excretion and blood-alcohol level. *Scandinavian Journal of Psychology, 16(4),* 303–310.

Nathan, P. E., Titler, N.A., Lowenstein, L. M., Solomon, P., & Rossi, A. M. (1970). Behavioral analysis of chronic alcoholism: Interaction of alcohol and human contact. *Archives of General Psychiatry, 22,* 419–430.

Noel, N. E., & Lisman, S. A. (1980). Alcohol consumption by college women following exposure to unsolvable problems: Learned helplessness or stress induced drinking? *Behaviour Research and Therapy, 18,* 429–440.

Pihl, R. O., & Smith, S. (1983). Of affect and alcohol. In L. A. Pohorecky & J. Brick (Eds.), *Stress and alcohol use* (pp. 203–228). New York: Elsevier.

Pihl, R. O., & Yankofsky, L. (1979). Alcohol consumption in male social drinkers as a function of situationally induced depressive affect and anxiety. *Psychopharmacology, 65,* 251–257.

Pohorecky, L. A. (1981). The interaction of alcohol and stress: A review. *Neuroscience and Biobehavioral Reviews, 5,* 209–229.

Pohorecky, L. A., & Brick, J. (Eds.). (1980). *Stress and alcohol use.* New York: Elsevier.

Pohorecky L. A., Rassi, E. Weiss, J. M., & Michalak, V. (1980). Biochemical evidence for an interaction of ethanol and stress: Preliminary studies. *Alcoholism: Clinical and Experimental Research, 4.* 423–426.

Polivy, J., Schueneman, A. L., & Carlson, K. (1976). Alcohol and tension reduction: Cognitive and physiological effects. *Journal of Abnormal Psychology, 85,* 595–600

Rimm, D., Briddell, D., Zimmerman, M., & Caddy, G. (1981). The effects of alcohol and the expectancy of alcohol on snake fear. *Addictive Behaviors, 6,* 47–51.

Rohsenow, D. J. (1983). Drinking habits and expectancies about alcohol's effects on self versus others. *Journal of Consulting and Clinical Psychology, 51,* 752–756.

Russell, J. A., & Mehrabian, A. (1975). The mediating role of emotions in alcohol use. *Journal of Studies on Alcohol, 36,* 1508–1536.

Schuckit, M. A., Engstrom, D., Alpert, R., & Duby, J. (1981). Differences in muscle tension response to ethanol in young men with and without family histories of alcoholism. *Journal of Studies on Alcohol, 42,* 918–924.

Sher, K. J., & Levenson, R. W. (1982). Risk for alcoholism and individual differences in the stress-response-dampening effect of alcohol. *Journal of Abnormal Psychology, 91,* 350–367.

Skurdal, A. J., Eckardt, M. J., & Brown, J. S. (1975). The effects of alcohol on escape learning and on regular and punished extinction in a self-punitive situation with rats. *Physiological Psychology*, *3*, 29–34.

Smail, P., Stockwell, T., Canter, S., & Hodgson, R. (1984). Alcohol dependence and phobic anxiety states: I. A prevalence study. *British Journal of Psychiatry*, *144*, 53–57.

Southwick, L., Steele, C, Marlatt, A., & Lindell, M. (1981). Alcohol-related expectancies: Defined by phase of intoxication and drinking experience. *Journal of Consulting and Clinical Psychology*, *49*, 713–721.

Steele, C. M., Southwick, L. L., & Critchlow, B. (1981). Dissonance and alcohol: Drinking your troubles away. *Journal of Personality and Social Psychology*, *41*, 831–846.

Steffen, J. J., Nathan, P. E., & Taylor, H. A. (1974). Tension-reducing effects of alcohol: Further evidence and some methodological considerations. *Journal of Abnormal Psychology*, *83*, 542–547.

Stockwell, T., Hodgson, R., & Rankin, H. (1982). Tension reduction and the effects of prolonged alcohol consumption. *British Journal of Addiction*, *77*, 65–73.

Stockwell, T., Smail, P., Hodgson, R., & Canter, S. (1984). Alcohol dependence and phobic anxiety states: II. A retrospective study. *British Journal of Psychiatry*, *144*, 58–63.

Sutker, P. B, Allain, A. N., Brantley, P. J., & Randall, C. L. (1982). Acute alcohol intoxication, negative affect, and autonomic arousal in women and men. *Addictive Behaviors*, *7*, 17–25.

Tabakoff, B., Jaffe, R. C., & Ritzmann, R. F. (1978). Corticosterone concentrations in mice during ethanol drinking and withdrawal. *Journal of Pharmacy and Pharmacology*, *30*, 371–374.

Tucker, J. A., Vuchinich, R. E., & Sobell, M. B. (1982). Alcohol's effects on human emotions: A review of the stimulation/depression hypothesis. *The International Journal of the Addictions*, *17*, 155–180.

Tucker, J. A., Vuchinich, R. E., Sobell, M. B., & Maisto, S. A. (1980). Normal drinkers' alcohol consumption as a function of conflicting motives induced by intellectual performance stress. *Addictive Behaviors*, *15*, 171–178.

Ullman, A. D. (1952). The psychological mechanism of alcohol addiction. *Quarterly Journal of Studies on Alcohol*, *13*, 602–608.

Van Thiel, D. (1983). Adrenal response to ethanol: A stress response? In L. A. Pohorecky & J. Brick (Eds.), *Stress and alcohol use* (pp. 23–27). New York: Elsevier.

Vogel, R. A., Frye, G. D., Wilson, J. H., Kuhn, C. M., Koepke, K. M., Mailman, R. B., Mueller, R. A., & Breese, G. R. (1980). Attenuation of the effects of punishment by ethanol: Comparisons with chlorodiazepoxide. *Psychopharmacology*, *71*, 123–129.

Vogel, W. H., & DeTurck, K. H. (1983). Effects of ethanol on plasma and brain catecholamine levels in stressed and unstressed rats. In L. A. Pohorecky & J. Brick (Eds.), *Stress and alcohol use* (pp. 429–438). New York: Elsevier.

Vuchinich, R. E., & Tucker, J. A. (1983). Behavioral theories of choice as a framework for studying drinking behavior. *Journal of Abnormal Psychology*, *92*, 408–416.

Williams, A. F. (1966). Social drinking, anxiety, and depression. *Journal of Personality and Social Psychology*, *3*, 689–693.

Wilson, G. T., & Abrams, D. (1977). Effects of alcohol on social anxiety and physiological arousal: Cognitive versus pharmacological processes. *Cognitive Therapy and Research*, *1*, 195–210.

Wilson, G. T., Abrams, D. B., & Lipscomb, T. R. (1980). Effects of intoxication levels and drinking pattern on social anxiety in men. *Journal of Studies on Alcohol*, *41*, 250–264.

Wilson, G. T., Perold, E. A., & Abrams, D. B. (1981). The effects of expectations of self-intoxication and partner's intoxication on anxiety in dyadic social interaction. *Cognitive Therapy and Research*, *5*, 251–264.

Woolfolk, A. E., Abrams, L. M., Abrams, D. B., & Wilson, G. T. (1979). Effects of alcohol on the nonverbal communication of anxiety: The impact of beliefs on nonverbal behavior. *Environmental Psychology and Nonverbal Behavior*, *3*, 205–217.

Yale Studies on Alcohol. (1945). *Alcohol, science and society*. Westport, CT: Greenwood Press.

# 3 Personality Theory and Research

## W. MILES COX

## Historical Overview

The practice of drinking alcoholic beverages for their pleasurable effects is very old, having been recorded before the birth of Christ. Problems associated with drinking alcohol are also very old, with incidents of alcoholism also having been recorded before the birth of Christ (Coleman, Butcher, & Carson, 1984, p. 398).

Despite the longevity of humankind's alcohol problems, it is only recently that people have begun to associate them with medical or psychological difficulties. Sporadic attempts to do so occurred during the 19th and early 20th centuries. For instance, the concept of alcoholism as a disease was first advocated by Benjamin Rush (1785/1843), who proposed that hospitals be established especially for the physical treatment of alcoholics. Also during the 19th century, scientists attempted to promote the view that alcoholism was a disease through the publication of the *Journal of Inebriety*, which continues to be published today as the *British Journal of Addiction* (Keller, 1976). The first published attempt to relate alcoholism and psychological difficulties apparently was Abraham's (1908/1954) article, in which he advocated that alcohol problems are interrelated with sexual difficulties.

These early attempts to promote medical and psychological views about the etiology of alcoholism notwithstanding, a prevalent view during the 19th and early 20th centuries was that alcoholism was a moral weakness and could therefore not appropriately be treated by medical or psychological interventions. Another common view was that "demon alcohol" was inherently addicting and could not be consumed by any person without substantial risk. According to the latter view, the way to eliminate alcoholism was to make

W. MILES COX. Veterans Administration Medical Center and Department of Psychiatry, Indiana University School of Medicine, Indianapolis, Indiana.

alcohol unavailable. This attitude gained widespread popular appeal through the temperance movement and eventually was put into law through the Eighteenth Amendment to the United States Constitution which became effective in 1920. Prohibition, of course, proved to be a disastrous failure and was repealed by the Nineteenth Amendment which became effective in 1933.

Following prohibition, medical and psychological views about the etiology of alcoholism were more seriously considered than before. In particular, interest was renewed in the disease concept of alcoholism because of the formation of Alcoholics Anonymous in 1935 (Alcoholics Anonymous, 1976). This self-help organization for alcoholics promoted the view that alcoholism is a disease and that alcoholics must abstain from alcohol completely in order to hold their disease in remission (Jellinek, 1960). Alcoholics Anonymous rapidly grew into a worldwide organization, and in North America it has become the primary means for treating alcoholism (Miller, 1983).

In addition to seeking help through Alcoholics Anonymous, alcoholics appear increasingly to have sought treatment from psychiatrists following prohibition. Psychiatrists utilized psychoanalytic theory in an attempt to understand the etiology of alcoholism and the techniques of psychoanalysis to treat their alcoholic patients. Psychoanalysts published case studies of their patients (Chassell, 1938; Knight, 1936, 1937, 1938), and the psychoanalytic view became the dominant professional view to account for the etiology of alcoholism.

According to the psychoanalytic point of view, personality plays a crucial role in the etiology of alcoholism. Alcoholism is said to be caused by premorbid personality disturbances, and alcoholics must undergo fundamental changes in their personality for successful treatment to occur. This view is not inconsistent with the disease concept of alcoholism that is advocated by Alcoholics Anonymous. Members of Alcoholics Anonymous seek to identify some basic defect in themselves (such as a faulty personality structure) to which the ultimate cause of their disease can be attributed. Alcoholics in Alcoholics Anonymous also assert that they must undergo a fundamental change in their personality and life-style in order to hold their disease in remission (Thoreson & Budd, 1986).

Apparently gaining impetus from the new emphasis on personality factors in alcoholism, the concept of the "alcoholic personality" was introduced during the 1940s (Landis, 1945; Seliger & Rosenberg, 1941). The alcoholic personality was presumed to be a unique constellation of personality characteristics that distinguished alcoholics from other individuals even before the onset of alcoholism. In order to identify what these characteristics were, clinicians administered a variety of personality tests to alcoholics (Hewitt, 1943; Machover & Puzzo, 1959; Machover, Puzzo, Machover, & Plumeau, 1959; Witkin, Karp, & Goodenough, 1959). These attempts to specify the nature of a single alcoholic personality proved unsuccessful (Armstrong, 1958; Bowman & Jellinek, 1942; Seliger & Rosenberg, 1941; Sutherland, Schroeder, & Tordella, 1950; Syme, 1957). Nevertheless, the general interest in personality factors in alcoholism continued unabated.

The degree of current interest in this topic is indicated by the fact that there are now more than 1000 entries in the PsychINFO database alone that relate to personality and alcoholism. In this chapter, I will discuss the major personality factors that are involved in the use and abuse of alcohol that have been identified through this prodigious research.

## Traditional Approaches to Understanding Personality Factors in Alcohol Use and Abuse

### Psychoanalysis

According to classical psychoanalysis, the etiology of alcoholism can be found in unresolved, unconscious conflicts that originated during early childhood. However, several different themes are apparent within this general point of view. For example, alcoholics have been seen by various psychoanalytic writers as fixated at, or regressed to, each of the three pregenital psychosexual stages of development: oral, anal, and phallic (Blum, 1966; Fenichel, 1945). Nevertheless, seeing alcoholics with some form of fixation at the oral stage is the most common point of view.

That alcoholics are orally fixated is inferred from several personality characteristics that have been commonly observed among adult alcoholics: dependency, immaturity, a low tolerance for frustration, and an inability to delay gratification. The alcoholic displaying these personality characteristics is likened to a young child who is presumed to have experienced severe frustrations during the oral stage of development. These frustrations propel such individuals to continue to seek oral gratification throughout their life, and they do so in an immature manner.

According to this view, imbibing alcohol is one means to achieve the gratification that persons who are fixated at the oral stage are seeking. That is, consuming alcohol not only is orally stimulating, but often provides an immediate feeling of psychological well-being. However, to drink alcohol in large quantities, as alcoholics typically do, is usually accompanied by a variety of adverse consequences. Thus, excessive drinking is an immature way to achieve oral gratification. In the section that follows, we will see why alcoholics are also regarded as dependent.

A second, less prominent theme among psychoanalytic writers (a variant of the oral frustration view) is that male alcoholics are characterized by homoeroticism, which is assumed often to be latent or not directly observable (Fenichel, 1945, p. 379). The homoeroticism of the alcoholic is presumed to have originated when the male child, frustrated by his mother during the oral stage of psychosexual development, develops an emotional attattchment for his father. However, the evidence offered by psychoanalysts that alcoholics are homoerotic is nebulous. As Lisansky (1960, p. 324) has pointed out, the psychoanalytic definition of "homosexuality" is unclear and has variously been described as "difficulties in adjusting to a stable heterosexual relationship, feminine identification and interests, strong mother attachment, an adolescentlike seeking out of male companionship, passivity, overt homosexual experience, misogyny, or a desire to form one's closest interpersonal ties with men."

Despite the lack of clarity of psychoanalysts' definition of homoeroticism, there is increasing evidence that many alcoholics do, in fact, have sexual difficulties, including difficulties with their sexual orientation (Benson & Wilsnack, 1983; Gomberg, 1986). Alcoholics' sexual problems include those related to gender roles, sexual abuse, and sexual dysfunction. Sometimes the sexual problems precede, and sometimes they follow, the alcohol problems. Whichever is the case, however, it seems that alcoholics' alcohol problems and their sexual problems often contribute reciprocally to each other.

A third psychoanalytic interpretation of alcoholism (another variant of the oral frustration view) has been promoted by Menninger (1938, p. 160ff). Menninger asserted that because of oral frustrations during infancy, young children become enraged with their parents, but since they are unable directly to express their hostile impulses to their more powerful parents, the impulses become self-directed. According to Menninger's point of view, alcohol serves two functions: It allows alcoholics to gratify both their oral cravings and self-destructive tendencies. That alcoholics are self-destruction is inferred from their ingrained habit of repeatedly imbibing alcohol despite the fact that the long-range consequences of doing so are distinctly negative (i.e., self-destructive).

Much pessimism has been expressed about the classical psychoanalytic interpretation of alcoholism, the major objections having been summarized by Lang (1983, p. 158). First, the evidence gathered by psychoanalysts to support their point of view is seen as a foregone conclusion, since psychoanalysts have operated under the assumption that personality difficulties are the basis for alcoholism—a premise that they held even prior to their actual observation of alcoholics. Second, the data that psychoanalysts have gathered on alcoholics' personalities have been seen as biased, since these data were gathered retrospectively from disturbed persons and only in the context of individual psychotherapy. Third, psychoanalysis is seen as basically an unscientific endeavor. Since psychoanalytic concepts are difficult, if not impossible, to operationalize it has been difficult to test their validity. Readers who want additional details about the psychoanalytic perspective on alcoholism and criticisms that have been leveled at it are referred to Barry's chapter (in press).

## Dependency Theories

As we saw above, dependency (which may be expressed directly or indirectly) is viewed by psychoanalytic writers as one of several prominent personality characteristics of male alcoholics that stem from their fixation at the oral stage of psychosexual development. Various writers have elaborated on how alcoholics' dependency manifests itself, the major views having been expressed by McCord and McCord (1960) and Blane (1968).

McCord and McCord (1960) view male alcoholics as having intense needs to be dependent on other people but equally strong needs to be independent of them. The need to be dependent is inferred from alcoholics' tendency to seek nurture and care from other people—a need that presumably arose from the frustration of oral needs during early childhood. The need to be independent is inferred from male alcoholics' masculine and aggressive personality characteristics—a role that is prescribed for males by American society. Thus, male alcoholics are caught in a conflict, and they attempt to satisfy their two opposing needs simultaneously through heavy drinking. That is, heavy drinking is clearly a masculine activity, but while they are intoxicated and incapacitated by alcohol, male alcoholics can allow themselves to indulge their dependency needs without suffering the strictures of society for having done so. Thus, they can be sentimental and close to other people, but can attribute these behaviors to alcohol rather than to their own motives.

Blane (1968), on the other hand, has asserted that male alcoholics' strong dependency needs can manifest themselves in several different ways. First, *openly dependent* alcoholics are blatantly dependent on other people; their primary style of interacting with other people is to seek their care and protectiveness. Second, *counterdependent* male alcoholics, although having intense, unconscious needs to be dependent on other people, assiduously avoid any conscious displays of dependency. Instead, they display an image that is directly opposite to their real needs: assertiveness, independence, and masculinity. Third, *dependent–independent* male alcoholics fluctuate between extreme dependence and independence, according to the particular circumstances in which they find themselves.

In summary, according to both McCord and McCord's (1960) and Blane's (1968) formulations, alcoholics' dependency often manifests itself in overt behavior that is opposite to their underlying motives.

## Tension Reduction

As we saw in the above Historical Overview, when the "alcoholic personality" concept was introduced, many attempts were made to identify alcoholics' distinctive personality characteristics. Tension was a characteristic that was commonly specified. The idea that alcoholics are tense originated from psychoanalysis, which asserted that alcoholics have high levels of tension or anxiety that stem from their oral frustrations and dependency conflicts and that they attempt to reduce by drinking alcohol. However, the view that tension produced by dependency conflicts was the primary motivation for excessive alcohol consumption, was supported by cross-cultural studies (Bacon, 1974; Horton, 1945) which found that the degree to which a society fostered dependency conflicts was correlated with the frequency of drunkenness in that society.

The effect of alcohol on resolving conflict was studied experimentally with laboratory animals during the 1940s and 1950s (Conger, 1951, 1956; Masserman & Yum, 1946). In these experiments, animals were placed in approach–avoidance conflict situations and were then administered alcohol. The alcohol caused them to approach the bivalent goal that they had previously avoided, presumably because the alcohol alleviated their tension.

Thus, these experiments were interpreted as providing empirical support for the tension reduction hypothesis of alcohol consumption: Alcohol reduces tension, and organisms drink alcohol in order to reduce their tension. As we will see in a later section, this hypothesis served as the impetus for subsequent research with human subjects.

## Reactions against Traditional Approaches

During the 1960s, major changes in the research on alcohol and alcoholism began to occur. Whereas the earlier research had largely involved administering psychological tests to alcoholics in an attempt to identify their unique personality characteristics, the new genre of research emphasized experimental techniques for identifying people's motivation for drinking. The changes that began during the 1960s were greatly advanced when the National Institute on Alcohol Abuse and Alcoholism was established during the early 1970s. The quantity of research increased rapidly (Cox & Thornton, 1986), and the results of the research caused strong dissatisfaction with traditional explanations of alcoholism.

## Power Theory

One of the very first research programs that led to a new theory about drinking was undertaken by David McClelland and his associates at Harvard. The primary focus of their research was to identify the motivations underlying people's drinking, and these investigators utilized several types of procedures in order to do so: cross-cultural analyses of folktales, naturalistic observation of drinking behavior, and laboratory experimentation to identify needs that drinking fulfills. The major findings of the research are summarized in a book, *The Drinking Man: A Theory of Human Motivation* (McClelland, Davis, Kalin, & Wanner, 1972). As the title of the book suggests, only male subjects (i.e., the drinking man) were tested in the research program, but as the subtitle suggests, the McClelland group felt that their findings would be applicable to both men and women (i.e., human motivation).

The McClelland group, like their predecessors, observed that male heavy drinkers are often independent, aggressive, and masculine. However, they did not interpret this observation to mean that these overt personality characteristics of heavy drinkers reflect counterdependence, that is, reactions against unconscious, unacceptable needs to be nurtured and cared for. Instead, they considered male drinkers' independence to reflect their need for power. The McClelland group believed that male heavy drinkers have a need to feel powerful because they have been socialized to believe that they should be powerful and that drinking is an activity that helps them satisfy their need for power.

McClelland's hypothesis that drinking satisfies needs for power was developed in part by analyzing male social drinkers' fantasies recorded from the Thematic Apperception Test before and after they had drunk alcohol in party settings. The primary effect of alcohol was to increase subjects' fantasies about being powerful. After drinking, they imagined themselves to be in positions of power and to exert control over other people, but the nature of this effect depended on the amount of alcohol consumed. When alcohol was consumed in small or moderate quantities, there were increases in fantasies about socialized power, or altruistic control over other people, such as being in a position to teach or help them. When alcohol was consumed in large quantities, there were increases in fantasies about personalized power, or self-aggrandizing control over other people that was often sexual or aggressive in nature. On the other hand, there was no evidence that alcohol affected anxious thoughts or thoughts about dependency.

## Theory of Womanliness

Wilsnack (1974) sought to determine whether McClelland's findings with male subjects were, in fact, applicable to women—that is, whether women have needs for power that alcohol allows them to satisfy. Wilsnack's (1974) methodology was similar to that of McClelland *et al.* (1972). During naturalistic parties, women's fantasies were measured with the Thematic Apperception

Test before and after they had imbibed alcohol. Wilsnack (1974) found no evidence that drinking alcohol increases fantasies of power among women. Instead, drinking *decreased* the frequency of women's fantasies about engaging in traditionally masculine activities and *increased* the frequency of their fantasies about engaging in traditionally feminine activities. Thus, Wilsnack concluded that drinking causes women to feel more womanly.

Wilsnack (1973) found that alcoholic women often have chronic doubts about their adequacy as women—doubts that appear to have arisen from assaults leveled at their feminine self-esteem, often in the form of interpersonal or gynocological problems. Thus, it appears that women who develop problems with alcohol have strong unmet needs to feel womanly, and they appear to be motivated to drink in order to acquire the feelings of womanliness that alcohol provides them (Wilsnack, 1976).

The results of McClelland *et al.*'s and Wilsnack's research taken together suggest that both men and women who develop problems with alcohol drink in order to experience traditional gender roles that are consistent with societal expectations but which they are unable to experience unless they drink alcohol (Benson & Wilsnack, 1983). This explanation of problem drinking is quite different from those arrived at through traditional approaches. Nevertheless, it is just one example among several new attempts to identify personality factors and life experiences underlying alcohol use and abuse (Cox, 1983).

### Recent Psychodynamic Approaches

The basic conceptualization of alcohol abuse that is currently advocated by psychoanalysts has not changed dramatically from the classical psychoanalytic point of view (Adams, 1978, p. 25). Nevertheless, there has been a shift in the concepts that are emphasized. For instance, there is a current emphasis on the ego functioning of alcoholics (and other drug abusers) that was not seen previously.

> I believe there is convincing evidence from several convergent lines of inquiry to support the point of view that significant impairments in ego structure predispose to alcoholism. Impairments in self-care leave individuals ill equipped to properly weigh, anticipate, and assess the consequences of risky and self-damaging behavior, but particularly in relation to the consequences of their alcohol involvement. The other area of ego impairment in alcoholics involves problems in recognizing, regulating, and harnessing feeling states to the point that conditions of immobilization or being overwhelmed with affects result, and alcohol is sought to overcome or relieve such dilemmas. (Khantzian, 1981, p. 168)

A second current emphasis is on the narcissistic conflicts that alcoholics and other drug abusers experience.

Narcissistic conflicts mean conflicts about self-esteem and self-worth, about power and self-love. They mean the wishes of massive overvaluation of the self and the pertinent other, the inevitable disillusionment, the consequent overwhelming affects (rage, shame, envy, loneliness), and the usually primitive defenses against these affects. Thereby they always also involve conflicts about limits, limitations and boundaries (Wurmser, 1978, p. 117).

[The narcissistic crisis] is obviously the starting point where the deeper conflicts about self-esteem and power get mobilized. Such a mobilization quite typically occurs at first during adolescence, rarely earlier, not too often later. Often the relapse from abstinence into drug use again is clearly marked by the recurrence of such a crisis. Most generally this crisis is the point in time where the conflicts and defects converge with a particular external situation and with the availability of the seeming means of solution: the drug. . . . In this narcissistic crisis the addictive search starts. (Wurmser, 1978, pp. 113–114).

Finally, forms of treatment that are alternative to classical psychoanalytic ones are currently being emphasized.

The individual suffering with a narcissistic disorder is characterized by an array of personality and character resistances (defenses) that are virtually impenetrable, therefore making the individual impervious to the usual methods of psychoanalytic intervention designed to produce personality and character change. . . . The use of specialized psychoanalytic techniques, which take into account the object striving of the patient and the analyst as the (transference) object towards whom he strives, and which are specifically geared to the systematic analysis of preoedipal resistances as they unfold in the transference, would resolve those resistances rendering the individual accessible to a more insight-oriented psychoanalytic approach resulting in his improvement and cure. (Adams, 1978, pp. 308–309)

## Empirical Research

There are several ways in which the research on the personality correlates of alcohol problems has changed during the last 50 years. First, whereas the focus of the original research was on characterizing the "alcoholic personality" among persons clinically diagnosed as alcoholic, the alcoholic personality is no longer regarded as a viable concept (Cox, 1983). Second, today the abuse of alcohol is not so sharply demarcated from the use of alcohol as previously, and the personality factors involved in the use of alcohol are considered valuable for understanding those involved in the abuse of alcohol. In a similar vein, the personality factors in alcohol use and abuse have been related to a variety of other addictive behaviors, including addiction to various psychoactive drugs as well as nondrug substances and activities (Cox, 1985). Third, alcohol problems are no longer attributed to a single cause (e.g., "demon alcohol," the "alcoholic personality," the "disease" of alcoholism). Instead, various biological, psychological (in addition to personality), and sociocultural variables are seen as interacting with one another to account for the development of alcohol problems. Several theories have been advanced to account for how these interactions take place (Blane & Chafetz, 1979; Huba & Bentler, 1982; Jessor & Jessor, 1977, 1978; Zucker, 1979, Zucker & Noll, 1982), and multidisiplinary approaches for understanding alcohol problems have been the topic of several books (Chaudron & Wilkinson, in press; Cox, in press; Galizio & Maisto, 1985).

Personality tests have been used to identify the personality factors involved in alcohol problems. Advocates of psychodynamic approaches have commonly used projective tests (Rorschach Inkblot Test, Thematic Apperception Test, Frank Drawing Completion Test) for measuring unconscious needs and impulses. More recently, other aspects of subjects' fantasy have been sampled with thought and imagery tests by researchers studying intrapsychic processes associated with the use of alcohol (Thought Sampling Questionnaire, Klinger & Cox, 1986; Imaginal Processes Questionnaire, Segal, Huba, & Singer, 1980). Conversely, researchers assessing differences between the personality characteristics of alcoholics and nonalcoholics have used various unidimensional tests (e.g., adjective checklists, Q-sorts, scales, and inventories) for measuring single personality characteristics and multidimensional tests (usually personality inventories) for providing comprehensive descriptions of subjects' personality. However, the Minnesota Multiphasic Personality Inventory (MMPI) has been the single most commonly used instrument for the multidimensional assessment of personality (Barnes, 1983; Cox, 1979) and we will frequently refer to results obtained with the MMPI in this chapter.

The empirical research discussed in this chapter is organized around three major issues that have concerned researchers investigating personality factors in alcohol use and abuse. The first issue concerns the personality precursors of alcohol use and abuse. That is, researchers have attempted to determine whether persons who in the future will drink alcohol and develop problems with it have personality characteristics that distinguish them from other individuals, and, if so, whether these distinctive personality characteristics help to account for the future use and abuse of alcohol. The second issue is whether or not diagnosed alcoholics have personality characteristics that distinguish them from nonalcoholic individuals. To identify the personality correlates of alcoholism not only has important theoretical implications for understanding the etiology of alcoholism but also practical implications for treating alcoholics. The third issue is to identify the immediate and long-term effects of alcohol on personality, both while the person is under the influence of alcohol and in the sober state. Identifying changes in personality produced by alcohol helps, of course, to understand people's motives for using alcohol.

## Personality Precursors of Alcohol Problems

The theoretical viewpoints described above see alcoholics and other problem drinkers as having personality characteristics that distinguish them from non-problem drinkers, even before the onset of the drinking problems. For example, psychoanalysts view alcoholics as having had oral personality characteristics from early childhood that led eventually to alcoholism or some other disorder involving psychological dependency. Similarly, the major reactions against psychoanalytic theory, McClelland *et al.*'s (1972) power theory and Wilsnack's (1976) theory of womanliness, each assumes that alcoholics' and other heavy drinkers' sex-role needs that they fulfill with alcohol were present prior to the onset of their problem drinking. In this section, we will discuss (1) the methods that have been used to evaluate whether problem drinkers have distinctive personality characteristics prior to the onset of their alcohol problems, and (2) the information about the personality precursors of alcohol problems that has been gathered with these methods.

### Methods of Study

It is very difficult to study the personality precursors of alcohol problems. As we will see, each method for doing so has major methodological or practical limitations.

The most valuable information about the personality precursors of alcohol problems would come from prospective longitudinal studies. A study would be prospective if it tested subjects who were expected to develop problems with alcohol at some future point in their lives, and it would be longitudinal if it followed them for an extended period of time. In order to clearly demonstrate whether or not personality is a precursor of alcoholism, it would be necessary for a prospective longitudinal study to follow subjects from an early point in their lives until some of the subjects had become alcoholic. Studies of this scope have generally been regarded as prohibitively costly and time-consuming to conduct. Nevertheless, a number of prospective longitudinal studies have reported results covering relatively brief periods of time (i.e., up to 5 years). Typically, these studies have followed adolescents from the time before they began to use alcohol (e.g., in junior high school) until the time when some subjects had developed drinking problems.

The value of longitudinal methodology notwithstanding, it is also considered valuable to test persons who are at risk for developing problems with alcohol, even if they can't be followed for extended periods of time. High-risk subjects include (1) the biological sons of male alcoholics (who are about four times as likely to become alcoholic as a person randomly drawn from the general population (Knop, Goodwin, Teasdale, Milkkelsen, & Schulsinger, 1984) and (2) persons with personality characteristics like those of alcoholics (Sher & Levenson, 1982). The benefits of high-risk studies are inevitable because they allow us to identify both the precursors of alcoholism (from those high-risk subjects who actually became alcoholic) and the factors that protect people from becoming alcoholic (from those high-risk subjects who do not become alcoholic). Nevertheless, because of the difficulties involved in studying subjects prospectively, various alternate, methodologically less desirable methods have often been resorted to.

Archival methodology (Cox, Lun, & Loper, 1983) provides one means for identifying the personality precursors of alcoholism. An archival study utilizes sources of information about alcoholics' personality characteristics that were recorded before they became alcoholic and without their having been identified as potential future alcoholics. When this information is gathered from more than one point in the alcoholic's prior life, the methodology is called *archival longitudinal*. Since archival data are available fortuitously, they provide less than optimal information about the personality precursors of alcoholism. One disadvantage, for example, is that samples of alcoholics on whom archival data have been available have been quite restricted, and caution must be exercised in generalizing beyond these samples. Another disadvantage is that the data themselves have been quite limited, often not including standardized measures of personality nor any information about drinking behavior.

Retropective methodolgy provides another alternate means for identifying the personality precursors of alcoholism. For example, clinical case studies of alcoholics have often included information about their prior personality characteristics that was recalled retrospectively. In other retrospective studies, alcoholics have been asked merely to recall what their personality was like before they became alcoholic and/or to indicate significant life experiences that may be related to the development of their problems with alcohol. The major difficulty with all retrospective methodology, of course, is that it is highly subjective and subject to distortions in memory by the respondents.

Research Findings

*Prospective Studies.* In the prospective longitudinal studies that have been completed to date, adolescents typically have been asked annually to complete various questionnaires, some of which provide information about their personality characteristics. Across the various studies, certain personality characteristics have been very consistently found among the adolescents who later developed problems with alcohol: independence, aggressiveness, nonconformity, rejection of societal values, antisocial behavior, impulsivity, and hyperactivity (Jessor, 1983; Jessor & Jessor, 1977, 1978; Kandel, 1978, 1980; Wingard, Huba, & Bentler, 1980; Zucker, 1979; Zucker & Noll, 1982). On the other hand, negative personality characteristics such as anxiety, depression, and low self-esteem have seldom been found to precede problems with alcohol. In contrast to adolescents who develop problems with alcohol, however, those who come to abuse "hard" illegal drugs do show various indications of psychopathology even before their use of drugs is initiated (Huba & Bentler, 1982; Wingard, Huba, & Bentler, 1980).

In short, the personality characteristics shown by adolescents who develop problems with alcohol suggest that they have less interest than other adolescents in working to achieve the long-range, enduring goals that are generally valued in our society. Instead, they find sources of positive reinforcement in immediately available, short-term incentives that they act impulsively to acquire. Drinking alcohol is one such incentive that brings them immediate reinforcement. However, as will be seen later in the chapter, heavy consumption of alcohol leads eventually to adverse negative consequences that no longer make it possible to achieve the positive reinforcement that initially was salient in the life of the problem drinker.

*Archival Studies.* Archival data available in Minnesota provided an unusual opportunity to compare persons who did and did not later in life become alcoholic on a standardized personality inventory, the Minnesota Multiphasic Personality Inventory. These data were available because the MMPI was routinely administered to incoming freshmen at the University of Minnesota from 1947 to 1961. Eventually, of course, some of the people who took the MMPI as college freshmen developed problems with alcohol and sought treatment for these problems. Thus, Loper, Kammeier, and Hoffmann (1973), inspecting patients' files at two treatment facilities in Minnesota, identified 38 patients who had earlier been students at the university. On the average, these patients had taken the MMPI as college freshmen 13 years prior to their entry into treatment. Comparing the patients' earlier profiles with those from a randomly chosen sample of their classmates who presumably did not later become alcoholic, Loper, Kammeier, and Hoffmann (1973) found that the prealcoholics were significantly higher than their classmates on three of the MMPI standard scales (*F. Pd*, and *Ma*) and on the MacAndrew (MAC) alcoholism scale and other MMPI-derived scales designed specifically to identify alcoholic personality characteristics. These differences suggested to the investigators that the prealcoholics were more impulsive, nonconforming, and gregarious than their classmates, although they were not more maladjusted.

The findings of the Minnesota study are supported by other archival studies of male alcoholics reviewed by Cox, Lun, and Loper (1983). The data from these studies consistently indicate that males who later in life become alcoholic are nonconforming, rebellious, independent, aggressive, impulsive, and undercontrolled prior to the time that their problems with alcohol develop. Thus, although the archival data indicate that there are personality precursors of alcoholism, the personality characteristics exhibited by male prealcoholics cannot be viewed as pathologic or even necessarily as undesirable.

On the other hand, an archival longitudinal study that included both sexes (Jones, 1968, 1971) found notable differences between males and females who later in life developed problems with alcohol. Whereas during high school males who later became problem drinkers were extraverted, rebellious, and masculine, females were pessimistic, withdrawn, and self-defeating and were less independent and self-satisfied than future moderate drinkers. Similarly, other studies that have acquired psychiatric diagnoses of alcoholics that were made before they became alcoholic have found a high incidence of sociopathy among future male alcoholics but a high incidence of affective disorders among future female alcoholics (Benson & Wilsnack, 1983).

*Retrospective Studies.* Retrospective studies of male prealcoholic personality characteristics have sometimes substantiated the findings of the archival studies. That is, male alcoholics have recalled themselves as having been impulsive, hyperactive, aggressive, masculine, and antisocial prior to their abuse of alcohol (Goodwin, Schulsinger, Hermansen, Guze, & Winokur, 1975; Tarter, McBride, Buonpane, & Schneider, 1977). Nevertheless, other studies have found that

> both alcoholic men and alcoholic women report high rates of disruption early in life. Parental absence or unavailability is frequently the source of this disruption, which includes loss of one or both parents through death, divorce, or separation and psychiatric problems, such as psychosis or alcoholism, in parents or other close relatives. Although both female and male alcoholics report higher rates of early family disruption than women and men in the general population do, alcoholic women appear to report even more such experiences than alcoholic men. (Benson & Wilsnack, 1983, p. 57)

In addition to the early life stressors, alcoholics frequently associate specific psychological crises with the beginning of their problem drinking. Such reports are far more common among female than male alcoholics and include problems such as abortions, the birth of a child, divorce, health problems, children leaving home, menopause, and death in the family (Benson & Wilsnack, 1983).

It is difficult to know exactly how to interpret alcoholics' retrospective self-reports. Retrospective reports cannot of course necessarily be taken at face value. It is entirely possible that the life crises that alcoholics recall having experienced represent their attempts to rationalize their problems with alcohol. These problems (especially alcohol problems among women) are still very much stigmatized in our society, and it is entirely plausible for alcoholics to attempt to absolve themselves of responsibility for their problems. At the same time, it is entirely possible that the different frequencies with which male and female alcoholics recall precipitating life crises accurately reflect different subtypes of alcoholism with different etiologies. One subtype, in which personality difficulties *precede* the development of alcohol problems, might occur more frequently among females. The other subtype, in which personality difficulties *follow* the onset of alcohol problems, might occur more frequently among males.

## Personality Correlates of Alcohol Use and Abuse

In this section, we will discuss the personality characteristics that have been found to distinguish persons who use and abuse alcohol from those who do not. As we will see, some of these characteristics seem to be antecedents of alcohol problems and to have contributed to their development, whereas other characteristics appear to be consequences of excessive use of alcohol.

### Methods of Study

As indicated previously, soon after professional therapists became actively involved in treating alcoholics, the concept of the "alcoholic personality" came into vogue. At that time, clinicians attempted to describe the personality characteristics of their alcoholic patients through clinical case studies, the published accounts of which often included results of projective testing. The emphasis at that time was on identifying alcoholics' intrapsychic needs and the motives that drinking alcohol served to fulfill.

Later, as formal treatment programs for alcoholics were developed, the standard practice was to administer a personality test to a group of patients and to compare their performance with that of group of nonalcoholics. This approach came to predominate, and alcoholic personality characteristics described in this section were largely derived in this manner.

Alcoholics in treatment afford readily accessible samples for studying alcoholic personality characteristics. Nevertheless, several caveats should be kept in mind when drawing inferences from these samples (Cox, 1983; Lang, 1983; Nathan & Lansky, 1978; Pihl & Spiers, 1978). First, alcoholics in treatment have been largely restricted to males of lower socioeconomic status who have presented themselves for treatment, and these samples may not represent alcoholics generally. Of particular concern is the customary underrepresentation of females. When female patients have been tested at all, their test scores have often been averaged with those from males, and it was assumed that the results could be generalized to all alcoholics (Benson & Wilsnack, 1983). Second, even *within* separate samples of males or females, various subtypes of alcoholic personalities are represented that are obscured by averaging the test scores of the entire sample (Jackson, 1983). Third, studies of alcoholics in treatment (like those of prealcoholics) have seldom measured drinking behavior. Hence, it has not been possible to establish typologies of drinking patterns that can be related to personality characteristics (Cox, Lun, & Loper, 1983). In spite of these weaknesses, the personality characteristics described in this section have been so commonly observed that they do appear to apply to a substantial subset of male alcoholics.

### Research Findings

*Nonconformity, Impulsivity, and Reward Seeking.* As indicated earlier, prealcoholics are distinguished from other individuals by their failure to value conventional societal mores and their tendency to act impulsively to acquire immediate gratification of their impulses. These same personality characteristics are apparent among alcoholics in treatment. The psychometric evidence for this conclusion has been gathered primarily with the MMPI and Zuckerman's Sensation Seeking Scale (SSS) (Zuckerman, 1979).

By far the most commonly observed feature in the *MMPI profiles* of alcoholics is their elevation on Scale 4 (Psychopathic Deviate). In fact, elevation by alcoholics on this scale is ubiquitous, having first been reported 43 years ago (Hewitt, 1943) and subsequently reported among alcoholics with a variety of demographic characteristics and backgrounds (Owen & Butcher, 1979; Patterson, Charles, Woodward, Roberts, & Penk, 1981; Uecher, Boutilier, & Richardson, 1980).

Rather than indicating full-fledged psychopathology, the degree to which alcoholics typically are elevated on Scale 4 is generally interpreted as reflecting their unconventionality and disregard for established social customs as well as their impulsivity and inability to tolerate frustration and profit from experience. Alcoholics' elevation on Scale 4, however, also reflects their manner of relating to other people. Although persons who are elevated on Scale 4 often are socially adroit (due at least partly to their lack of concern about social stricture), they generally have difficulty forming committed, enduring relationships with other people. More specifically, Scale 4 deals

> in the main with general social maladjustment and absence of strongly pleasant experience. These include complaints against family, feelings of having been victimized, boredom, and feelings of alienation from the group—

of not being in on things. High 4 people are generally characterized by angry disidentification with recognized conventions; their revolt may be against family or society or both. Many high 4s exhibit an apparent inability to plan ahead, if not a reckless disregard of the consequences of their actions, and unpredictability is a feature of their behavior. Usually social relationships are shallow; the individual rarely develops strong loyalties of any kind. These people sometimes make a good impression at first, but on longer acquaintance their essential unreliability, moodiness, and resentment become apparent . . . . High 4 is associated with inability to profit from experience. (Carson, 1969, pp. 287–288)

Despite the frequency with which alcoholics are elevated on Scale 4, neither this scale nor any other of the clinical scales from the MMPI was developed specifically to identify alcoholic personality characteristics. On Scale 4, other diagnostic categories are elevated besides alcoholics. For this reason, MacAndrew (1965) set out to derive a scale from the MMPI specifically for identifying alcoholics (i.e., one that would measure alcoholics' distinctive personality characteristics apart from their psychological maladjustment). As a consequence of administering the MMPI to alcoholic inpatients and nonalcoholic psychiatric inpatients, MacAndrew identified 49 items (exclusive of 2 items that pertain directly to the use of alcohol) to which the two groups responded differently. This set of items has come to be known as the MacAndrew Alcoholism Scale. Since the majority of male alcoholics (about 85%) score high on the MAC scale, MacAndrew calls them *primary alcoholics*. Their personality is characterized by reward seeking. They are bold, aggressive, and hedonistic, and they use alcohol actively and impulsively.

Although its high rate of detection is impressive, the MAC scale does misclassify about 15% of nonalcoholics as alcoholics (false-positives) and 15% of alcoholics as nonalcoholics (false-negatives). Thus, some nonalcoholics have personality characteristics that resemble those of alcoholics, and some alcoholics have personality characteristics that resemble those of nonalcoholics. It is a mistake, therefore, to use the MAC scale as a definitive diagnosis of alcoholism.

In addition to the MAC scale, MacAndrew (1979, 1980) has isolated a set of 18 MMPI items that measure the personality characteristics of the approximately 15% of alcoholics who are not identified by the MAC scale. MacAndrew describes alcoholics who score high on these items as *secondary alcoholics*. They are punishment avoiders who are characterized by fear, reticence, and constricted interests. They use alcohol to cope with their tension and depression.

Zuckerman's (1979) *Sensation Seeking Scale* has not been used as extensively with alcoholics as has the MMPI, but it substantiates findings with the MMPI regarding alcoholics' unconventionality and reward seeking.

Although young problem drinkers and older alcoholics both score high on Zuckerman's scale, the two age groups show different patterns of sensation seeking (Zuckerman, 1979). Young heavy alcohol users score high on the Disinhibition Subscale of the SSS, endorsing items indicating that they enjoy a lot of fun and excitement and that their behavior tends to be unconventional or even illegal. Older alcoholics, on the other hand, tend to receive their highest scores on the Boredom Susceptibility Subscale. They endorse items indicating that they like excitement and unpredictability and tend to become restive and lose patience when things are boring, dull, or uninteresing.

The high scores achieved by alcoholics on the Pd and MAC scales from the MMPI and on the SSS indicate that they have an unconventional attitude toward the world and that they impulsively seek excitement and other rewards for themselves. Alcoholics' unconventionality, impulsivity, and reward seeking were apparent even before they begin to abuse alcohol, since prealcoholics and other young problem drinkers score high on all three scales. The personality characteristics measured by these scales appear to be a permanent feature of alcoholics' personality, since alcoholics maintain their elevated scores even following the termination of treatment.

*Negative Affect and Low Self-Esteem.* Upon entering treatment, alcoholics have strong negative affect, the intensity of which is positively correlated with the degree of their dependence on alcohol (Skinner & Allen, 1982). In fact, it is very common for alcoholics to be diagnosed as having a depression or anxiety disorder in addition to being alcoholic (Bowen, Cipywnyk, D'Arcy, & Keegan, 1984; Schuckit, 1979).

In addition to their primary elevation on Scale 4 (Psychopathic Deviate) of the MMPI, alcoholics characteristically show secondary elevations on Scale 2 (Depression) and Scale 7 (Psychasthenia) of the MMPI. Scale 2 measures "worry, discouragement, self-esteem, and general outlook. Scale 2 . . . tends to be fairly unstable, being highly sensitive to mood changes . . . . In general, it is the best single—and a remarkably efficient—index of immediate satisfaction, comfort, and security; it tells something of how the individual evaluates himself and his role in the world" (Carson, 1969, p.285). Scale 7 measures "anxiety symptoms, inability to resist, irrational fears, and self-devaluation. This scale is a general measure of anxiety and ruminative self-doubt. High scorers tend to be obsessionally worried, tense, indecisive, and unable to concentrate" (Carson, 1969, p. 292).

Alcoholics' negative affect that is reflected by MMPI Scales 2 and 7 has also been measured by a variety of other tests, including mood scales and inventories, adjective checklists, and multidimensional personality inventories besides the MMPI. For instance, on the neuroticism scales of the Eysenck Personality Inventory and Eysenck Personality Questionnaire, alcoholics have consistently scored higher than nonalcoholics (Cox, 1985). Alcoholics' elevations on these scales reflect their general emotionality, tension, and worry.

Despite the intensity of alcoholics' negative affect when they enter treatment, as they go through treatment and remain abstinent from alcohol, their depression and anxiety attenuate considerably. Thus, it appears that alcoholics' intense negative affect when they enter treatment is a consequence rather than a precursor of their excessive drinking. Further evidence for this conclusion comes from the fact that problem drinkers whose problems with alcohol are not severe enough for them to be diagnosed as alcoholic typically are not severely depressed and anxious (Midanik, 1983).

It is to be expected that alcoholics who feel anxious and depressed would also feel negative about themselves, that is, would have low self-esteem. In order to evaluate alcoholics' self-esteem, a variety of adjective checklists, Q-sorts, scales, and inventories have been administered to them. Two of these instruments are the Baron Ego Strength Scale, a scale derived from the MMPI, and the Tennessee Self-Concept Scale, which yields scores on five different aspects of self-concept.

Alcoholics upon entering treatment have consistently shown feelings of low self-esteem and lack of self-worth on these instruments, and they show wide discrepancies between the way they view themselves and the way they ideally would like to be (i.e., between self and ideal self). Although the feelings of low self-esteem are commonly reported among both male and female alcoholics, these feelings appear to be especially acute among female alcoholics (Benson & Wilsnack, 1983).

Two sources of evidence suggest that feelings of low self-esteem, like depression and anxiety, are a consequence rather than an antecedent of the drinking problems. First, in spite of the pervasiveness of low self-esteem among alcoholics, these feelings are not shared by prealcoholics or persons in the early stage of alcohol abuse. Second, therapeutic strategies for enhancing alcoholics' feelings of self-confidence and self-esteem at the same time that their alcohol problems are being dealt with have been successful (Cooper, 1983; Curry & Marlatt, 1986).

**Cognitive–Perceptual Style.** By "cognitive–perceptual style," we mean the manner in which people characteristically think about and perceive the world around them. There are three dimensions along which alcoholics' cognitive/perceptual style has been studied: stimulus intensity modulation, field dependence–independence, and locus of control. On all three dimensions, alcoholics have been found to differ from nonalcoholics.

From her work on people's perception of painful and other stimuli, Petrie (1967) concluded that three categories of people can be distinguished according to the intensity with which they characteristically perceive these stimuli: (1) stimulus moderates accurately perceive stimuli, (2) stimulus reducers perceive stimuli as less intense than they actually are, and (3) stimulus augmenters perceive stimuli as more intense than they actually are.

Although the work on alcoholics' *stimulus intensity modulation* has not been extensive, alcoholics have on several occasions been found to be stimulus augmenters (Barnes, 1983; Petrie, 1967). Furthermore, studies investigating the effects of alcohol on stimulus intensity modulation have found that alcohol causes augmenters to be less sensitive than they normally are, while alcohol leaves moderates and reducers unaffected (Petrie, 1967). The later finding suggests that alcoholics might drink alcohol in order to achieve a stimulus modulating effect. Among college students, stimulus augmenters, in fact, have been shown to use alcohol for its analgesic, medicating effect (Brown & Cutter, 1977).

The work on stimulus intensity modulation and alcohol consumption clearly points to a possible reason why alcohol is more reinforcing for those persons who develop problems with it than it is for other persons. Recently, other lines of research have been initiated to further elucidate why alcohol is especially reinforcing for people who develop problems with it (Sher, Chapter 7, this volume; Sher & Levenson, 1982).

Working from the basic premise that the manner in which people perceive the world around them covaries with their basic personality characteristics, Witkin and his associates (Witkin, Lewis, Hertzman, Machover, Meissner, & Wapner, 1954; Witkin, Dyk, Faterson, Goodenough, & Karp, 1962) studied relationships between people's perceptual processes and their personality. The Witkin group also devised tests to measure these relationships, including the Body Adjustment Test, Rod and Frame Test, and Embedded Figures Test.

Witkin *et al.* (1954) identified *field dependence–independence* as a basic dimension along which people perceive the world around them. Field–dependent persons utilize cues from the external world, while field–independent persons utilize cues within themselves. Witkin hypothesized that in their interpersonal relationships field–dependent people depend on other people and they are predisposed to develop psychological disorders (such as alcoholism) that involve exaggerated needs for dependency.

Consistent with this hypothesis, Witkin, Karp, and Goodenough (1959) discovered that alcoholics are field dependent. This finding has been replicated many times; in fact, alcoholics have often been found to be extremely field dependent (Goldstein, 1976; Sugerman & Schneider, 1976). Nevertheless, field–dependent persons do not evince general psychological dependence as the Witkin group originally thought, although field–dependent and field–independent people do function differently in their interpersonal relationships (Witkin & Goodenough, 1977).

How is alcoholics' field-dependent perceptual style related to their problems with alcohol? There are no longitudinal data to evaluate directly whether field dependence is a precursor or a consequence of alcoholism. Moreover, various indirect tests (such as whether people's field dependence–independence is affected by ingestion of alcohol or related to the length of their drinking history or sobriety) have yielded conflicting results (Danahy & Kahn, 1981; Goldstein, 1976; Sugerman & Schneider, 1976). Another possibility for accounting for alcoholics' field dependence is that it reflects their brain damage caused by alcohol. Brain-damaged individuals as well as alcoholics are field dependent. However, neuropsychological testing of alcoholics has shown that they have very specific mental deficits, unlike the general deficits of individuals with brain damage (Goldstein, 1976).

Alcoholics' specific mental deficits seem to be associated with their inability to realize the long-range negative consequences of their immediate actions. It is very reasonable that persons with this inability would be prone to drink alcohol excessively, although it seems unlikely that such a specific cognitive deficit would be caused by the deleterious effects of alcohol.

*Locus of control* refers to the location from which people perceive that the source of their reinforcement comes. Locus of control has usually been measured by Rotter's (1966) Internal–External (I-E) Locus of Control Scale, which places people on a continuum from extreme internality (perceiving that they themselves are in control of their lives) to extreme externality (perceiving that their lives are controlled by factors external to themselves such as fate, luck, or fortune). However, other locus of control scales, including drinking related ones, have been used as well (see Rohsenow, 1983a).

Since alcoholics are able to control neither their intake of alcohol nor other aspects of their lives, it seems reasonable to expect them to be external in their perception of control. Alcoholics have, in fact, consistently been found to be more externally controlled than nonalcoholics whenever they have been carefully matched with nonalcoholics on demographic variables that covary with locus of control (Rohsenow, 1983a; Wright & Obitz, 1984). Similarly, among social drinkers, direct relationships have been established between degree of externality and the quantity and frequency of alcohol habitually consumed (Barnes, 1983; Naditch, 1975a; Rohsenow, 1983a). Nevertheless, social drinkers, like alcoholics, vary widely in their locus of control according to various demographic variables and patterns of drinking (Cox & Baker, 1982a, 1982b; Rose, Powell, & Penick, 1978).

From the evidence reviewed in this section, it is apparent that alcoholics have a cognitive/perceptual style that is different from that of nonalcoholics. It has been shown that the distinctive cognitive style of alcoholics is shared by prealcoholics and others at risk for becoming alcoholic (Tarter & Alterman, in press). It has been argued, moreover, that alcoholics' distinctive cognitive style reflects a specific neural dysfunction that is inherited (Tarter & Alterman, in press).

*Alcoholic Personality Subtypes.* The possibility that there might be various alcoholic personality subtypes instead of a single "alcoholic personality" has been recognized for some time, and specific subtypes of alcoholic personalities have been proposed (Knight, 1937; Levine & Zigler, 1973, 1981; Rudie & McGaughran, 1961).

Empirical identification of alcoholic personality subtypes has involved the application of multivariate classification techniques to alcoholics' scores on personality inventories, including the MMPI, Differential Personality Inventory, Personality Research Form, and Sixteen Personality Factor Questionnaire (Cox, 1979; Jackson, 1983; Morey & Blashfield, 1981; Nerviano & Gross, 1983; Skinner, 1982). Various alcoholic personality subtypes have been identified in this manner and have been related to alcoholics' demographic characteristics, cognitive functioning, drinking practices, and responsiveness to treatment (Jackson, 1983; Nerviano & Gross, 1983). Nevertheless, two principal subtypes, each with distinctive drinking styles and problems, have been found repeatedly (Morey & Blashfield, 1981; Skinner, 1982). These two subtypes include (1) psychopathic alcoholics, whose excessive drinking seems to reflect their lack of impulse control, and (2) distressed, neurotic alcoholics, who appear to drink excessively in an attempt to cope with their psychological distress.

We have already seen that MacAndrew (1983) refers to these two principal subtypes as *primary* and *secondary* alcoholics, respectively. We have also seen that the ratio of primary to secondary alcoholics appears to be quite different among male and female alcoholics.

## Motivational Determinants of Alcohol Use and Abuse

We have noted previously that, according to the tension reduction hypothesis, the primary reason why organisms (animals and humans) are motivated to drink alcohol is to reduce their tension. It follows from this hypothesis that alcoholics are persons who have the greatest need to achieve the tension-reducing effects of alcohol.

We have also seen that the initial laboratory studies with animals were interpreted as providing empirical support for the tension reduction hypothesis. However, whether or not the subsequent research with animals also supports the hypothesis is a more controversial matter (Cappell & Greeley, Chapter 2, this volume). In the present section, we will briefly summarize the research with human subjects, which we will see also lends equivocal support to the tension reduction hypothesis and indicates some alternative reasons why people are motivated to drink alcohol.

## Methods of Study

The research to test the tension reduction hypothesis with human subjects was initiated during the 1960s. The first study was conducted by Diethelm and Barr (1962) and was followed by studies from the laboratories of Mayfield (e.g., see Mayfield & Allen, 1967), Mello and Mendelson (e.g., Mendelson & Mello, 1966), and Nathan (e.g., Nathan, Titler, Lowenstein, Solomon, & Rossi, 1970). In these studies, various procedures were used to test the effect of alcohol on tension. The procedures varied with regard to the subjects who were tested, the method for administering alcohol, and the length of the testing session.

The first studies tested the effect of alcohol on hospitalized alcoholics, thus violating the dictum established by the disease concept of alcoholism that persons diagnosed as alcoholic should never have alcohol to drink. Subsequent studies, however, tested social drinkers as well as alcoholics. Several methods have been used for administering alcohol. In the first studies, alcohol was infused directly into subjects' bloodstream. In subsequent studies, subjects were usually provided with alcoholic beverages to drink, but there were several ways in which the beverages were delivered. In some cases, single beverages (i.e., fixed doses of alcohol) were given, whereas in other cases, fixed doses were given at fixed time intervals. In other studies, subjects were required to perform operant tasks successfully in order to receive an alcoholic beverage. In still other studies, subjects were allowed to drink on an ad lib basis. Drinking sessions have included acute ones that tested the effects of a single dose of alcohol, and chronic ones in which subjects have been observed drinking for as long as several weeks. Finally, whereas changes in mood as a function of amount of alcohol consumed have usually been the focus of interest, the amount of alcohol consumed as a function of setting or subject characteristics has been studied as well.

## Research Findings

Studies administering alcohol to human subjects have not provided uniform support for the tension reduction hypothesis (see Cappell & Greeley, Chapter 2, this volume). The most general conclusion that can be drawn from these studies is that initial consumption of alcohol tends to result in positive affective reactions, but that further consumption, especially if it occurs over extended intervals of time, gives rise to negative affective reactions. Nevertheless, the particular affective reaction that results from drinking alcohol depends on a number of additional independent variables that have been summarized recently (Adesso, 1985, Cox, 1985; Langenbucher & Nathan, 1983). Hence, our goal here is briefly to summarize these variables.

One important consideration is the amount of alcohol that is consumed. In small quantities (e.g., one or two drinks) alcohol is likely to give rise to positive feelings. When drunk in larger quantities (e.g., three or more drinks) alcohol is more likely to lead to negative feelings. A second consideration is whether the blood alcohol level is ascending or descending when the drinker's affect is measured. Positive emotions are more likely to be experienced on the ascending limb of the blood alcohol curve. Negative emotions are more likely to be experienced on the descending limb. Another consideration is the situation in which the alcohol is consumed. For example, in a happy, convivial party setting where a person normally experiences positive affect, drinking alcohol is likely to enhance the positive emotions. Conversely, when subjects are alone in a sterile laboratory environment, drinking alcohol is likely to cause them to feel worse. It is also important to consider the gender of the drinker. One study (Konovsky & Wilsnack, 1982) in which males and females were served alcoholic beverages in a naturalistic party setting found that the male drinkers tended to have more positive self-concepts at the end of the party than they had at the beginning, whereas the self-concepts of the female drinkers became significantly more negative during the course of the party. It seems plausible that this gender difference in the effect of alcohol on self-concept was due to the different attitudes that society holds toward drinking by males and females. Males in our society are strongly encouraged to drink heavily in order to uphold their masculine self-image. On the other hand, drinking (especially heavy drinking) by females has been considered "unladylike."

It is also important to consider how people's affective reactions to alcohol are related to their enduring personality characteristics. In this regard, Sher and Levenson (1982) found that male college students who had personality characteristics like those of future alcoholics (outgoing, aggressive, impulsive, and antisocial) had more intense affective reactions to alcohol, that were different from those of other male college students. Specifically, when subjects were placed in a stressful situation (involving either electric shock or a self-disclosing speech), those subjects with personality characteristics resembling future alcoholics derived a greater stress buffering effect from drinking alcohol (in terms of cardiovascular responses and self-reported level of tension) than did the other subjects.

In conclusion, although drinking alcohol does reduce tension under certain circumstances, it can give rise to various other affective reactions. Drinkers' positive affect can be enhanced or their negative affect can be either palliated or intensified.

### Synthesis of the Empirical Findings: A Personality and Motivational Model of Why People Use and Abuse Alcohol

It is apparent from the preceding discussion that affective change plays a crucial role in people's motivation for using and abusing alcohol. Although the actual affective consequences of drinking alcohol can be quite variable, alcohol can enhance positive emotional states under some circumstances and counteract negative emotional states under other circumstances. People develop strong expectations that alcohol will have one or the other of these positive effects on them, and they regularly use alcohol to achieve these effects.

We propose that the affective consequences of alcohol use change during the course of people's drinking career, especially among those people who develop problems with alcohol. As a consequence, the use that people make of alcohol in controlling their affective states also changes during the course of their career with alcohol. In the present section, we will explore the separate roles of alcohol in controlling positive and negative affect, with special attention to the changes that occur in these roles across time. Developmental models of alcohol use have been proposed by other writers (Pandina, Labouvie, & White, 1984; Zucker, 1979).

#### The Role of Alcohol in Controlling Positive Affect

The use of alcohol to regulate positive affect appears to be most salient early in the drinking career of people who eventually develop problems with alcohol. This conclusion is drawn from two sources of information about prealcoholics and others who later develop drinking problems: (1) their enduring personality characteristics and (2) their affective reactions to alcohol.

##### Personality Characteristics

Prealcoholics and other future problem drinkers are nonconforming, gregarions, and impulsive. They seek sources of reinforcement for themselves that most people in our society do not customarily pursue: exciting and unusual sensations that are easily and quickly obtained instead of more difficult to obtain incentives that provide a more lasting source of satisfaction. Drinking alcohol impulsively and in excessive quantities is an example of an activity that satisfies the sensation-seeking needs of such individuals. The fact that impulsive and excessive drinking violates societal mores is not an impeding factor.

On the other hand, prealcoholics and other future problem drinkers typically are not characterized by negative affect such as depression, anxiety, and low self-esteem. Hence, they do not drink alcohol in an attempt to counteract these negative affective states. Prealcoholics' personality characteristics strongly suggest, therefore, that persons who will develop drinking problems use alcohol initially to enhance their positive affect rather than to reduce their negative affect.

## Effects of Alcohol

There are two sources of evidence to suggest that persons who are prone to develop drinking problems obtain a more intense reaction from drinking alcohol than do other people: (1) alcoholics' anecdotal descriptions of their early drinking experiences, and (2) laboratory research on the affective reactions to alcohol of persons who are at risk for becoming problem drinkers.

When alcoholics recall their early drinking experiences, they frequently describe them as having been profoundly reinforcing. The very first drinking occasion is often recalled as an event that transformed the prealcoholic into an entirely different individual. Future problem drinkers appear to be motivated to drink in order to continue to obtain the reinforcing effect from alcohol that their earliest drinking experiences allowed them to achieve. With regard to the laboratory research with high-risk subjects, we have seen that the research by Sher and Levenson (1982; Sher, Chapter 7, this volume) indicated that male college students who are outgoing, aggressive, impulsive, and antisocial (i.e., their personality characteristics are the same as those of prealcoholics) derive a stronger affective reaction to drinking alcohol than do male college students with different personality characteristics. These results indicate that persons who are at risk for developing alcohol problems derive greater reinforcement from alcohol than persons not at risk.

In conclusion, we have evidence both from anecdotal reports and laboratory research suggesting that alcoholics derive special affective reaction from alcohol that other people do not achieve. The personality characteristics of prealcoholics suggest that the special effect they derive from alcohol is used to enhance their positive affect. Thus, it seems that for persons who will develop problems with alcohol, early in their drinking career the role of alcohol in regulating positive affect is more salient than its role in regulating negative affect.

## Consequences of Habitual Excessive Consumption of Alcohol

Whereas future problem drinkers' initial reactions to drinking alcohol are quite positive and drinking alcohol represents a salient source of positive reinforcement in their lives, the changes that occur eventually reduce the salience of alcohol as a source of positive reinforcement for them.

Tolerance for the pharmacologic effects of alcohol is one such change. As habitual drinkers continue to consume alcohol, a given acute dosage comes progressively to have less and less of an effect on them. Thus, it becomes increasingly difficult for people to enhance their positive affect with alcohol. However, since people persist in expecting that alcohol will enhance their positive affect (Beckman, 1980; Brown, Goldman, Inn, & Anderson, 1980; Christiansen, Goldman, & Inn, 1982; Rohsenow, 1983b; Southwick, Steele, & Marlatt, 1981), they try harder and harder to derive this effect, and a recurrent cycle develops.

When drinking alcohol becomes a less salient means for enhancing problem drinkers' positive affect, they have fewer alternative sources of positive reinforcement to turn to than do other people. We have seen that future alcoholics are distinguished by their impulsivity, need for immediate gratification of their impulses, and lack of value for enduring incentives that are difficult to obtain. As a consequence of these personality characteristics, future alcoholics do not work as hard as other people to achieve difficult-to-obtain incentives that can serve as enduring sources of positive affect.

## The Role of Alcohol in Controlling Negative Affect

As future alcoholics' drinking experiences continue, their chronic affect changes, the effect of alcohol on them changes, and their motivation for using alcohol changes. As a result of these changes, alcohol's control of negative affect comes to be more salient than its control of positive affect. What are these changes, and why do they occur?

### Cumulative Affective Consequences of Alcohol Consumption

Alcohol does not affect people only when they are intoxicated; its effects also extend into the sober state. Coinciding with the greater difficulty in achieving a positive affective reaction to an acute dose of alcohol, the cumulatvie effects of alcohol on the drinker's chronic affective state become progressively more negative.

In a study by Birnbaum, Taylor, and Parker (1983), one group of female social drinkers maintained their usual level of drinking for 6 weeks, while another group who customarily drank at the same level as the maintenance group abstained for 6 weeks. During the course of the 6 weeks, the maintenance group showed significant increases while the abstinence group showed significant decreases in their negative affect (depresion, anger, and confusion). There are other clear indications that the long-term consequences of alcohol consumption are to intensify drinkers' chronic feeling of dysphoria (Aneshensel & Huba, 1983; Rohsenow, 1982).

It will also be recalled that whereas alcoholics are significantly depressed and anxious when they enter treatment, they become much less so as they become abstinent from alcohol (Edwards, Bucky, & Schuckit, 1977; Ornstein, 1981; Pettinati, Sugerman, & Maurer, 1982; Sutker & Archer, 1979). Similarly, although prealcoholics show little or no negative affect, the same individuals have developed significant anxiety and depression by the time they enter treatment (Kammeier, Hoffmann, & Loper, 1973), presumably as a direct consequence of their excessive consumption of alcohol.

## Disruptive Life Situation

We have seen that persons who develop problems with alcohol have fewer sources of positive affect to enjoy than less impulsive individuals who place greater value on obtaining difficult-to-acquire incentives. In addition, however, the alternative sources of positive affect that the problem drinker does have (e.g., family, friends, and employment) are likely to become seriously disrupted as a direct consequence of their excessive drinking.

## Self-Medication

As alcoholics have fewer and fewer means of enhancing their positive affect and their negative affect continues to mount, they begin to use alcohol in an effort to counteract their negative affect. When psychoactive drugs are used for self-medication in this manner, serious negative consequences are likely to occur (Naditch, 1975b). A vicious circle is likely to occur, with increased negative affect leading to increased alcohol consumption, which in turn further intensifies the negative affect.

## *Summary and Conclusions*

According to the model we have proposed, people are motivated to drink alcohol in order to control their positive and negative affective states. For certain people, drinking alcohol is especially reinforcing, and affective control with alcohol is very salient for them. However, when people habitually drink alcohol in large quantities in order to control their affect, negative affective consequences occur. Besides the negative acute reactions alcohol causes in heavy drinkers, alcohol causes the drinkers' chronic negative affect to mount when they are sober. Thus, as these individuals' drinking careers continue, drinking alcohol to regulate positive affect becomes progressively less salient, whereas drinking alcohol to regulate negative affect becomes progressively more salient.

This analysis is not intended to apply to all persons who develop problems with alcohol. There are multiple pathways to becoming alcoholic, and different factors have different salience for different people. Nevertheless, the model that we have proposed seems to be the typical one for a substantial subset of male alcoholics. Far fewer data are available on the personality correlates of alcohol use and abuse among females than among males, but we conclude tentatively that a different model applies to males and females.

## Evaluation of the Approach

In this chapter, we have presented evidence that personality factors are antecedent to, concomitants of, and consequences of alcohol use and abuse. Nevertheless, personality factors interact with biological determinants (such as a person's inherited biochemical reactivity to alcohol), other psychological determinants (such as a person's expectations about the effects of alcohol), environmental factors (such as peer pressure to drink), and sociocultural determinants (such as the attitudes about drinking that prevail in the culture in which the drinker lives).

In spite of the demonstrated importance of personality as a determinant of alcohol use and abuse, much work remains to be done if we are to fully understand the role of personality. In particular, there is a need to study persons with drinking problems other than alcoholics who are enrolled in formal treatment programs, and attention should be given to various minority groups (such as blacks, elderly, gays and lesbians, and women) who have been neglected in previous research. It would be productive to follow these subjects longitudinally and to give close attention to their motivation for using and abusing alcohol, and the temporary and permanent changes in their personality that are brought about by their use of alcohol. Finally, we need to consider not only the personality factors that make people vulnerable to having problems with alcohol, but also the personality factors that protect some individuals from developing these problems.

# References

Abraham, K. (1954). The psychological relations between sexuality and alcoholism. In *Selected papers of Karl Abraham, M.D.* (pp. 80–89). New York: Basic Books. (Original work published 1908)

Adams, J. W. (1978). *Psychoanalysis of drug dependence.* New York: Grune & Stratton.

Adesso, V. J. (1985). Cognitive factors in alcohol and drug use. In M. Galizio & S. A. Maisto (Eds.), *Determinants of substance abuse: Biological, psychological, and environmental factors.* New York: Plenum Press (pp. 179–208).

*Alcoholics Anonymous* (3rd ed., 1976). New York: Alcoholics Anonymous World Services, Inc.

Aneshensel, C. S., & Huba, G. J. (1983). Depression, alcohol use, and smoking over one year: A four-wave longitudinal causal model. *Journal of Abnormal Psychology, 92,* 134–150.

Armstrong, J. D. (1958). The search for the alcoholic personality. *Annals of The American Academy of Political and Social Sciences, 315,* 40–47.

Bacon, M. K. (1974). The dependence-conflict hypothesis and the frequency of drunkenness: Further evidence from a cross-cultural study. *Quarterly Journal of Studies on Alcohol, 35,* 836–876.

Barnes, G. E. (1983). Clinical and prealcoholic personality characteristics. In B. Kissin & H. Begleiter (Eds.), *The biology of alcoholism: Vol. 6. The pathogenesis of alcoholism: Psychosocial factors* (pp. 113–196) New York: Plenum Press.

Barry, H. (in press). Psychoanalytic theory. In C. D. Chaudron & D. A. Wilkinson (Eds.), *Theories of alcoholism.* Toronto: Addiction Research Foundation.

Beckman, L. J. (1980). Perceived antecedents and effects of alcohol consumption in women. *Journal of Studies on Alcohol, 41,* 518–530.

Benson, C. S., & Wilsnack, S. C. (1983). Gender differences in alcoholic personality characteristics and life experiences. In W. M. Cox (Ed.), *Identifying and measuring alcoholic personality characteristics* (pp. 53–68). San Francisco: Jossey-Bass.

Birnbaum, I. M., Taylor, T. H., & Parker, E. S. (1983). Alcohol and sober mood state in female social drinkers. *Alcoholism: Clinical and Experimental Research, 7,* 362–368.

Blane, H. T. (1968). *The personality of the alcoholic: Guises of dependency.* New York: Harper.

Blane, H. T., & Chafetz, M. E. (Eds.). (1979). *Youth, alcohol, and social policy.* New York: Plenum Press.

Blum, E. M. (1966). Psychoanalytic views of alcoholism. *Quarterly Journal of Studies on Alcohol, 27,* 259–299.

Bowen, R. C., Cipywnyk, D., D'Arcy, C., & Keegan, D. (1984). Alcoholism, anxiety disorders, and agoraphobia. *Alcoholism: Clinical and Experimental Research, 8,* 48–50.

Bowman, K. M., & Jellinek, E. M. (1942). Alcohol addiction and chronic alcoholism. In E. M. Jellinek (Ed.), *Alcohol addiction and its treatment* (Vol. 1, pp. 3–80). New Haven, CT: Yale University Press.

Brown, R. A., & Cutter, H. S. G. (1977). Alcohol, customary drinking behavior, and pain. *Journal of Abnormal Psychology, 86,* 179–188.

Brown, S. A., Goldman, M. S., Inn, A., & Anderson, L. R. (1980). Expectations of reinforcement from alcohol: Their domain and relation to drinking patterns. *Journal of Consulting and Clinical Psychology, 48,* 419–426.

Carson, R. C. (1969). Interpretative Manual to the MMPI. In Butcher, J. N. (Ed.), *MMPI: Research developments and clinical applications* (pp. 279–296). New York: McGraw-Hill.

Chassell, J. (1938). Family constellation in the etiology of essential alcoholism. *Psychiatry, 1,* 473–503.

Chaudron, D. C., & Wilkinson, D. A. (in press). *Theories of alcoholism.* Toronto: Addiction Research Foundation.

Christiansen, B. A., Goldman, M. S., & Inn, A. (1982). Development of alcohol-related expectancies in adolescents: Separating pharmacological from social-learning influences. *Journal of Consulting and Clinical Psychology, 50* 336–344.

Coleman, J. C., Butcher, J. N., & Carson, R. C. (1984). *Abnormal psychology and modern life.* Glenview, IL: Scott, Foresman.

Conger, J. J. (1951). The effects of alcohol on conflict behavior in the albino rat. *Quarterly Journal of Studies on Alcohol, 12*, 1–29.

Conger, J. J. (1956). Alcoholism; Theory, problem and challenge. II. Reinforcement theory and the dynamics of alcoholism. *Quarterly Journal of Studies on Alcohol, 17*, 296–305.

Cooper, S. E. (1983). The influence of self-concept outcomes of intensive alcoholism treatment. *Journal of Studies on Alcohol, 44*, 1087–1092.

Cox, W. M. (1979). The alcoholic personality: A review of the evidence. In B. A. Maher (Ed.), *Progress in experimental personality research* (Vol. 9, pp. 89–148). New York: Academic Press.

Cox, W. M. (Ed.). (1983). *Identifying and measuring alcoholic personality characteristics.* San Francisco: Jossey-Bass.

Cox, W. M. (1985). *Personality correlates of substance abuse*: In M. Galizio & S. A. Maisto (Eds.), *Determinants of substance abuse: Biological, psychological, and environmental factors* (pp. 209–246). New York: Plenum Press.

Cox, W. M. (in press). *Why people drink: Parameters of alcohol as a reinforcer.* New York: Gardner Press.

Cox, W. M., & Baker, E. (1982a). Are male, heavy wine drinkers more internally controlled than others? *Bulletin of the Society of Psychologists in Substance Abuse, 1*, 165–168.

Cox, W. M., & Baker, E. (1982b). Sex differences in locus of control and problem drinking among college students. *Bulletin of the Society of Psychologists in Substance Abuse, 1*, 104–106.

Cox, W. M., Lun, K., & Loper, R. G. (1983). Identifying prealcoholic personality characteristics. In W. M. Cox (Ed.), *Identifying and measuring alcoholic personality characteristics* (pp. 5–17). San Francisco: Jossey-Bass.

Cox, W. M., & Thornton, A. (1986). Some recent trends in the quantity of alcohol and other drug publications. Unpublished manuscript.

Curry, S. G., & Marlatt, G. A. (1986). Building self-confidence, self-efficacy, and self-control. In W. M. Cox (Ed.), *Treatment and prevention of alcohol problems* (pp. 117–137). Orlando: Academic Press.

Danahy, S., & Kahn, M. W. (1981). Consistency of field dependence in treated alcoholics. *International Journal of the Addictions, 16*, 1271–1275.

Diethelm, O., & Barr, R. M. (1962). Psychotherapeutic interviews and alcohol intoxication. *Quarterly Journal of Studies on Alcohol 23*, 243–251.

Edwards, E., Bucky, S. F., & Schuckit, M. (1977). Personality and attitudinal change for alcoholics treated at the Navy's alcohol rehabilitation center. *Journal of Community Psychology, 5*, 180–185.

Fenichel, O. (1945). *The psychoanalytic theory of neurosis.* New York: Norton.

Galizio, M., & Maisto, S. A. (1985). *Determinants of substance abuse: Biological, psychological, and environmental factors.* New York: Plenum Press.

Goldstein, G. (1976). Perceptual and cognitive deficit in alcoholics. In G. Goldstein & C. Neuringer (Eds.), *Empirical studies of alcoholism* (pp. 115–152). Cambridge, MA: Ballinger.

Gomberg, E. L. (1986). Alcohol, gender, and sexual problems: An interface. In W. M. Cox (Ed.), *Treatment and prevention of alcohol problems* (pp. 235–259). Orlando: Academic Press.

Goodwin, D. W., Schulsinger, F., Hermansen, L., Guze, S., & Winokur, S. (1975). Alcoholism and the hyperactive child syndrome. *Journal of Nervous and Mental Disease, 160*, 349–353.

Hewitt, C. C. (1943). A personality study of alcohol addiction. *Quarterly Journal of Studies on Alcohol, 4*, 368–386.

Horton, D. (1945). The functions of alcohol in primitive societies. In Yale Studies on Alcohol, *Alcohol, science and society* (pp. 153–178). Westport, CT: Greenwood Press.

Huba, G. J., & Bentler, P. M. (1982). A developmental theory of drug use: Derivation and assessment of a causal modeling approach. In P. B. Baltes & O. G. Brim (Eds.),

*Life-span development and behavior* (Vol. 4, pp. 147–201). New York: Academic Press.

Jackson, D. N. (1983). Differential Personality Inventory types among alcoholics. In W. M. Cox (Ed.), *Identifying and measuring alcoholic personality characteristics* (pp. 87–100). San Francisco: Jossey-Bass.

Jellinek, E. M. (1960). *The disease concept of alcoholism.* New Haven, CT: Hillhouse Press.

Jessor, R. (1983). *Adolescent problem drinking: Psychosocial aspects and developmental outcomes.* Unpublished manuscript, University of Colorado Institute of Behavioral Science, Boulder.

Jessor, R., & Jessor S. (1977). *Problem behavior and psychosocial development: A longitudinal study.* New York: Academic Press.

Jessor R., & Jessor, S. (1978). Theory testing in longitudinal research on marijuana use. In D. Kandel (Ed.), *Longitudinal research on drug use,* (pp. 41–71), Washington, DC: Hemisphere.

Jones, M. C. (1968). Personality correlates and antecedents of drinking patterns in adult males. *Journal of Consulting and Clinical Psychology, 32,* 2–12.

Jones, M. C. (1971). Personality antecedents and correlates of drinking patterns in women. *Journal of Consulting and Clinical Psychology, 36,* 61–69.

Kammeier, M. L., Hoffmann, H., & Loper, R. G. (1973). Personality characteristics of alcoholics as college freshmen and at time of treatment. *Quarterly Journal of Studies on Alcohol, 34,* 390–399.

Kandel, D. B. (1978). *Longitudinal research on drug use: Empirical findings and methodological issues.* Washington, DC: Hemisphere.

Kandel, D. B. (1980). Drug and drinking behavior among youth. In A. Inkeles, N. J. Smelser, & R. H. Turner (Eds.), *Annual review of sociology* (Vol. 6, pp. 235–285). Palo Alto, CA: Annual Review.

Keller, M. (1976). The disease concept of alcoholism revisited. *Journal of Studies on Alcohol, 37,* 1694–1717.

Khantzian, E. J. (1981). Some treatment implications of the ego and self disturbances in alcoholism. In M. H. Bean & N. E. Zinberg (Eds.), *Dynamic approaches to the understanding and treatment of alcoholism* (pp. 163–206). New York: Free Press.

Klinger, E., & Cox, W. M. (1986). Thought flow, frustration, and the impulse to drink alcohol. Unpublished manuscript.

Knight, R. P. (1936). Psychodynamics of chronic alcoholism. *Journal of Nervous and Mental Disease, 86,* 538–548.

Knight, R. P. (1937). The psychodynamics of chronic alcoholism. *Journal of Nervous and Mental Disease, 86,* 538–548.

Knight, R. P. (1938). The psychoanalytic treatment in a sanatorium of chronic addiction to alcohol. *Journal of the American Medical Association, 3,* 1443–1448.

Knop, J., Goodwin, D., Teasdale, T. W., Mikkelsen, U., & Schulsinger, F. (1984). A Danish prospective study of young males at high risk for alcoholism. In D. W. Goodwin, K. T. Van Dusen, & S. A. Mednick (Eds.), *Longitudinal research in alcoholism,* (pp. 107–124). Boston: Kluwer-Nijhoff.

Konovsky, M., & Wilsnack, S. C. (1982). Social drinking and self-esteem in married couples. *Journal of Studies on Alcohol, 43,* 319–333.

Landis, C. (1945). Theories of the alcoholic personality. In Yale Studies on Alcohol, *Alcohol, science and society* (pp.129–142). Westport, CT: Greenwood Press.

Lang, A. R. (1983). Addictive personality: A viable construct? In P. K. Levison, D. R. Gerstein, & D. R. Maloff (Eds.), *Commonalities in substance abuse and habitual behavior* (pp. 157–235). Lexington, MA: Lexington Books.

Langenbucher, J., & Nathan, P. E. (1983). The "wet" alcoholic: One drink. . . then what? In W. M. Cox (Ed.), *Identifying and measuring alcoholic personality characteristics* (pp. 21–33). San Francisco: Jossey-Bass.

Levine, J., & Zigler, E. (1973). The essential–reactive distinction in alcoholism: A developmental approach. *Journal of Abnormal Psychology, 81,* 242–249.

Levine, J., & Zigler, E. (1981). The developmental approach to alcoholism: A further investigation. *Addictive Behaviors, 6,* 93–98.

Lisansky, E. S. (1960). The etiology of alcoholism: The role of psychological predisposition. *Quarterly Journal of Studies on Alcohol, 21*, 314–343.

Loper, R. G., Kammeier, M. L., & Hoffmann, H. (1973). MMPI characteristics of college freshmen males who later become alcoholics. *Journal of Abnormal Psychology, 82*, 159–162.

MacAndrew, C. (1965) The differentiation of male alcoholic outpatients from nonalcoholic psychiatric outpatients by means of the MMPI. *Quarterly Journal of Studies on Alcohol, 26*, 238–246.

MacAndrew, C. (1979). Evidence for the presence of two fundamentally different, age-independent characterological types within unselected runs of male alcohol and drug abusers. *American Journal of Drug and Alcohol Abuse, 6*, 207–221.

MacAndrew, C. (1980). Male alcoholics, secondary psychopathy and Eysenck's theory of personality. *Personality and Individual Differences, 1*, 151–160.

MacAndrew, C. (1983). Alcoholic personality or personalities: Scale and profile data from the MMPI. In W. M. Cox (Ed.), *Identifying and measuring alcoholic personality characteristics* (pp. 73–85). San Francisco: Jossey-Bass.

Machover, S., & Puzzo, F. S. (1959). Clinical and objective studies of personality variables in alcoholism: I. Clinical investigation of the "alcoholic personality." *Quarterly Journal of Studies on Alcohol, 20*, 505–527.

Machover, S., Puzzo, F. S., Machover, K., & Plumeau, F. (1959). Clinical and objective studies of personality variables in alcoholism: III. An objective study of homosexuality in alcoholism. *Quarterly Journal of Studies on Alcohol, 20*, 528–542.

Masserman, J. H., & Yum, K. S. (1946). An analysis of the influence of alcohol and experimental neurosis in cats. *Psychosomatic Medicine, 8*, 36–52.

Mayfield, D., & Allen, D. (1967). Alcohol and affect: A psychopharmacological study. *American Journal of Psychiatry, 123*, 1345–1351.

McClelland, D. C., Davis, W. N., Kalin, R., & Wanner, E. (1972). *The drinking man: A theory of human motivation.* New York: Free Press.

McCord, W., & McCord, J. (1960). *Origins of alcoholism.* Stanford, CA.: Stanford University Press.

Mendelson, J., & Mello, N. (1966). Experimental analysis of drinking behavior of chronic alcoholics. *Annals of the New York Academy of Sciences, 133*, 828–845.

Menninger, K. A. (1938). Man against himself. New York: Harcourt.

Midanik, L. (1983). Alcohol problems and depressive symptoms in a national survey. In B. Stimmel (Ed.), *Psychological constructs of alcoholism and substance abuse* (pp. 9–28). New York: Haworth Press.

Miller, W. R. (1983). Alcoholism American style: A view from abroad. *Bulletin of the Society of Psychologists in Addictive Behaviors, 2*, 11–41.

Morey, L. C., & Blashfield, R. K. (1981). Empirical classifications of alcoholism: A review. *Journal of Studies on Alcohol, 42*, 925–937.

Naditch, M. P. (1975a). Locus of control and drinking behavior in a sample of men in Army basic traning. *Journal of Consulting and Clinical Psychology, 43*, 96.

Naditch, M. P. (1975b). Relations of motives for drug use and psychopathology in the development of acute adverse reactions to psychoactive drugs. *Journal of Abnormal Psychology, 84*, 374–385.

Nathan, P. E., & Lansky, D. (1978). Common methodological problems in research on the addictions. *Journal of Consulting and Clinical Psychology, 46*, 713–726.

Nathan, P., Titler, N., Lowenstein, L., Solomon, P., and Rossi, A. (1970). Behavioral analysis of chronic alcoholism. *Archives of General Psychiatry, 22*, 419–430.

Nerviano, V. J., & Gross, H. W. (1983). Personality types of alcoholics on objective inventories. *Journal of Studies on Alcohol, 44*, 837–851.

Ornstein, P. (1981). Psychometric test changes following alcohol inpatient treatment and their relationships to posttreatment drinking behaviors. *International Journal of the Addictions, 16*, 263–271.

Owen, P., & Butcher, J. (1979). Personality factors in problem drinking: A review of the evidence and some suggested directions. In R. Pickens & L. Heston (Eds.), *Psychiatric factors in drug abuse.* New York: Grune & Stratton.

Pandina, R. J., Labouvie, E. W., & White, H. R. (1984). Potential contributions of the life span developmental approach to the study of adolescent alcohol and drug use: The Rutgers Health and Human Development Project, a working model. *Journal of Drug Issues, 14*, 253-268.

Patterson, E. T., Charles, H. L., Woodward, W. A., Roberts, W. R., & Penk, W. E. (1981) Differences in measures of personality and family environment among black and white alcoholics. *Journal of Consulting and Clinical Psychology, 49*, 1-9.

Petrie, A. (1967). *Individuality in pain and suffering.* Chicago: University of Chicago Press.

Pettinati, H. M., Sugerman, A. A., & Maurer, H. S. (1982). Four year MMPI changes in abstinent and drinking alcoholics. *Alcoholism: Clinical and Experimental Research, 6*, 487-494.

Pihl, R., & Spiers, P. (1978). The etiology of drug abuse. In B. A. Maher (Ed.), *Progress in experimental personality research* (Vol. 8, pp. 93-195). New York: Academic Press.

Rohsenow, D. J. (1982). The Alcohol Use Inventory as predictor of drinking by male heavy social drinkers. *Addictive Behaviors, 7*, 387-395.

Rohsenow, D. J. (1983a). Alcoholics' perceptions of control. In W. M. Cox (Ed.), *Identifying and measuring alcoholic personality characteristics* (pp. 37-48). San Francisco: Jossey-Bass.

Rohsenow, D. J. (1983b). Drinking habits and expectancies about alcohol's effects for self versus others. *Journal of Consulting and Clinical Psychology, 51*, 752-756.

Rose, G. S., Powell, B. J., & Penick, E. C. (1978). Determinants of locus of control orientation in male alcoholics. *Journal of Clinical Psychology, 34*, 250-251.

Rotter, J. B. (1966). Generalized expectancies for internal versus external control of reinforcement. *Psychological Monographs: General and Applied, 80* (1, Whole No. 609).

Rudie, R. R., & McGaughran, L. S. (1961). Differences in developmental experience, defensiveness, and personality organization between two classes of problem drinkers. *Journal of Abnormal and Social Psychology, 62*, 659-665.

Rush, B. (1943). An inquiry into the effects of ardent spirits upon the human body and mind, with an account of the means of preventing and of the remedies for curing them. *Quarterly Journal of Studies on Alcohol, 4*, 324-341. (Original Work published 1785)

Schuckit, M. A. (1979). Diagnostic confusion. In D. W. Goodwin & C. K. Erickson (Eds.), *Alcoholism and affective disorders: Clinical, genetic, and biochemical studies* (pp. 9-19). New York: SP Medical and Scientific Books.

Segal, B., Huba, G. J., & Singer, J. L. (1980). *Drugs, daydreaming, and personality: A study of college youth.* Hillsdale, NJ: Lawrence Erlbaum.

Seliger, R. V., & Rosenberg, S. J. (1941). Personality of the alcoholic. *Medical Record, 54*, 418-421.

Sher, K. J., & Levenson, R. W. (1982). Risk for alcoholism and individual differences in the stress-response-dampening effect of alcohol. *Journal of Abnormal Psychology, 91*, 350-367.

Skinner, H. A. (1982). Statistical approaches to the classification of alcohol and drug addiction. *British Journal of Addiction, 77*, 259-273.

Skinner, H. A., & Allen, B. A. (1982). Alcohol dependence syndrome: Measurement and validation. *Journal of Abnormal Psychology, 91*, 199-209.

Southwick, L., Steele, C., & Marlatt, G. A. (1981). Alcohol-related expectancies: Defined by phase of intoxication and drinking experience. *Journal of Consulting and Clinical Psychology, 49*, 713-721.

Sugerman, A. A., & Schneider, D. U. (1976). Cognitive styles in alcoholism. In R. E. Tarter & A. A. Sugerman (Eds.), *Alcoholism: Interdisciplinary approaches to an enduring problem* (pp. 395-434). Reading, MA: Addison-Wesley.

Sutherland, E. H., Schroeder, H. G., & Tordella, C. L. (1950). Personality traits and the alcoholic: A critique of existing studies. *Quarterly Journal of Studies on Alcohol, 11*, 547-561.

Sutker, P. B., & Archer, R. P. (1979). MMPI characteristics of opiate addicts, alcoholics, and other drug abusers. In C. S. Newmark (Ed.), *MMPI: Current clinical and research trends* (pp. 105-148). New York: Praeger.

Syme, L. (1957). Personality characteristics of the alcoholic: A critique of current studies. *Quarterly Journal of Studies on Alcohol, 18,* 288–301.

Tarter, R. E., & Alterman, A. I. (in press). Neurobehavioral theory of alcoholism etiology. In C. D. Chaudron & D. A. Wilkinson (Eds.), *Theories of alcoholism.* Toronto: Addiction Research Foundation.

Tarter, R. E., McBride, H., Buonpane, N., & Schneider, D. U. (1977). Differentiation of alcoholics. *Archives of General Psychiatry, 34,* 761–768.

Thoreson, R. W., & Budd, F. C. (1986). Self help groups and other group procedures for treating alcohol problems. In W. M. Cox (Ed.), *Treatment and prevention of alcohol problems* (pp. 157–181). Orlando: Academic Press.

Uecker, A. E., Boutilier, L. R., & Richardson, E. (1980). "Indianism" and MMPI scores on men alcoholics. *Journal of Studies on Alcohol, 41,* 357–362.

Wilsnack, S. C. (1973). Sex role identity in female alcoholism. *Journal of Abnormal Psychology, 82,* 253–261.

Wilsnack, S. C. (1974). The effects of social drinking on women's fantasy. *Journal of Personality, 42,* 43–61.

Wilsnack, S. C. (1976). The impact of sex roles on women's alcohol use and abuse. In M. Greenblatt & M. A. Schuckit (Eds.), *Alcoholism problems in women and children* (pp. 37–63). New York: Grune & Stratton.

Wingard, J. A., Huba, G. J., & Bentler, P. M. (1980). A longitudinal analysis of personality structure and adolescent substance use. *Personality and Individual Differences, 1,* 250–272.

Witkin, H. A., Dyk, R. B., Faterson, H. F., Goodenough, D. R., & Karp, S. A. (1962). *Psychological differentiation.* New York: John Wiley & Sons.

Witkin, H. A., & Goodenough, D. R. (1977). Field dependence and interpersonal behavior. *Psychological Bulletin, 84,* 661–689.

Witkin, H. A., Karp, S. A., & Goodenough, D. R. (1959). Dependence in alcoholics. *Quarterly Journal of Studies on Alcohol, 20,* 493–504.

Witkin, H. A., Lewis, H. B., Hertzman, M., Machover, K., Meissner, P. B., & Wapner, S. (1954). *Personality through perception.* New York: Harper.

Wright, M. H., & Obitz, F. W. (1984). Alcoholics' and nonalcoholics' attributions of control of future life events. *Journal of Studies on Alcohol, 45,* 138–143.

Wurmser, L. (1978). *The hidden dimension.* New York: Jason Aronson.

Zucker, R. A. (1979). Developmental aspects of drinking through the young adult years. In H. T. Blane & M. E. Chafetz, (Eds.), *Youth, alcohol, and social policy* (pp. 91–146). New York: Plenum Press.

Zucker, R. A., & Noll, R. B. (1982). Precursors and developmental influences on drinking and alcoholism: Etiology from a longitudinal perspective. In *Alcohol consumption and related problems* (Alcohol and Health Monograph 1, Department of Health and Human Services Publication No. ADM 82-1190, pp. 289–330). Washington, DC: Government Printing Office.

Zuckerman, M. (1979). *Sensation seeking: Beyond the optimal level of arousal.* New York: John Wiley & Sons.

# 4 Interactional Theory

## STANLEY W. SADAVA

The extent to which behavior is consistent across structures or is specific to situations is an issue that concerned psychological theorists in the 1970s. To a large extent, the issue concerned the locus of causality of behavior as residing within the person or in the situation. This, of course, mirrored the two parallel methodologies of psychology: experimental manipulation of situations in which responses are measured and individual differences treated as error variance, and correlational studies of cross-situational traits or other individual differences (Bowers, 1973; Cronbach, 1957). The existence of stable, intraorganismic dispositions was both challenged and affirmed (e.g., Alker, 1972; Hogan, DeSoto, & Solano, 1977; Mischel, 1968). The controversy eventually subsided with an implicit consensus that both sides were largely correct.

Coincident with, and perhaps causally related to this confrontation, has been the revival of interactionism, a framework within which "neither the person per se nor the situation per se is emphasized, but the interaction of these two factors is regarded as the main source of behavioral variation" (Ekehammar, 1974, p. 1026). Endler and Magnusson (1976) describe four features of modern interactionism: (1) a continuous process of feedback between the person and situation determines the behavioral response; (2) the person is conceived as an intentional, active agent, not merely the passive recipient of present contingencies, past reinforcement schedules, or psychosexual development; (3) the person is represented by affective, motivational, and cognitive factors, although, consistent with the current *Zeitgeist*, cognitive factors are considered to be dominant (Endler, 1983); and (4) the situation is to be conceived in terms of its psychological meaning to the person, rather than its physical or experimenter-defined meaning. In their own writings and in an important series of edited volumes, Endler and Magnusson have stimulated keen interest and a rethinking of theoretical positions (Endler & Mag-

STANLEY W. SADAVA. Department of Psychology, Brock University, St. Catharines, Ontario, Canada.

nusson, 1976; Magnusson & Endler, 1977; Magnusson, 1981; Magnusson & Allen, 1983).

One must consider the following regarding this very positive development. First, the principle of interactionism is eminently sensible if not self-evident; in the normal course of human existence, a given action generally occurs by someone with a disposition to act in a situation in which such an action is possible, even probable, if not desirable. Second, the principle is not novel to psychology. Ekehammar (1974) has traced the deep historical roots of interactionism in the work of Kantor, Lewin, Murray, Sullivan, and others. Finally, perusal of the edited books cited above shows interactionism to be consistent and compatible with a wide range of theoretical positions, including psychodynamics, behaviorism, developmental psychology, individual differences, experimental social psychology, social learning, and so forth. Apart from the rigid Freudian and behavioristic orthodoxies, interactionism appears to be a theoretical dimension that is relatively orthogonal to other dimensions and assumptions.

It is evident that, in terms of generally accepted criteria, interactionism must be seen at present as "a model but not yet a theory" (Endler, 1983). However, it does represent a distinct paradigm, characterized by a "deliberate, conscious inclusion" of both person and environment, as well as attempts to delineate interrelationships between aspects of person and environment. It must be noted that the various theories, including those reviewed in the present chapter, may not have originated from an explicitly interactionist framework. However, they have emerged within the same period of time with features consistent with this perspective.

Much of what is described as "modern interactionism" has been dominated by two-factor analysis of variance (ANOVA) models (e.g., see Endler, 1983). As applied to a specific phenomenon such as anxiety, it contrasts the intraorganismic disposition (a "trait") with situationally elicited variation (a "state") and tests the interactionist hypothesis by means of its trait-by-state ANOVA analogue. While useful as a means of demonstrating interaction, the approach has been criticized on several grounds, for example, individual and situational variation in the relative weights of the person (P), situation (S), and $P \times S$ components; the unidirectional nature of the model; the focus on a mechanistic, time-limited product of interaction, rather than upon a dynamic interactive process. Particularly relevant to the present chapter are two problems. A two-factor, trait–state model per se presents an impoverished view of the complexity and multidimensionality inherent in both human personality and the environment as construed and experienced by the individual. And, the focus upon specific, discrete responses is inappropriate to the study of complex, relatively consistent patterns of behavior over time. For example, consider that alcohol abuse, alcoholism, or problem drinking imply a relative consistency over time and situations in drinking behavior, whether as manifested in loss of control over quantity consumed, inability to abstain, or a pattern of drinking inappropriate to personal needs or situational demands. Edwards (1974) describes substance dependence in terms of a loss of "behavioral plasticity," an inability to adapt behavior to situation.

Thus a molar interactional psychology is appropriate to the study of complex, temporally extended behavioral patterns and problems (Sadava, 1980). Several general principles can be specified. Personality is represented by a multivariate system, in which variables may be grouped into logical sets or domains, for example, aspects of the self, personal controls, attitudes and values, and so forth. Environment is described in terms of temporally extended characteristics which are relatively consistent across situations; for example, we would be interested in aspects of the climate rather than situation-specific weather reports. In both person and environment, variables can be further described as proximal or distal to the behavior of interest. For example, certain variables proximal to drinking would be highly predictive, such as drinking by close friends, availability of alcohol, and attitudes toward drinking. Others represent predispositions toward drinking in both person and environment, for example, capacity to control impulsivity, unconventional values and attitudes, deprivation of opportunity within the social class structure, and stressful life circumstances. Of course, more of the variance will be "accounted for" by psychosocial variables proximal to drinking behavior. However, models restricted to proximal variables tend to state the self-evident: people who drink heavily tend to have alcohol readily available, have heavy-drinking friends, and have more positive attitudes toward alcohol. The distal variables represent increased probability of a particular outcome, along with others; for example, those with inadequate control of impulses may drink too much, eat too much, have uncontrolled temper tantrums, drive recklessly, gamble excessively, steal—or all of the above. The distal level of analysis provides the necessary context in which an enriched explanaation of problem drinking and its psychosocial concomitants becqmes possible.

It must be noted at the onset that, while these models include both person (P) and environment (E) characteristics, the conception of *interactionism* per se is problematic (Braucht, 1983; Southwood, 1978). The original Lewinian equation: B = f(P, E), in which B = behavior does not preclude an additive main-effects model, and certainly does not rule out clearly distinguishable effects of personality and environment; for example, the differences between ethnic groups in drinking problems and the role of certain personality dispositions need not and cannot be disregarded. However, the concept of interactionism implies combinations that are not reducible to separate person and environment components. For example, person and environment may combine multiplicatively (e.g., personal attitudes and social norms amplify each other's effect), subtractively (e.g., the gap between personal expectancy and environmental accessibility), or proportionately (the "fit" between person and environment). Person and environment may influence each other (e.g., an individual with certain attitudes may join groups with compatible norms, which may subsequently strengthen those attitudes). Finally, a fully reciprocal model posits feedback effects of behavior upon person and environmental attributes; clearly, alcohol abuse can cause changes in individuals and their life situations. We will consider how the theories are interactional in their treatment of codetermination and reciprocal effects among person, environment, and behavior.

In the area of alcohol and other substance abuse, considerable advances have been made in the development of a molar interactionism. Perhaps the reason is rather simple. Many theories of alcohol and drug abuse have emerged (see Lettieri, Sayers, & Pearson, 1980). The source of drinking patterns has been sought in the structure or dynamics of personality, cognitive structures, situational factors, sociocultural characteristics, and in the psychopharmacology of alcohol and possible genetically based differences. However, as the data base has expanded rapidly and methodology has improved, the inadequacy of "a simple and sovereign theory" has become increasingly evident. Thus, a major trend has been a shift toward theories that are overarching, integrating various concepts, data, and subdisciplines. The framework of interactionism, particularly as it implies the deliberate inclusion of both person and environment variables, has proven to be both useful and necessary in bringing some sense of order to the reality of many interrelated variables.

There is no single, widely used interactionist theory of alcohol use. Rather, a number of researchers have developed their own models, all of which pertain to drinking as jointly determined by aspects of the person and of the social environment. In that the various models have both areas of convergence and of divergence, it is appropriate to examine several. Thus, in the present chapter, we will review the models of Richard Jessor, George Huba and Peter Bentler, and Robert Zucker. Each of these models is to be outlined in turn, with particular attention to their interactionist orientation. Research generated by each model will be reviewed briefly. Then the three models, individually and collectively, will be critically evaluated, and several practical implications will be explored.

## Explication of the Models

The models developed by R. Jessor (R. Jessor, 1983; R. Jessor, Graves, Hanson, & S. L. Jessor, 1968; R. Jessor & S. L. Jessor, 1975, 1977, 1978), Huba and Bentler (1982a, 1982b, 1984, in press), Zucker (Zucker, 1979;

Zucker & DeVoe, 1975; Zucker & Noll, 1982), and their respective colleagues are to be reviewed. Note that these models contain both aspects in common and features distinctive to each. All three focus on the entire range of "normal" drinking patterns (i.e., not including clinically defined or diagnosed alcoholism). They conceive of problem drinking within a larger context of functionally equivalent behavioral patterns and thus are not specific theories of drinking. All focus on adolescence, and on precursors, sequelae, and developmental stages pertaining to this stage of life. And of course, all are interactionist as defined previously and as described by the theorists themselves [albeit constituting "early-stage interactionist explanations" (Zucker, 1979) in dealing with complex networks of psychosocial variables]. The models diverge in how they delineate and define various subgroupings or systems of variables, the specific variables selected for inclusion in the model, and in the nature of hypotheses generated and problems investigated.

Thus, the following discussion will demonstrate both the common trends and the heterogeneity inherent in the framework of interactionism. It is crucial to note that each of these models serves three complementary functions: as examples of interactionist theories, as theories of drinking, and as theories pertaining to adolescence. It is important to examine how each of these functions are served.

### The Tri-Ethnic Project (R. Jessor)

The focus of this study was a small town in Colorado, consisting of substantial communities of Anglo-Americans, Ute Indians, and Hispano-Americans. R. Jessor, Graves, Hanson, and S. L. Jessor (1968) set out to explain both intergroup differences and intragroup individual differences in deviant behavior within one integrated theoretical framework. Differences in ethnic group *rates* of problem drinking and other deviance are to be explained in terms of a set of group characteristics: a sociocultural system. Differences between individuals (adolescents) in problem drinking, apart from their group membership, are explained in terms of a set of relevant individual characteristics: a personality system. Finally, the linkages between characteristics of groups and individual personality are explained through relevant characteristics and practices of the parents: a socialization system. In terms of overall design, parental socialization is conceived as the process by which a sociocultural system is transmitted to the adolescent and becomes incorporated within the individual as a system of personality. Note that socialization at the group level combines with the sociocultural system to influence group differences in problem drinking rates, while socialization at the level of the individual family combines with the personality of the adolescent to influence individual differences in problem drinking. Thus, by a set of logical linkages, person and environment are combined to form a field theory of problem drinking.

Interactionism is also evident in this theory by conceiving of analogous variables *across* the three systems. In abstraction, both individual and group differences in problem drinking are seen as outcomes of two sets of forces: (1) instigation toward deviant behavior resulting from denial of opportunity to gain valued rewards (i.e., frustration) by nondeviant means, and (2) reduced controls against deviance, in terms of beliefs regarding "right and wrong" and other controls against impulsive behavior. R. Jessor and his colleagues have borrowed liberally and explicitly from several theories, including anomie theory (Merton, 1957), differential opportunity theory (Cloward & Ohlin, 1960), social learning theory (Rotter, 1954), and a broad literature in developmental psychology. While the concepts and variables are not novel, and their individual relationships to problem drinking and deviant behavior are well established, their integration into a coherent multidisciplinary theory represented a considerable tour de force.

Consider a few examples of lateral, cross-system linkages. Instigation toward a deviance is conceived as a logical goal-directed behavioral response to the frustration of nondeviant or conventional goal-directed behavior. At the group level, this is represented as a value-access disjunction, the extent to which the group is disadvantaged within the American socioeconomic structure. At the personal level it is represented as a disjunction or gap between valued adolescent goals (social affection, academic recognition) and expectancies of attaining satisfaction. At the socialization level, parental behavior was assessed in terms of affection and rewarding good behavior—an opportunity structure within the family. Linkages between these concepts and with problem drinking are established.

Consider the aspect of controls against deviance. At the level of the group, these include exposure to problem drinking models, an absence of sanctions by the group against deviance, and opportunities to engage in deviance, for example, availability of alcohol and locations for undetected drinking. This may be reflected in parental controls, such as an alcoholic parent as a model, limit-setting, and supervision. At the level of personality, self-controls are represented in attitudes toward deviance, and an inability to delay gratification.

Two interesting issues must be noted. First, in a contrast with his subsequent work, Jessor conceives and measures the environment as external to the perception of the individual. A survey of community adults and interviews with parents provides the data for the ethnic group and family environment. Subsequently, Jessor (1981) makes an emphatic case for the conceptualization of environment in terms of the subjective experience of the actor. He notes that the sociocultural system of this study describes environment in "perceiv*able* but not perceiv*ed* terms," and as more distal to experience. Clearly, as Lewin (1951) explained, one cannot properly explain behavior if one does not understand how the person views and interprets a world in which opportunities seem to be denied or where models for heavy drinking exist. Yet, the richness of explanation provided by this interdisciplinary perspective remains impressive. Perhaps multiple conceptions of environment can coexist within the same framework, and conceptions of the environment as socially defined and as perceived need not be considered mutually exclusive.

It must also be noted that the specific variables are predispositional, with probabilistic relationships with problem drinking. That is, an adolescent with low impulse control or low expectancies for doing well in school would be more likely to manifest problem drinking, as well as other responses such as generalized delinquency, emotional disturbances, even intensified efforts to acquire self-control and enhance achievement. Several subsequent studies show how the personal meanings or functions of alcohol serve as theoretical linkages, relating predispositional characteristics to the specific response of problem drinking. Jessor, Carman, and Grossman (1968) showed that drinking in relation to low expectancies for need satisfaction occurs in relation to the "personal effects" function of alcohol-drinking in an attempt to cope with frustration. In a significant comparative study of Italian youth residing in Italy and the United States, R. Jessor, H. Young, E. Young, and Tesi (1970) showed that drinking in relation to frustration and alienation occurs only among persons and cultures where alcohol carries this meaning. Another study showed small but significant relationships between problem drinking and the stress related to life changes and the job (Sadava, Thistle, & Forsyth, 1978). In the latter study, this relationship was observed in persons to whom drinking does not tend to be accompanied by a fear of negative consequences and where drinking is seen as a coping strategy.

### Problem Behavior Theory (R. Jessor)

Problem behavior theory (PBT) considers drinking behavior within a broad context of psychosocial variables and behaviors (see Figure 4.1). The concept of problem behavior itself pertains to "those actions of youth that are considered by the larger society to be inappropriate or undesirable, to depart from widely shared and institutionalized legal or social norms, and to warrant the exercise of social controls (R. Jessor & S. Jessor, 1977, p. 34). Thus, the concept of problem drinking rests ultimately upon social definition, rather than signs of dependence, physical consequences, or other clinical criteria. Problem behavior is also to be conceived as a generalized disposition and a

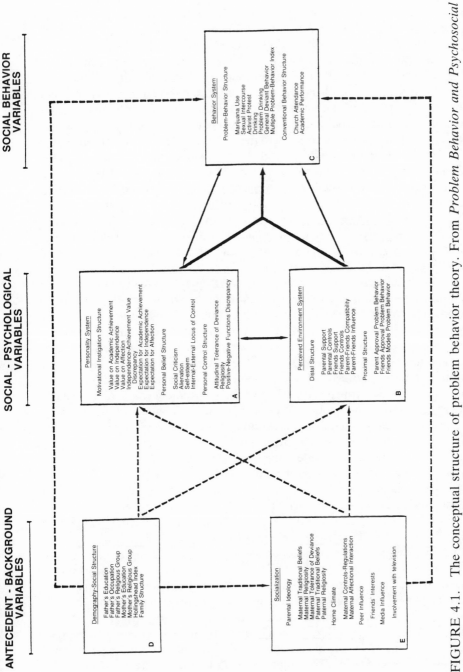

**SOCIAL BEHAVIOR VARIABLES**

**SOCIAL - PSYCHOLOGICAL VARIABLES**

**ANTECEDENT - BACKGROUND VARIABLES**

**Behavior System**

Problem-Behavior Structure

Marijuana Use
Sexual Intercourse
Activist Protest
Drinking
Problem Drinking
General Deviant Behavior
Multiple Problem-Behavior Index

Conventional Behavior Structure

Church Attendance
Academic Performance

C

**Personality System**

Motivational Instigation Structure

Value on Academic Achievement
Value on Independence
Value on Affection
Independence-Achievement Value Discrepancy
Expectation for Academic Achievement
Expectation for Independence
Expectation for Affection

Personal Belief Structure

Social Criticism
Alienation
Self-esteem
Internal-External Locus of Control

Personal Control Structure

Attitudinal Tolerance of Deviance
Religiosity
Positive-Negative Functions Discrepancy

A

**Perceived Environment System**

Distal Structure

Parental Support
Parental Controls
Friends Support
Friends Controls
Parent-Friends Compatibility
Parent-Friends Influence

Proximal Structure

Parent Approval Problem Behavior
Friends Approval Problem Behavior
Friends Models Problem Behavior

B

**Demography-Social Structure**

Father's Education
Father's Occupation
Father's Religious Group
Mother's Education
Mother's Religious Group
Hollingshead Index
Family Structure

D

**Socialization**

Parental Ideology

Maternal Traditional Beliefs
Maternal Religiosity
Maternal Tolerance of Deviance
Paternal Traditional Beliefs
Paternal Religiosity

Home Climate

Maternal Controls-Regulations
Maternal Affectional Interaction

Peer Influence

Friends Interests
Media Influence
Involvement with television

E

FIGURE 4.1. The conceptual structure of problem behavior theory. From *Problem Behavior and Psychosocial Development: A Longitudinal Study of Youth* (p. 38) by R. Jessor and S. L. Jessor. New York: Academic Press. Copyright 1977 by Academic Press, Inc. Reprinted by permission.

class of behaviors which tend to covary as a syndrome. Thus the findings regarding problem drinking are not conceived as unique to problem drinking.

Social-structural variables and socialization are to be considered as antecedent and background to the psychosocial problem patterns. The former refer to aspects of social class as relevant to opportunity, while the latter focus on aspects of socialization similar to those considered in the tri-ethnic project. As aspects of the environment derived external to the person, they are considered rather parenthetically in explaining aspects of personality and perceived environment, in contrast to their central role in the tri-ethnic model.

The heart of the model is a interaction among three systems located within the individual: personality, perceived environment, and behavior. In each, structures and variables representing *problem proneness* or *nonconventionality* are elaborated, all as outcomes of social learning and experience. The greater the degree of "proneness" within each system, the more likely is the occurrence of problem behavior. Overall proneness toward problem drinking is thus seen as a consistent profile of personality, environmental, and behavior attributes.

Clearly underlying the behavior, personality, and perceived environment systems is the notion of a dynamic relationship between factors conducive to problem behavior and those which constrain it. With regard to behavior, the dynamic is between dispositions toward problem behavior and conventional behavior; a zero-sum model is implied where engaging in one serves as both a constraint and an alternative to the other. Within personality, the dynamic relation is between pressures to engage in problem behavior and self-control mechanisms which constrain it. Within the environment, a similar dynamic exists between the perception of models, reinforcements, and opportunities for problem behavior and the perception of social controls against it. While measure have not been derived that directly assess the balance between pressures and constraints, the underlying logic provides another consistent thread linking personality, environment, and behavior.

Within the personality system, three component structures are identified. A motivational–instigational structure represents pressures toward problem behavior, for example, low expectancies and values for academic recognition, high expectancies and values for independence, and the *relative* values of academic recognition and independence. Constraints are represented by personal beliefs (alienation, low self-esteem, external locus of control) and of personal controls (attitudinal tolerance of deviance, low religiosity, more positive than negative functions or reasons for engaging in problem behavior). In the perceived environment system, problem behavior proneness refers to the perception that significant social constraints and supports are lacking and that opportunities for problem behavior are present. At a more distal level, parents are perceived by their adolescents as less supportive, less influential and less consistent or compatible with their friends. At a proximal level, the adolescent reports more approval, presure, and models for drinking, particularly among friends. Finally, in the behavior system, proneness to problem drinking is related to involvement with other problem behaviors (e.g., marijuana and other illicit drug use, sexuality, general deviant/delinquent acts) and less involvement with conventional, approved activities in church and school. The rationale and empirical bases for these variables are provided in detail (R. Jessor & S. L. Jessor, 1977).

Several important features of the model must be noted. With regard to alcohol use, drinking per se and problem drinking (although not alcoholism) are understood as continuous; that is, the same psychosocial system distinguishes among problem drinkers, nonproblem social drinkers, those who drink minimally, and those who abstain absolutely. The model is not specific to alcohol use but to problem behavior, although personal functions and social variables are defined specific to problem drinking, drug use, sexual precociousness, and so forth. As PBT is a social-psychological theory, the psychopharmacology of alcohol is relevant only insofar as its effects are reflected in the personal meanings or functions of drinking to the individual.

While the research generated by PBT will be reviewed subsequently, the theory has several implications for research that must be noted here. One is the necessity for multivariate design and appraisal. Each individual variable should have a predictable relationship with problem behavior, whether correlational (e.g., with quantity–frequency index of alcohol consumption), or comparative (e.g., mean scores for problem drinkers vs. nonproblem drinkers), and whether cross-sectional or predictive over time. However, the essence of the theory is a consistent pattern of personality, environmental, and behavioral nonconventionality, as shown both in increased instigative pressures and reduced constraints. This implies multivariate analyses within overall systems of variables where theoretical consistency becomes empirical covariation. This creates serious problems, which will be addressed below.

Relevant to this is R. Jessor's thoughtful and cautious position regarding causal inference. As will be described subsequently, the centerpiece of PBT is a major longitudinal study, now in its second decade. R. Jessor astutely warns that causal inference is ultimately a matter of logic and theory, not simply an inevitable outcome of any research design. Longitudinal design provides unique, and compelling kinds of data regarding the temporal ordering of events and the processes of change in personal environmental and behavioral attributes. However, unlike Huba and Bentler, he has generally abstained from specific statements of causality.

Rather, converging lines of evidence are used to assess the validity of the person–environment–behavior syndrome of nonconventionality or problem proneness. The following provides some of the flavor of this strategy: (1)

replication across time, across sex, across school levels, across cohorts, and across various problem behaviors; (2) use of various criteria of problem drinking; (3) consistencies across univariate and multivariate cross-sectional relationships; (4) description of parallel changes in personality, environment, and behavior; (5) psychosocial predictors of the *onset* of drinking and of problem drinking, and concomitant changes in the psychosocial system; and (6) prediction of the *timing of onset* of drinking, and its relation to changes in psychosocial variables. While these various lines of evidence are not independent, their covergence adds compellingly to support for the theory.

The model as represented in Figure 4.1 is one of fully reciprocal interaction among person, environment, and behavior. Much of the research has been directed to the correlates and predictors of certain behavioral *criteria* such as problem drinking, or the onset of drinking. However, it is clear in the model and in the research that changes in drinking status or drinking pattern may be accompanied by changes in the direction of psychosocial nonconventionality. This again demonstrates a clear sense of limits in linear causal inferences.

Finally, it must be emphasized that R. Jessor's PBT is a theory of adolescent development. Psychosocial proneness to problem behavior increases during adolescence as a function of normal psychosocial development. Thus, drinking will also increase, again as normal development. Indeed, R. Jessor suggests that coming to terms with the use of alcohol (and other drugs) is a developmental task during the adolescent stage. Its easy availability and impact as a symbol of adult status make drinking decisions both inescapable and significant to the adolescent. Note that the model of psychosocial development implies linear progression toward proneness to problem behavior, transition to drinking, and problem drinking, with no implications of pathology. Indeed, data obtained from these subjects a decade after their adolescence show a generalized reversal, toward conventionality and away from problem behavior, as typical of psychosocial development during that period of life (Donovan, R. Jessor, & J. L. Jessor, 1983).

## Domain Model (Huba and Bentler)

The primary concern of these investigators is the investigation of patterns of causal influence, particularly by means of structural equation models. Consider, for example, the role of drinking by the adolescent's peer group. Whereas most investigators (e.g., R. Jessor) treat this as one of a set of predictor variables to be entered in a linear, additive regression equation, Huba and Bentler are interested in comparing causal paths by which peer drinking influences drinking behavior by the individual. For example, they can ask whether the influence on behavior is direct, or through changes in personal attitudes toward drinking. Or, they can ask how peer influences might be mediated by parental influences. With longitudinal data, they can determine the extent to which drinking behavior tends to "cause" changes in peer group selection or influence. Of course, in order to derive relatively reliable estimates of the relative causal influence of one variable or a set of variables, all of the major sources of influence must be included. Thus, they have developed a model that is explicitly comprehensive in its intended scope, from which they can derive and evaluate models involving subsystems of variables.

The domain model concerns adolescent behavioral styles. That is, drinking behavior is embedded in a larger set of general behavioral tendencies or life-styles, which show some generality or consistency over time and situational contexts, and which may include recreational activities, drug use, other illicit or criminal acts, compulsive eating, or gambling. They note that behavioral alternatives may be mutually substitutable within and between individuals and functionally equivalent with respect to psychosocial causes and personal consequences. Thus, the model is not specific to alcohol use or to substance use per se.

The model is interdisciplinary, including biological, intrapersonal, interpersonal, and sociocultural influences (see Figure 4.2). It incorporates the theoretical and empirical findings of psychopharmacology, psychology, sociology, and other biological and social sciences, all of which have had important things to say about alcohol use and other adolescent behavioral styles. Thus, without any reductionist assumptions, Huba and Bentler have evolved a framework sufficiently comprehensive for their purposes, and including the effects of alcohol as a drug.

Turning to the specific domains, the biological system is defined in terms of genetically determined anatomical, physiological, and developmental characteristics, as well as the physical organismic status at the time, particularly with resepct to the acute or chronic states of health or illness of various systems. A domain of psychophysiology represents mind–body interactions, such as responsiveness and reactivity to stress, psychosomatic disease, and arousal levels. The intrapersonal system includes a domain of psychological status, consisting of various attributes of cognitive and perceptual style, experiences of consciousness, and other personality traits. It also includes a domain of socioeconomic resources, representing the individual's capacity to acquire what is desired (e.g., discretionary income). A domain of self-perceived behavioral pressure includes the expectancies of rewards and costs of a particular action to the actor, judgments of morality regarding the behavior, and the perception of the values and actions of significant others (social support) regarding the behavior. Note that this domain is explicitly psychosocial, in combining the intrapersonal and the interpersonal. The interper-

BIOLOGICAL          INTRAPERSONAL          INTERPERSONAL          SOCIOCULTURAL

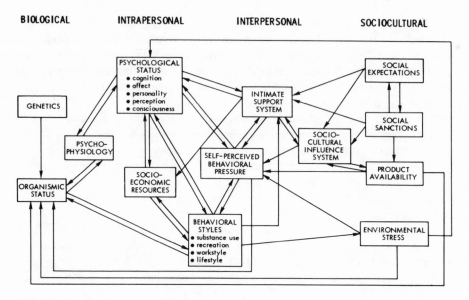

FIGURE 4.2.    Huba and Bentler's domain theory. From "A Developmental
Theory of Drug Use: Derivation and Assessment of a Causal Modeling Approach." In P. B. Baltes & O. G. Brim (Eds.), *Life-span development and
behavior* (Vol. 4, pp. 147–203). New York: Academic Press. Copyright 1977
by Academic Press, Inc. Reprinted by permission.

sonal system is represented by a domain of intimate support, providing proximal sources of relevant valued models and reinforcement for various behaviors
from significant others, as well as a sense of identity and belonging. The
sociocultural systems consists of domains of social expectations or norms for
various roles, social sanctions (formal and informal) for certain actions or
life-styles, product availability relevant to certain behavioral styles (e.g., price,
licensing, and age restrictions regarding use of alcohol), and generalized levels
of environmental stress confronting the individual. Finally a domain of sociocultural influence is located at the intersection of the interpersonal and
sociocultural systems, representing the individual's immediate experience of
his or her culture, including nonintimate others, mass media, and other source
of norms, models, and values.

　　Several observations must be noted. At a higher level of abstraction,
biological, intrapersonal, interpersonal, and sociocultural systems are delineated. These must be seen as categorical descriptions within which various
domains are differentiated—as, indeed, the domains are categorical descriptions of related sets of subsystems of variables. It is significant to note that

three domains—psychophysiology, self-perceived behavioral pressure, and sociocultural influence—are located across the boundaries, between systems. Thus, the model represents a logically defensible, empirically supportable heuristic description, a mapping of the major sources of causal influence. Huba and Bentler note that it is a first approximation, from which successive versions will evolve through causal analyses of empirical data.

Causality is, of course, crucial to the model. In general, the various domains are seen as mutually interrelated, particularly those located in contiguous systems. Some are conceived as directly linked to behavior, others influence behavior indirectly through other domains, while other exert both direct and indirect influences. For example, psychophysiology influences behavior only through organismic and psychological status, self-perceived behavioral pressure has a direct influence on behavior, and psychological status may influence behavior both directly and indirectly through causing changes in other domains. Note also that, in many cases, behaviors such as alcohol use will also influence organismic status, intimate supports, and environmental stress. Finally, Huba and Bentler (1982a) note that a dimension of time is implicit in their framework. Various patterns of causal influence can be expected at different stages of use (e.g., initiation vs. maintenance vs. abuse vs. cessation vs. relapse) and at different stages of developemnt before, during, and after adolescence. Superimposed upon this, of course, will be broad patterns of historical change and cultural distinctiveness.

As noted, this framework has been developed to enable a microanalysis of causality in subsystems of variables. This research will be reviewed below, in Evaluation of the Model. In general, as noted earlier, multidirectional causality is taken as given with regard to these phenomena and this model. However, the research can begin to delineate the *relative* influence of various domains and the paths by which such influence occurs.

## Developmental Model (Zucker)

Most of the research on adolescent drinking traces the acquisition of drinking patterns to the home, and then out to peer-dominated social contexts. However, apart from earlier psychoanalytic formulations, there has been little effort directed toward understand *how* the family environment of the child influences later drinking. Zucker and his colleagues have delineated a developmental model by which the direct and indirect influences of parents, in relation to other personal and social factors, can be explored. One purpose of this model is to provide an organizational framework for the multivariate array of determinants that are already empirically well established. The other is to provide a heuristic model for the study of changes over time, particularly those of psychosocial development before, during, and after adolecence. In addition to providing a basis for his own research, the model has also been utilized as a conceptual framework for several excellent analytic reviews of the literature on adolescent drinking (Zucker, 1976; Zucker, 1979; Zucker & Noll, 1982).

Zucker defines three levels of variables (see Figure 4.3): (1) sociocultural and community influences, (2) group influences, and (3) intraindividual influences. Group influences are further differentiated into those concerning the family of origin (parents) and those concerning peers and other intimate family. Within each of the four classes of variables, a further differentiation is made between those specific to drinking and those that are not drinking-specific but predispositional to it. Class I influences, concerning the impact of the immediate community and the general culture, include social class, ethnic, and religious influences, and neighborhood values, as well as the availability of alcohol and values concerning its use. Classes II and III, concerning the influence of primary and intimate secondary groups, include personalities and interaction patterns of parents and peers, child-rearing patterns, peer socialization, and the attitudes and actions of parents and peers with respect to alcohol (e.g., modeling processes). The intraindividual influences of Class IV include possible genetic influences concerning both alcohol and temperament, attitudes and other cognitive structures, and relevant patterns of personality.

With regard to causality or direction of influence, Zucker conceives of drinking behavior as directly influenced *only* through intraindividual factors. These in turn are influenced by the social variables, directly through intimate groups, and both indirectly and directly by the sociocultural and community environment. Finally, drinking behavior is expected to influence intraindividual attributes, which in turn will influence the primary and intimate secondary groups. Thus, the model includes both the notions of direct and indirect causation and of feedback as the consequences of drinking behavior.

Zucker is also concerned with the developmental implications in the patterns of causation or influence. That is, the relative impact of classes of variables (and, one must suppose, of specific variables within each class) will shift as the individual matures, in ways interpretable through the logic of development. For example, peer group influences will be virtually nonexistent in early childhood but very significant in adolescence, while family influences may decline during the adolescent stage. Similarly, possible genetic influencs may produce neurologic or attentional abnormalities in childhood that may, directly or indirectly, predispose adolescent drinking problems. Zucker (1979) reviews research evidence that illustrates and supports the developmental dimension of this model.

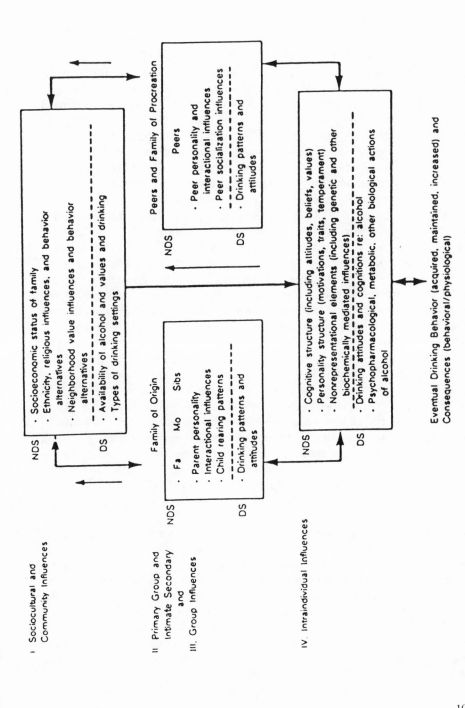

FIGURE 4.3. Zucker's structure for classes of influence upon drinking behavior. From Zucker and Noll (1982).

## Empirical Research

One important test of the practicability of a good theory is the quality of research generated by it. In this sense, all three models are impressive. The following is a brief overview of important aspects of the design, methods, and findings of the research reported by the Jessor, Zucker, and Huba and Bentler groups. Note that these must be viewed as significant and representative contemporary findings from ongoing projects. While there are important points of divergence, the research shares several fundamental features. All focus on problem drinking as one aspect of adolescent behavior. All have generated important longitudinal research, in order to test the notions of development and causal priority implicit in the theories.

The basic source of data is the self-report of the adolescent, by means of various questionnaire and interview methods. With regard to alcohol use, research progress has been retarded by a proliferation of concepts, nonstandardized criteria, and measures (Walizer, 1975). Certainly, measurement difficulties are possible, if not likely; these may include self-presentation tendencies, defensive denial, even a cognitive bias toward overestimating consistency over time. Although these studies adopt some useful strategies, such as multiple measures, alternative criteria and "error-free" latent variables, their data would be strengthened by behavioral observations, collateral reports by significant others, official records, or laboratory tests. In general, the validity studies (reviewed in Midanik, 1982; Pernanen, 1974) show some tendencies toward underreporting of heavy drinking—which would suggest that the findings and interpretations likely err on the side of caution in relation to problem drinking. While these issues are important, the literature does not lead one to a sense of discouragement with regard to self-report measures of alcohol use and alcohol problems. Indeed, the so-called "objective" or external measures are not free of problems, such as observer biases, time sampling biases, and so forth. Psychology as a discipline has not yet discovered a pipeline to the soul of the drinker, and self-report measures are not inherently inferior to alternatives.

It must be noted that few of the univariate findings are novel or surprising in themselves. A number of excellent reviews document the significance of certain personality, peer, and familial characteristics in relation to problem drinking, particularly in adolescence (e.g., Braucht, 1981; Gorsuch & Butler, 1976; Kandel, 1978; Sadava, 1978; Zucker, 1979). Rather, it is in the integration of these various replicated findings within a coherent conceptual framework that these studies are significant. Thus, for example, it will come as no great shock that peer group drinking is important in relation to the drinking of the adolescent. However, in these studies, we can examine peer influences in relation to, and in combination with, adolescent personality vulnerabilities or relationships with parents. This is clearly a step forward.

The research utilizes an impressive array of multivariate analytic techniques. It is beyond the scope of this chapter to provide a detailed, critical review of the various approaches to factor analysis, multiple discriminant analysis, multiple regression analyses, canonical analysis and structural/path analysis using latent variables (LISREL). Suffice it to assert that competence in these methods has become a *sine qua non* for the capacity to do research in this area. Given the fact that experimental methods are neither accessible nor appropriate to study time-extended patterns of drinking behavior, multivariate analyses are fundamental in testing theories which are essentially multivariate (see Bentler, Lettieri, & Austin, 1976).

### Problem Behavior and Problem-Prone Syndrome (R. Jessor)

In the earlier tri-ethnic project, R. Jessor, Graves, Hanson, and S.L. Jessor (1968) reported data from various sources on the three systems. A community survey interview provided data concerning the relative sociocultural systems of the Anglo-American, Hispanic, and Ute communities. Questionnaire data from the entire high school population provided data on the personality system, supplemented by some intensive subsample interviews. Intensive interviews with subsamples of mothers of adolescents from each group provided the socialization system data. Teacher, parent, and court reports provided validation data for deviant behavior.

In general, the data provided impressive support for the model. Sociocultural system variables differentiated between groups of *rates* of deviant behavior, although less impressively among adolescents than among adults. Similarly, personality variables, singly and in combination, were related to individual differences in deviant behavior. Moreover, the relative position of members of the three ethnic groups on personality variables corresponded to the relative positions of these groups with regard to the analogous sociocultural variables. Thus, Anglos-Americans had both the greatest objective access to valued goals by legitimate means, and the *perception* of greatest opportunity. Socialization system variables were shown to be related to the family's ethnic position in the opportunity structure, and to the personality and behavior of the adolescent.

While impressive in conception and design, the study suffered from several important limitations. Some of the measures, particularly in the socialization study, were not adequately developed. The sample was drawn from a single, small southwestern U.S. town, thus limiting generality. Certain variables which are demonstrably related to adolescent behavior, particularly peer group influences, were not included. Multivariate appraisal of the model was limited to dichotomous "pattern analyses," which fail to account for continuity and covariation among predictors. Prediction of deviance was relatively less successful within the Ute Indian group, perhaps reflecting inadequacies in measurement, theory, and/or in understanding this cultural group. Finally, the study attempts to test an essentially longitudinal model by cross-sectional data.

R. Jessor subsequently turned to a culturally homogeneous sample for the intensive, longitudinal study of problem drinking. It began with 432 high school students in grades 7–9, and 205 first-year university students, all in one small city in the midwestern United States. Of the subjects, 403 of the high school students and 193 of the university students were retested at annual data-gathering points over the following 3 years. After a 7-year hiatus, 384 individuals from the high school sample and 184 from the university sample have been recontacted and retested annually. Thus, with overlapping cohorts, the study covers a modal age range from 13 to 30 years, and 90% of the subjects have been retained over six data points and 12 yeas (R. Jessor, 1983).

To review the findings from such a complex and rich data base is a daunting task. As noted earlier, Jessor adopts a strategy of pervasive replication in order to build a case in support of PBT, across time, sex cohorts, and school grade samples. Findings from cross-sectional correlations are replicated and strengthened by longitudinal evidence of prediction and of concurrent patterns of changes. Findings regarding the onset of drinking are replicated by those concerning the onset and maintenance of problem drinking. Findings regarding alcohol are replicated by those concerning the use of marijuana and other illicit drugs, sexual behavior, deviant behavior, and dissenting social activism (the latter findings were not particularly conclusive), and behaviors related to church, school, and family. Findings regarding behavioral nonconventionality are replicated by the data showing concurrent and consistent nonconventionality in personality and in the perceived social environment.

One important concern is validation of the concept of "problem behavior" itself. The data show strong covariation among various adolescent problem behaviors: alcohol use, marijuana and other illicit drug use, sexual behavior, and general deviant behavior including cheating, lying, petty theft, and vandalism. Precocious onset of drinking is related to the onset of other behaviors and to later problem drinking, as well as other problem behaviors. With regard to scalogram analyses of the sequence or progression in the onset of various substance-use behaviors (Kandel, 1975), Donovan and R. Jessor (1983) show that problem drinking tends to occur *after* initial marijuana use, and *before* the onset of other illicit drug involvement.

Furthermore, the data that problem behaviors tend also to occur along with lesser involvement with conventional behaviors related to school and church. In a more extensive study, Hundleby, Carpenter, Ross, and Mercer

(1982) also found tendencies toward the clustering of problem behaviors in opposition to conventional behaviors. One exception: "activist protest" was included as one of the drugs–sex–radicalism triad that characterized the "youth counterculture" of the era in which the study was initiated. However, while this behavior can be considered as nonconventional, it was virtually irrelevant to the incidence of problem behaviors. Indeed, a multiple problem behavior index was constructed, consisting of dichotomous items representing problem drinking, marijuana use, nonvirginity, general deviance, and activism. Scale homogeneity and reliability was adequate in the high school sample, even though activism was only marginally related to other item and total scale score.

While univariate relationships with person and social environment variables are generally substantial, these data are not crucial to the theory. It is an explicitly multivariate model that posits a *syndrome* or *pattern* of interrelated psychosocial risk factors which may be labeled as problem proneness or transition proneness. Thus, the most direct and relevant support for the model derives from cross-sectional and longitudinal multivariate prediction, such as multiple regression and multiple discriminant analyses. Several general patterns are evident: (1) sets of personality or environment variables provide substantial increments in prediction over that provided by single variables; (2) sets of person and environment predictors together increase prediction somewhat over subsets of variables representing only personality or social environment; (3) distal variables provide some increments over the more proximal variables, for example, the general pattern of parental controls and supports for the adolescent are not simply reflected in parental disapproval for heavy drinking. In general, multiple $R$'s obtained range from the .40's to the .70's, including those extending over several years.

Let us examine several patterns of results in more detail, particularly in relation to criteria of drinking behavior. A number of multiple regression runs are reported of predictor sets on the multiple problem behavior index (R. Jessor & S.G. Jessor, 1977). With some variation by sex, cohort, and sample, multiple regression coefficients obtained in the high school samples were as follows: (1) .57–.58 for the personality system, including variables from various structures; (2) .67 and .69 for the perceived environment; (3) .72 and .74 for the "field pattern" of person and environment combined; and (4) .74–.77 for the overall set, including 14 person, environment, and behavior variables. In the university sample, prediction was somewhat lower. Similar runs are reported with individual criteria, including problem drinking; multiple $R$'s obtained for that criterion were .45–.59 for the adolescents, and .25–.48 for the university students. Similar findings are reported in the U.S. national sample (Donovan & R. Jessor, 1978).

R. Jessor and S. Jessor (1975) focus on the onset of drinking in adolescence, particularly as "an age-graded, normatively regulated, transition-marking behavior" (p. 31). Over the 4 years, subjects are classified into five groups in terms of *when* they began to drink (including those who abstained throughout that period). Univariate and multivariate analyses showed psychosocial problem proneness differentiated among groups, both before and after the 4-year period. Initial-year scores yielded predictive multiple $R$'s of .37–.47, while final-year scores yielded multiple $R$'s of .68–.74. In particular, beginning to drink is accompanied by and, to some extent, preceded by less value on academic recognition, greater value on independence, greater tolerance of deviant behavior, less religiosity, less involvement with parents and with friends whose general outlook is similar to that of the parents, more friends who drink and who approve of drinking, less involvement with organized religion, and a tendency toward deviant transgressions. Furthermore, earlier onset was accompanied by a more rapid rate of change toward nonconventionality in some of these attributes. Thus, transition to drinker status was accompanied by a generalized psychosocial transition.

Donovan, Jessor, and Jessor (1983) report on the follow-up study tracing subjects' development into young adulthood. Overall, the trend was away from problem drinking, including most of those individuals who manifested problem drinking in adolescence. This was accompanied by a trend back to conventionality in psychosocial variables. Interestingly, subjects classified as problem drinkers as adults tended, as adolescents, to have greater personal instigations and reduce personal controls relevant to problem behavior, more models and social approval for problem behavior, less involvement with schools and church, and deeper personal involvement in problem behavior *other than drinking itself*. That is, adolescents who will be problem drinkers as young adults do not show specific predispositions toward problems with alcohol but do show a generalized proneness toward problem behavior such as generalized deviant behavior and heavy marijuana use.

A final feature of R. Jessor's data is worthy of consideration. The model is explicitly developmental in nature. That is, normal adolescent psychosocial development is viewed as a process characterized by certain symbolic status transitions, such as becoming a drinker on becoming a nonvirgin. Coincident with these transitions are changes in the psychosocial attributes in the direction of "problem proneness," including lower value for academic recognition, higher value for independence, higher alienation, more tolerant attitudes toward deviance, less religiosity, and more peer models for problem behavior. These trends or "growth curves" tend to level off during subjects' time in university and to reverse in the direction of greater conventionality during the third decade of life. Indeed, the most problem-prone adolescents show the greatest "regression toward the mean" in the direction of postadolescence conventionality. As a stage of life, adolescence is shown to be characterized developmentally by a consistent, time-bounded pattern of problem proneness in personality, perceived environment, and behavioral tendencies. Indeed, R. Jessor (1983) suggests that coming to terms with problems such as alcohol must be viewed as a developmental task confronting the contemporary adolescent in our society and culture. Other research has been generated within PBT. R. Jessor and his colleagues incorporated measures of a subset of PBT variables in two national surveys of U.S. adolescents ($N$ = 13,122 and 839), which included a 4-year follow-up of one subsample (Donovan & R. Jessor, 1978; R. Jessor, Chase, & Donovan, 1980; R. Jessor, Donovan, & Widmer, 1980). In addition to providing large data sets for replication, these studies provide an opportunity to test the generality of the theory across samples of various ethnic groups within the United States. Utilizing various subsets of predictor variables and alcohol criterion measures, consisitent levels of overall prediction were obtained; average multiple correlation coefficients were .53 for white Anglos-Americans, .53 for Hispanics, .52 for blacks, .48 for American Indians, and .57 for Asian-Americans (Donovan & R. Jessor, 1978). However, variation was reported in the relative importance of specific predictor variables in the different groups, particularly among females. For example, in predicting times drunk among females, peer models were more important than personality variables (tolerance of deviance, expectancies for academic achievement) in the Anglo-Americans, American Indian, and Hispanic samples, but relatively less important among the black and Asian-American samples. It is impossible to determine whether the source of such variation is in the theory, measures, or instabilities of mutlivariate analyses.

Sadava has conducted 1-year longitudinal studies of first-year students in two Canadian universities, and a cross-sectional study of working adults (Sadava, 1973, 1977, 1984, Sadava & Forsyth, 1977a, 1977b; Sadava, Thistle, & Forsyth, 1978). Although these longitudinal studies focused on illicit drug use, several findings are of interest in the present context. In general, overall levels of prediction obtained were consistent with those reported by R. Jessor's group. In Sadava's longitudinal analysis, both antecedent scores on psychosocial variables and residual gain scores, representing change over time in these variables, were utilized. One set of multiple discriminant analyses obtained relatively high levels of prediction for the onset of marijuana use among nonusers, cessation of use among users, and relapse among former users (accuracy of classification from 78 to 90%). A similar strategy yielded particularly high, cross-validated multiple correlations for subsequent multiple drug use (.75) and adverse consequences (.71). Canonical analyses revealed distinctive subsets of psychosocial predictors for composites representing moderate use (a long time since initial use, low adverse consequences) and problem use (high in adverse consequences and frequency of use). The moderate pattern was predicted by increasingly high social support for use, tolerance of deviance, and decreasing concerns with negative functions of use, while problem use was predicted by low expectations for social sanctions against use, high coping functions, and high concern with the negative meanings of use. In several cases, cross-product terms (e.g., social support and functions of use) added significantly to regression equations, suggesting possibilities for genuine interactive models. The study of working samples included measures of job stress and life-change stress, and satisfaction in various ares of life, providing some low-level increment in prediction. Overall multiple correlations obtained were .64 for quantity–frequency, .52 for frequency of intoxication, .60 for problem drinking, and .58 for adverse consequences. These data provide some support for the generality of the model beyond adolescence, although the selection of psychosocial variables cannot be limited to the construct of nonconventionality.

Schlegel has conducted a large-sample longitudinal study of Canadian high school students, with annual data points over 6 years (DiTecco & Schlegel, 1982; Schlegel, Crawford, & Sanborn, 1977; Schlegel, d'Avernas, & Manske, 1984). In general, his data are consistent with those of R. Jessor in predicting drinking onset, levels, and transitions to excessive patterns. However, Schlegel reports different predictor subsets for different criterion measures and at different levels of the drinking continuum. That is, personality variables differentiated between moderate and excessive drinkers but not between moderate drinkers and abstainers, while the perceived environment variables more successfully predicted moderate drinking onset from nondrinking. Schlegel also raises the interesting question as to whether R. Jessor's extensive multivariate set may be replaced by a more parsimonious model such as Fishbein and Ajzen's (1979) two-factor theory of intentional behavior (attitude and perceived norms). He concludes that, while the latter model can be highly successful in predicting alcohol use, it is less so with a more "deviant" criterion indicating problem drinking. Furthermore, a finding that people who drink more have more favorable attitudes toward drinking and perceive others as favorable to drinking, does not provide the richness in explanation afforded by R. Jessor's multivariate model.

While the overall trend of these data provide important and impressive support for the model, they are not free of problems. Some inconsistencies are evident in both univariate and multivariate results that cannot be explained by the theory. For example, among the univariate correlations with the frequency of having been drunk in the male and female high school samples, the following were *not* statistically reliable: value for independence, expectancies for independence, expectancies for academic recognition (females), alienation, religiosity, parental controls, and approval for drinking (females) (R. Jessor & S. Jessor, 1977). In comparisons of initial-year scores of groups constituted on the base of *when* they began to drink, value for independence, alienation, parental controls, parental–friend compatibility, and church attendance were all nonsignificant (R. Jessor & S. Jessor, 1975). In the adult follow-up study, Donovan, R. Jessor, and S. Jessor (1983) compared adolescent problem drinkers and nonproblem drinkers who maintained or changed problem-drinker status as young adults. The following adolescent psychosocial attributes did *not* differentiate significantly between groups as predicted: value for independence, religiosity, alienation, all personal functions of drinking, peer drinking models, parental controls, and approval of problem behavior.

Multivariate analyses reveal similar troublesome inconsistencies. Overall levels of multiple correlations obtained are rather unstable between various sets of predictors, various criterion measures, cohorts, years, and samples. In general, prediction is higher in the high school sample than in the university sample, a fact easily explained, since this is a theory of addolescent development. In most cases, prediction is higher for males than for females, perhaps reflecting inadequacies in the theory to explain important gender and sex role differences in the nature and causes of problem drinking. Prediction levels are also higher for certain behavioral criteria (marijuana use, overall deviant behavior) than for others (sexual activity, problem drinking).

It is not clear whether these inconsistencies represent limitations of the theory itself or problems in the data and their analyses. Indeed, the succeeding section Evaluation of the Models, below, will suggest that both explanations are likely true. Notwithstanding these reservations, one must consider that accounting for up to 50% of the variance over time in adolescent problem behavior represents a significant contribution. Given the complexity of such problems, and difficulties inherent in measurement and multivariate analyses, the extent of cross-validation within subsamples of Jessor's study and in the other replications is impressive. One may reasonably conclude that the data support PBT as an interactionist working model, and that the glass is half-full, rather than half-empty. Subsequent discussion will suggest possibilities for filling more of the glass.

## Causal Modeling (Huba and Bentler)

As noted in Domain Model, above, the major interest of these investigators is in the analysis of causality. To do so, they have adopted the techniques of confirmatory causal modeling techniques (structural and covariance structure equation models), using latent variables (i.e., "error-free" variables) to determine the pattern of causal influence (Bentler, 1980). Latent variables consist of the factor scores derived from multiple measures of observed variables. For example, a latent variable of "alcohol use" is derived from measures of the frequency of drinking and of the typical quantity consumed (Aneshensel & Huba, 1984), while a latent variable of "peer culture involvement" is derived from measures of time spent with friends and in activities with peers. With these variables, various structural or path equations can be tested for "goodness of fit," in comparison with alternative paths (Jöreskog & Sörbom, 1978). Particularly where longitudinal data are available, the ways in which various subsystems or combinations of variables influence adolescent behavioral styles (including alcohol use) can thus be assessed.

Several reported analyses will illustrate the flavor of such analyses and their findings. Aneshensel and Huba (1984) investigate the patterns of influence among latent variables representing depression, stress, social supports, physical illness, and alcohol use, utilizing data collected at four points over a 1-year period. They found that alcohol use tended to be followed by a short-term alleviation of depression, but there was a subsequent increase over the 1-year time period. Depression in turn was followed by slight, short-term increases in stress and alcohol consumption. While illness and depression were mutually influential, stress effects on depression were mediated by other variables, particularly social support and physical illness.

Huba and Bentler (1982a) report similar analyses among latent variables representing intimate supports for deviant behavior, rebelliousness, perceived peer pressure to drink, and alcohol use. Behavioral pressure was directly related to alcohol. Rebelliousness was also related directly to drinking, and also exerted a causal influence through behavioral pressure (i.e., rebellious adolescents tend to choose or perceive friends who are heavily involved with alcohol). Finally, intimate support for deviance influenced drinking only through perceived behavioral pressures to drink.

The relative impact of peer and parental models has been studied intensively. Newcomb, Huba, and Bentler (1983), utilizing data gathered directly from parents and from adolescents' perceptions, examined the extent to which parental modeling of substance use influenced substance intake by the adolescent, independent of the perceptions and interpretations of the latter. In the case of both alcohol and "pills" (tranquilizers, amphetamines, sedatives), the pattern of use by the mother influenced use by the adolescent only to the extent that the mother's use influenced the adolescent's perception of how adults in general use alcohol or pills. However, in the case of marijuana, a direct parental modeling effect improved prediction beyond that accounted for by cognitive mediation. Using longitudinal data, Huba, Dent, and Bentler (1980) found that adolescents with many adult drinking models are predisposed to seek out and/or perceive heavy-drinking peers. Peer drinking models influence alcohol consumption directly and are influenced by it. Finally, Huba and Bentler (1984) found that initial rebelliousness and a tendency to disobey laws, when combined with peer involvement, influences alcohol and cannabis use. Alcohol and cannabis involvement, when accompanied by a poor self-concept, predicted involvement with "hard drugs."

It must be noted that this approach is not free of controversy. Martin (1982) questions whether the latent variables are constructed from adequate observable operational variables, whether the "causal analyses" are appropriate, particularly with cross-sectional data, and whether, indeed, this has been proven to be superior to more conventional approaches. In their rejoinder, Huba and Bentler (1982b) both defend their position and caution that it is not a panacea. Clearly, as Baumrind (1983) warns, one cannot and must not "compensate for bad measurement practices with powerful statistical methods." For example, latent variables representing alcohol involvement are constituted from quantities and frequencies of drinking. More intensive measurement strategies, including assessment of alcohol problems, would certainly strengthen their data and clarify their meaning.

### Familial Antecedents (Zucker)

Utilizing data from both the adolescents and their parents, Zucker and his colleagues have examined the influence of the family environment, and the characteristics and behavior of the parents. Zucker and Barron (1973) found that both parents of the heavy-drinking adolescent boys tended to drink heavily, were more antisocial, and utilized social isolation and deprivation as disciplinary techniques. Heavy-drinking boys tended to have mothers who worried about their own drinking and fathers who denied being worried about their own drinking. The boys perceived their fathers as emotionally distant, unrewarding, and uncaring about their accomplishments. With respect to adolescent girls, Zucker and DeVoe (1975) found that the mothers of heavy drinkers tended to be heavy drinkers themselves, and were characterized as having an aggressively sociable style of interaction. These mothers also used isolation and withdrawal of praise or affection as disciplinary techniques. The girls' fathers tended to be heavy drinkers and were often physically absent from the home. Early findings from the high-risk study are consistent with these findings (Zucker et al., 1984).

Thus, the family environments of adolescent problem drinkers tend to be relatively harsher and more negative in affect, and characterized by parental detachment and tense interactions. Their findings, which were consistent with those of R. Jessor's group; with those of Kellam, Brown, Rubin, and Emsminger (1983), and with those of other investigators, indicate that there seems to be disturbances in three areas: (1) parental deviant or antisocial behavior, including alcohol abuse, (2) parental disinterest and lack of involvement with their child, and (3) lack of affectionate and supportive interaction between parents and children. Of course, causality cannot be directly inferred from the findings of familial disturbances concurrent with adolescent problem drinking; indeed, one can expect that the latter will influence the former. However, Zucker (1978) argues convincingly that such familial conditions and parental behaviors are likely to have begun early in childhood, before the onset of drinking. His current childhood antecedent study and that of Kellam's group can be expected to provide valuable evidence in relation to this contention.

**Evaluation of the Models**

In the present chapter, we have reviewed three models. All are multivariate, all are consistent with the broad framework of psychosocial interactionism, and all are, to a greater or lesser extent, models of adolescent development. The theories are not, however, specific to alcohol problems or drinking behavior. Indeed, both Jessor and Zucker distinguish between "distal" variables which are predispositional to adolescent antisocial and problem behavior and the "proximal," drinking-specific variables such as expectancies, attitudes, personal meanings, availability, and models. Repeatedly in the history of research in psychopathology, one can observe a dialectic between approaches that differentiate particular syndromes or problems and approaches that attempt to determine common bases for different problems. Thus, for example, recent genetic evidence suggests a common basis for certain subtypes of alcoholism and sociopathy or depression, mediated by sex and gender roles (Stabenau, 1984; Goodwin, 1979). A strength of these models is their attempt to explore and synthesize both the convergent and divergent nature of problem drinking, relative to other phenomena.

The three models were selected because of their impact, the quality of research generated, and because they illustrate some important alternatives in approaches to explanation and to data analysis. It is important to note that other significant research on alcohol and drug use has been conducted within a psychosocial, interactionist perspective. As noted above, in Problem Behavior Theory, R. Jessor's PBT has stimulated other studies (e.g., DiTecco & Schlegel, 1982; Sadava & Forsyth, 1977a, 1977b; Schlegel et al., 1984). Other significant psychosocial work includes that of Cahalan, Room, and colleagues on problem drinking (e.g., see Cahalan & Room, 1974), Kandel's longitudinal study of adolescent substance abuse, particularly in relation to peer socialization (e.g., Kandel, Kessler, & Margulies, 1978), as well as other longitudinal research (J. Brook, Whiteman, D. Brook, & Gordon, 1981; Kaplan, 1982, Pulkkinen, 1983).

It is difficult to evaluate these models as theories. Hypotheses are essentially devised as composites of univariate findings from the literature, whether as a linear composite of Jessor's variables, a composite of variables weighted by developmental stage (Zucker), or a "best fit" among alternative structural equations (Huba and Bentler). Clearly, substantial multivariate prediction has been demonstrated, and some causal paths "fit" better than others. The adequacy of these findings, apart from statistical confidence levels, must be judged in the context of the relative level of development of contemporary social sciences. One may well be impressed by such success, and yet recognize that these are "not yet" at the stage of formal theory.

The construction of the models reveals their pretheoretical character. Broad constructs are defined in very general terms as representing sets of variables: a domain of intimate support (Huba and Bentler), nondrinking-specific family influences (Zucker), or a motivational–instigation personality structure (R. Jessor). Such constructs have heuristic value in providing structure and organization to the mélange of observable, empirically validated variables that are relevant to adolescent drinking behavior. In turn, the variables included in a given study are to be, by implication, representative of certain systems, classes, or domains. For example, R. Jessor's motivational–instigation structure is to be represented by expectancies and values for academic achievement, independence, and affection, and a discrepancy between values for independence and achievement. What is lacking is a theoretically derived specification of what would adequately describe or represent a motivational–instigation structure or a domain of intimate support. R. Jessor's notion of an overarching dimension of conventionality/nonconventionality provides some guidance to the specification of variables—yet nonconventionality in a motivational–instigation structure is left to pure empiricism and face validity.

While less than satisfactory in terms of the requisites of formal scientific theory, these models represent a significant advance. Indeed, their pretheoretical character is, arguably, advantageous at the present stage of development in this area. The extensive empirical literature provides us with a "grab-bag" of empirical findings and relevant variables, many of them well established. For example, one review of personality predispositions relevant to alcoholism describes six broad constructs or themes, each of which is represented by many measures: problems with dependency, defensive denial, depression, sex-role identity problems, inadequate impulse control, and subjective dissatisfaction (Sadava, 1978). The inclusive and integrative functions of interactionist frameworks is preferable, at this stage, to a narrowing of focus imposed by formal theory, which would ignore much of what has been painfully acquired in research. The models bring some sense of coherence to the multivariate reality of problem drinking. Within a framework within which predictive/explanatory variables can be investigated in a context of organized structures, evolution toward theory can be expected to proceed.

As regards interactionist theories, much remains to be done. In particular, they are, for the most part, based upon linear mathematical models that assume purely additive effects of variables. In several ways, this limits our understanding of drinking behavior and drinking problems. First, the assumption of a linear, monotonic criterion of drinking levels is likely invalid. At one polarity, there is considerable evidence that the abstainer category is unique, often including both "reformed" problem drinkers, those who abstain for religious reasons that are part of their culture, and those adolescents who have experienced psychosocial developmental difficulties (Goldman & Najman, 1984; Knupfer, 1961). At the other polarity, problem drinking/alcoholism must not be assumed to be continuous with other levels of moderate or light drinking. A second problem is that linear additive models do not allow for nonadditive interaction effects. Although these are exceedingly complex, such effects can be of considerable significance. For example, the impact of peer models upon drinking behavior may depend upon factors such as prior normative beliefs, and involvement with nondrinking, church-going family and peers (Britt & Campbell, 1977). While interaction terms can be used in linear regression models (Southwood, 1978) and have been used in studies of drug use (Sadava & Forsyth, 1977a), they are difficult to identify theoretically and equally difficult to interpret. Categorical systems can be adopted within ANOVA designs, but here one would encounter the problem of the definition of category boundaries. Clearly, the expansion to nonadditive interactions must begin at the level of the theories themselves.

Another limitation to linear additive models is that they provide little insight into the dynamics by which person and environmental factors modify and shape each other. For example, we know that peer influence, relationships with parents, and certain personality attributes representing a rebellious–nonconventional disposition all influence adolescent drinking behavior—but we know little of *how* these variables interrelate and influence each other. While we can make probability statements regarding the increased risk of these variables, singly, in combination and, as a "best fit," in sequence, we cannot explain why some adolescents with heavy-drinking friends do not follow suit, why some adolescents in well-functioning families manifest problem drinking, and why some adolescents find nonalcoholic ways to express rebelliousness or nonconventionality. While the work of Huba and Bentler and other investigators is beginning to provide some insight into such questions, it has not as yet had an impact upon theory.

It is clear that these psychosocial variables tend to be highly interrelated. In itself, this poses no problem for the theories. Indeed, Jessor's construct of "nonconventionality" specifies an underlying consistency among personal and environmental attributes. Similarly, within Zucker's model of familial influences, one would expect that parental deviance, lack of parental involvement, and a poor quality of interaction between parent and child would covary. However, as one must use multivariate analyses to test multivariate models, the problem of multicollinearity is rather acute. While the intercorrelations among predictor variables are not so high as to abort analyses entirely, they do cause considerable instability in the inverted matrices.

In particular, as the regression coefficients become unreliable, it becomes impossible to assess the relative impact of different variables or classes of variables. For example, in various reports of R. Jessor's problem behavior research, we find impressive overall multiple correlation coefficients, determined by equations that generally include variables representative of various subsystems and of the general construct of nonconventionality. However, it is not possible to determine the relative importance, for example, of reinforcement values for independence upon adolescent problem drinking. While replication across samples, cohorts, years, and criterion measures is impressive at the macro level of analysis, instabilities in particular regression coefficients are evident. Indeed, given the fact that multicollinearity is an inevitable outcome of the theory itself, replications and stabilities may reflect more of the peculiar psychometric properties of variables within the matrix rather than the impact of a given construct. Failure to replicate may reflect the inherent instability of the matrices and/or genuine differences in samples, cohorts, or criteria.

Tabachnick and Fidell (1983) suggest several possible solutions, none of which is entirely satisfying. Use of stepwise, setwise, or hierarchical entry procedures will reduce or eliminate multicollinear variables; however, entry will be unreliable across samples. One can, after examining the matrix, eliminate offending collinear variables from the analyses. However, from the perspective of theory, the choice of variables to delete would be troublesome. Note also that in most cases, more than two variables are involved. One can create a new composite variable of factor scores after principle components analysis. Indeed, Huba and Bentler (1982a, 1982b) suggest strongly that such "error free latent variables" should largely replace observed scores within domains. However, this does not solve the problem of multicollinearity domains. In general, one might simply toss all predictor scores into the factor matrix, and hope to derive interpretable factors, represented by factor scores. However, the factors may not correspond to the systems or domains defined by the theory—and the theory would then become untestable.

If none of the alternative solutions are entirely adequate, then using several analytic strategies can only contribute to the persuasiveness of the "weight of evidence." The existence in these models of interdependent predictors and multicollinearity may not be simply a matter of theoretical and operational inadequacies. Indeed, we may have to accept that there is a considerable degree of *inherent* unreliability in these regression analyses, reflecting interacting systems as well as individual, sample, and historical variability. Unless one is to retreat to using only simple sovereign theories, multicollinearity is a reality that must be recognized and accepted. Recall that contemporary interactionism posits full, reciprocal influence among person, environment, and behavior (Endler & Magnusson, 1976a, 1976b). The notion of predictors–criteria model is a convenience that allows explanation of a phenomenon such as problem drinking, and does not imply a simple linear, unidirectional model of causality.

Bry (1983) challenges all of these approaches that seek to "account for" a given percentage of variance or to establish "best fit" equations in combining predictors. She identifies a number of psychosocial "risk factors" from a review of the literature, including distant family relationships, low self-esteem peer and family models for abuse, high sensation seeking, and so on. For each psychosocial variable, scores are collapsed into high- and low-risk "regions" on the bases of extensive epidemiologic data. Then, abuse of alcohol or other drugs is predicted solely by the *number* of high-risk factors, without assumptions regarding covariation, the subset involved, weightings, and so on. As a practical method for identifying high-risk drinkers, this approach has considerable merit, as shown in the epidemiology of various health problems. Without doubt, Bry is correct in assuming multiple etiologies or "pathways" among and even within populations. Only extensive comparative research will show in the end whether Huba and Bentler, as well as Zucker and R. Jessor, are excessively optimistic about the explanatory possibilities of theory in this area.

One other strategic imperative is to search for other psychosocial predictor constructs that are relatively independent of those in the models. This must entail close examination of the criteria. In general, with regard to alcohol use, there is some reason for confusion as to what the theories are about. Clearly, none pertain directly to clinical syndromes of alcoholism, and one must be constrained from generalizing to these problems (Nathan & Lansky, 1978). R. Jessor's work suggests that the same psychosocial syndrome of problem proneness can predict onset of drinking, precocious early drinking, quantity and frequency of drinking, adverse consequences, and frequent drunkenness—and, to a considerable extent, it does. Huba and Bentler construct a latent variable for alcohol use consisting of frequencies for beer, wine, and liquor, and quantities consumed. Zucker employs a variety of alcohol consumption and problem drinking measures. As argued earlier, in Problem-Prone Behavior and Problem-Prone Syndrome, it is questionable whether the same set of variables can be expected to predict along the entire continuum of alcohol use patterns. In particular, it would seem to be necessary to distinguish more clearly between alcohol drinking behavior and alcohol-related problems. I have argued elsewhere that the literature shows surprisingly modest relationships between individual consumption levels and alcohol problems (Sadava, 1984; Sadava, 1985). While psychosocial patterns representing non-conventionality may predict increased consumption levels, they may predict problems only to the extent that the consumption represents increased risk. Thus, other personality, familial, environmental, and behavior variables (including concurrent multiple drug use) may explain differences in vulnerability to problems at the same consumption levels.

Kandel's (1975) work merits an additional note from the perspective of criterion definition. Her scalogram analyses, subsequently well replicated, established a set of stages, a sequence in which adolescent drug involvement occurs: (1) beer/wine, (2) liquor/cigarettes, (3) marijuana, and (4) other illicit drugs (Kandel, 1975). Then, Kandel provides evidence that different social psychological factors predict initiation into different stages of drug use (Kandel et al., 1978). for example, parental influence accounted for 41% of the explained variance in initiation to liquor, but for only 12% for marijuana and other illicit drugs. Personal beliefs and values accounted for 2% for liquor, 26% for marijuana, and 15% for hard drugs. For peer influences, the corresponding figures were 34%, 48%, and 33%, respectively, and for minor delinquent behavior, the figures were 23%, 14%, and 40%, respectively. Thus, prior involvement with minor delinquency and with beer and wine, high levels of sociability with friends, and exposure to peer and parental drinking models predicted the onset of hard liquor use. In contrast, the onset of hard drug use was preceded by poor interpersonal relationships, a variety of social models using a variety of drugs, and psychological distress, including depression. Recall that Donovan and Jessor (1983) showed that the onset of problem drinking tends to occur after marijuana and prior to other illicit drugs. It would be of considerable interest to ascertain the relative weightings of predictors for this criterion.

One fascinating issue emerges, particularly in the work of R. Jessor. Various criteria are used interchangeably as indicators of problem behavior. In particular, the *onset* of drinking and *problems* with drinking are treated as two indicators of the same underlying construct. They are explained within the same pattern of personal, social, and behavioral attributes, called "non-conventionality" or a "problem-prone" psychosocial syndrome. Further, normal adolescent development is shown as involving increasing psychosocial nonconventionality, implying increased risk of problem drinking and other problem behaviors. Thus, adolescence represents a paradox: normal (i.e., normative) psychosocial development implies risk of increasingly abnormal behavior.

Certainly it is defensible to conceive of adolescence as a critical, high-risk stage of life. Indeed, in his young-adult follow-up study, R. Jessor (1983) reports some continuity over that time in problem proneness, but an overall tendency of a shift toward conventionality and away from problem behavior—especially among those groups highest in nonconventionality or problem proneness during adolescence. Problem drinking in general populations tends to be reversible and is often reversed over time (Clark, 1976; Donovan, R. Jessor, & S. Jessor, 1983). In another longitudinal study, Verhofstad-Denève (1984) found that, among an institutionalized delinquent sample, those who manifested more emotional conflicts in adolescence exhibited fewer psycho-social complications in adulthood. This suggests a perspective on adolscence in which problems such as alcohol abuse may, in certain psychosocial and intrapsychic contexts, enhance maturation in the long run.

On the other hand, one must caution against the assumption that psy-chosocial conventionality and nonproblem, nonprecocious alcohol use (or abstinence) represent arrested development. Some current research on ad-olescence challenges the notion that it is necessarily or preferably a period of excessive turmoil (e.g., Rutter, Graham, Chadwick, & Yule, 1976). Zucker (1979) raises important questions regarding the concept of psychosocial non-conventionality. First, a strong case can be made that the significance of adolescent problem drinking lies, not in its "transgressive" or problem nature, but in that it facilitates autonomy, particularly from the family and established institutions that dominated childhood. Assuming this ambiguity, the design and model does not specify the variables that are primary to the process of independence, as distinct from antisocial, deviant, or problem predispositions. Zucker suggests that the transition proneness in adolescence may center on the recognition that "greater freedom is possible." While problem drinking is certainly consistent with notions of independence and freedom in adoles-cence, it is not directly implicated. Indeed, nonproblem alternatives become quite possible.

While nonconventionality/problem proneness may be one characteristic of adolescent development, there are likely others which may attenuate the risks. For example, Pandina, Labouvie, and White (1984) suggest five de-velopmental tasks of adolescence: (1) development and maintenance of phys-ical health, (2) development of a sense of identity, including sex roles, values, personality traits, and psychological well-being as well as self-concept, (3) preparation for occupational goals, including education, (4) development of social interactions, including friendship groups, peers, adults, and (5) prep-aration for marriage or other committed relationships, which includes dating and sexuality. Within this framework, variables both proximal and predis-positional to substance abuse can be identified, and their major interactional longitudinal study has been initiated.

   In summary, we have examined several interactional models, all of which have generated significant research and represent important advances. In order to evolve toward a more general theory, research and analyses should now be designed to provide clear comparisons and possible integration of alternative models. For example, it is important to evaluate the relative efficacies of structural equation causal models, linear additive regression models, and summated epidemiologic risk factor models. It is important to determine the generality of models as well as how they may be specific to level or stage of consumption (e.g., Kandel), to developmental stage (e.g., Zucker), to ethnic/cultural group (e.g., R. Jessor's tri-ethnic project), as well as to gender and other sample characteristics. It is important to determine the generality of models and how they may be specific to alcohol use itself, and to initiation to drinking, casual or moderate drinking, heavy consumption, and various types of problem drinking and alcoholism.

   Several other directions can be suggested in which both the theories may evolve and research may be designed. First, one might ask how one can improve on 50% of the variance. A likely answer is a clearer conceptual and operational separation between the normal levels of increased risk in the drinking patterns characteristic of adolescence, and the patterns clearly indicative of present problems and clinical prognosis of alcohol abuse. One possibility that emerges in the literature is a clear deficit in social skills, often combined with aggressive, antisocial behavior (O'Leary & O'Leary, 1976). The literature suggests several correlates and precursors of alcholism including dependency conflicts, sex-role identity confusion, and inadequate impulse controls (Sadava, 1978) that can be incorporated into the framework.

   While the work has focused on adolescence, the implications clearly cover the entire life-span, and the theories can readily be broadened. Several longitudinal studies have identified a number of important familial and personal variables predictive of later alcohol/drug problems (e.g., see Jones, 1968, 1971; Kellam et al., 1983; McCord & McCord, 1962; Vaillant, 1983; Vicary & Lerner, 1983). Others, including those under the direction of Jessor, Kandel, and Schlegel, follow the adolescents into young adulthood and, one hopes, beyond (see also Newcomb & Bentler, 1985). The perspective of life-span development is ideally suited to the modification and expansion of interactionist models. For example, psychosocial variables relevant to themes of commitment, intimacy, and productivity (in work, relationships, and family) might well become more relevant to problem drinking in adulthood. Conceptualization or reconceptualization of etiologically relevant variables within this framework of life-span development will be a major challenge.

   The meaning of alcohol and its use must be considered carefully within this framework. While heavy drinking implies increased risk of problems, and problem drinking implies increased risk of alcoholism, they are neither synonymous nor inevitably progressive. Indeed, as discussed in Evaluation of Models, above, heavy drinking implies only a modest probability of problem behavior, and problem drinking tends to be self-correcting and reversed well short of clinical syndromes of alcoholism. Within a culture where alcohol carries such strong symbolic representation of adult status, masculinity, sociability, and tension relief, drinking may represent benign, even positive psychosocial development and functioning. To focus exclusively on the malignant, problem aspects of alcohol use in this context is to miss much in the explanation of drinking behavior.

## Implications for Intervention and Prevention

The models outlined in the present chapter have not (as yet) had a discernible impact on treatment and prevention. This is entirely understandable in terms of the nature and purposes of these models. They do not pertain directly to specific methods or strategies of treatment or prevention. As well, they do not pertain directly to alcohol abuse or alcoholism. Albee (1982) observes cogently that, while about 15% of the U.S. population represents persons in lower socioeconomic groups, who are at high risk of developing "hard-core" debilitating psychopathology, the mental health system, including prevention, is directed primarily to helping middle-class individuals cope with "problems in living." It is crucial that interactional models and research be directed toward the higher-risk groups and the risk aspects inherent in both social class structure and organic/genetic predispositions. Important beginnings are evident in strategies such as Jessor's tri-ethnic project, Zucker's high-risk families, and Huba and Bentler's inclusion of various socioeconomic/ethnic groups. It is equally crucial that conceptual and empirical linkages be established between the "problem" drinking addressed in these studies and syndromes of alcohol abuse and dependence.

Interactionism can impact primarily in the definition of goals for intervention and prevention rather than in techniques. In particular, one is compelled to think in terms of changes in systems of interacting psychosocial and behavioral attributes, rather than on a narrow focus on change in drinking behavior or in attitudes. For example, Perry and R. Jessor (1983) suggest a strategy of complementary health-promoting interventions aimed at changing personality dispositions that sustain health-compromising behavior (e.g., values, sensation-seeking, tolerance of deviance) and environmental aspects relevant to such behavior (e.g., exposure to excessive drinking models, access to alcohol, and so on. Interestingly, they put equal emphasis upon strengthening behavioral alternatives that serve similar functions and promote health (e.g., physical activity, new hobbies, and so forth) and on those that promote the development of social skills and other behavioral competencies. Personality and social attributes that increase the likelihood that preferred behavioral alternatives to drinking would be strengthened include, for example, increasing the value of health and fitness, strengthening health-related locus of control, and providing access to physical activities and to influential models. Clearly the implication is that a narrow focus on drinking, to the exclusion of other problem behaviors and preferable alternatives, is futile.

R. Jessor (1983) discusses the problem of prevention in the context of alcohol/drug involvement as part of normal adolescent development. While the promotion of functionally equivalent alternatives is possible, some level of involvement with alcohol is unlikely to be prevented in contemporary Western societies. However, a strategy of *minimization* may seek to limit involvement to experimentation or moderation, and specifically to prevent chronic, heavy drinking. A strategy of *insulation* would be directed specifically against serious adverse consequences, such as family disruption, drunk driving, violence, or vandalism while drunk. A strategy emphasizing *delay of onset* would seek to postpone initial or regular drinking, in the expectation that the adolescent will become more mature and skilled in dealing with alcohol in a responsible way. All of these begin with the recognition of psychosocial reality of adolescence in contemporary society.

Zucker and Noll (1982) suggest several implications from their work. Their research with children shows the impact of early cognitive development upon attitudes toward alcohol itself and toward adult models who drink. Thus, they advocate early education about alcohol, designed to be suited to the developmental cognitive capacity of the child. Of course, as a logical outcome of their work, Zucker and Noll suggest that more effort be directed to early intervention with regard to family interaction patterns, particularly in high-risk families (those with parental alcoholism). Finally, within a more general perspective of life-span development, they suggest that prevention and intervention might be targeted more specifically to periods of significant transition, particularly in social roles. For example, programs might be designed that focus specifically on the first year of high school, the graduation from high school to college/university or work, the period around college graduation and/or marriage, and the midlife transitional phase as observed by Levinson (1978). Note that the data of R Jessor and S. Jessor (1977) and others show that the *incidence of problem behavior*, including that related to alcohol, tends to increase through high school, reach asymptote during university, and then decline through the twenties age period. However, the periods of maximum vulnerability may be during these transitions.

In general, the relative empirical success of the research within the framework of psychosocial interactionism is encouraging. It may also be discouraging in that it provides eloquent testimony to the complexity of the problems.

One must feel constrained against "premature closure" regarding the efficacy of various programs. The field of alcoholism is replete with new directions, programs, and controversies: behavior modification for controlled drinking, alcohol "awareness" school programs, group supports and self-help fellowships, changes in consumption levels by pricing policies, employee assistance programs, health promotion and physical fitness, and even simple advice about excessive drinking from a physician. All report their victories and experience their defeats. Psychosocial interactionism can offer a framework and a context in which we can begin to evaluate and understand how, why, when, and where all of these treatment modalities may be effective.

## References

Albee, G. W. (1982). Preventing psychopathology and promoting human potential. *American Psychologist, 37*, 1043–1050.

Alker, A. (1972). Is personality situationally specific or intrapsychically consistent? *Journal of Personality, 40*, 1–16

Aneshensel, C. S., & Huba, G. J. (1984). An integrative causal model of the antecedents and consequences of depression over one year. In J. R. Greenley (Ed.), *Research in community and mental health*, (Vol. 1, pp. 35–72). Greenwich, CT: JAI Press.

Baumrind, D. (1983). Specious causal attributions in the social sciences: The reformulated stepping-stone theory of heroin use as exemplar. *Journal of Personality and Social Psychology, 45*, 1289–1298.

Bentler, P. M. (1980). Multivariate analysis with latent variables: Causal modeling. *Annual Review of Psychology, 31*, 419–456.

Bentler, P. M., Lettieri, D. J., & Austin, G. A. (Eds.). (1976). *Data analysis strategies and designs for substance abuse research*. National Institute on Drug Abuse. Washington, DC: Government Printing Office.

Bowers, K. S. (1973). Situationism in psychology: An analysis and a critique. *Psychological Review, 80*, 307–336.

Braucht, G. N. (1981). Problem drinking among adolescents: A review and analysis of psychosocial research. In *Special Population Issues* (Alcohol and Health Monograph 4, Department of Health and Human Services Publication No. ADM 82-1193, pp. 143–164). Washington, DC: Government Printing Office.

Braucht, G. N. (1983). How environments and persons combine to influence problem drinking. In M. Galanter (Ed.), *Recent developments in alcoholism* (pp. 237–264). New York: Plenum Press.

Britt, D. W, & Campbell, E. Q. (1977). A longitudinal study of alcohol use, environmental conduciveness, and normative structure. *Journal of Studies on Alcohol, 38*, 1640–1647.

Brook, J. S., Whiteman, M., Brook, D. W., & Gordon, A. S. (1981). Paternal determinants of male adolescent marijuana use. *Developmental Psychology, 17*, 841–847.

Bry, B. H. (1983). Predicting drug abuse: Review and reformulation. *International Journal of Addictions, 18*, 223–233.

Cahalan, D., & Room, R. (1974). *Problem drinking among American men*. New Brunswick, NJ: Rutgers Center of Alcohol Studies.

Chassin, L., Presson, C. C., Bensenberg, M., Corty, E., Olshavsky, R. W., & Sherman, S. J. (1981). Predicting adolescents' intentions to smoke cigarettes. *Journal of Health & Social Behavior, 22*, 445–455.

Clark, W. B. (1976). Loss of control, heavy drinking and drinking problems in longitudinal study. *Journal of Studies on Alcohol, 37*, 1256–1290.

Cloward, R. A., & Ohlin, L. E. (1960). *Delinquency and opportunity*. New York: Free Press.

Cronbach, L. J. (1957). The two disciplines of scientific psychology. *American Psychologist, 12*, 674–684.

DiTecco, D., & Schlegel, R. P. (1982). Alcohol use among young males: An application of problem behavior theory. In J. R. Eiser (Ed.), *Social psychology and behavioral medicine*, (pp. 193–233). Chichester, England: J. R. Wiley.

Donovan, J. E., & Jessor, R. (1978). Adolescent problem drinking: Psychosocial correlates in a national sample study. *Journal of Studies on Alcohol, 39*, 1506–1524.

Donovan, J. E., & Jessor, R. (1983). Problem drinking and the dimension of involvement with drugs: A Guttman Scalogram analysis of adolescent drug use. *American Journal of Public Health, 73*, 543–552.

Donovan, J. E., Jessor, R., & Jessor, S. L. (1983). Problem drinking in adolescence and young adulthood. A follow-up study. *Journal of Studies on Alcohol, 44*, 109–137.

Edwards, G. (1974). Drugs, drug dependence and the concept of plasticity. *Quarterly Journal of Studies on Alcohol, 35*, 176–195.

Ekehammar, B. (1974). Interactionism in personality from a historical perspective. *Psychological Bulletin, 81*, 1026–1048.

Endler, N. S. (1983). Interactionism: A personality model but not yet a theory. In M. M. Page (Ed.), *Nebraska Symposium on Motivation, 1982: Personality—current theory and research* (pp. 155–200) Lincoln: University of Nebraska Press.

Endler, N. S., & Magnusson, D. (Eds.). (1976a). *Interactional psychology and personality*. Washington, DC: Hemisphere Publications.

Endler, N. S., & Magnusson, D. (1976b). Toward an interactional psychology of personality. *Psychological Bulletin, 83*, 956–974.

Fishbein, M., & Ajzen, I. (1974). Attitudes toward objects as predictors of single and multiple behavioral criteria. *Psychological Review, 81*, 59–74.

Goldman, E., & Najman, J. M. (1984). Lifetime abstainers, current abstainers and imbibers: A methodological note. *British Journal of Addiction, 79*, 309–314.

Goodwin, D. (1979). Alcoholism and heredity: A review and a hypothesis. *Archives of General Psychology, 36*, 57–61.

Gorsuch, R. L., & Butler, M. (1976). Initial drug abuse: A review of predisposing social psychological factors. *Psychological Bulletin, 83*, 120–137.

Hogan, R., DeSoto, C. B., & Solano, C. (1977). Traits, tests and personality research. *American Psychologist, 32*, 255–264.

Huba, G. J., Dent, C, & Bentler, P. M. (1980, September). *Causal models of peer–adult support and youthful alcohol use*. Paper presented at the 88th Annual Convention of the American Psychological Association, Montreal, Quebec, Canada.

Huba, G. J., & Bentler, P. M. (1982a) A developmental theory of drug use: Derivation and assessment of a causal modeling approach. In P. B. Baltes & O. G. Brim (Eds.), *Life-span development and behavior*, (Vol. 4, pp. 147–203). New York: Academic Press.

Huba, G. J., & Bentler, P. M. (1982b). On the usefulness of latent variable causal modeling in testing theories of naturally occurring events (including adolescent drug use): A rejoinder to Martin. *Journal of Personality and Social Psychology, 43*, 604–611.

Huba, G. J., & Bentler, P M. (1984). Causal models of personality, peer culture characteristics, drug use and crucial behavior over a five-year span. In D. W. Goodwin, K. T. VanDusen, & S. A. Mednick (Eds.), *Longitudinal research in alcoholism* (pp. 73–95). Boston: Kluwer-Nijhof.

Huba, G. J, & Bentler, P. M. (in press). *Antecedents and consequences of adolescent drug use: A psychosocial study of development using a causal modeling approach*. New York: Plenum Press.

Huba, G. J., Wingard, J. A., & Bentler, P. M. (1980). Longitudinal analysis of the role of peer support, adult models and peer subcultures in beginning adolescent substance use: An application of setwise canonical correlation methods. *Multivariate Behavioral Research, 15*, 259–280.

Hundleby, J. D., Carpenter, R. A., Ross, R. A. J., & Mercer, G. W. (1982). Adolescent drug use and other behaviors. *Journal of Child Psychology and Psychiatry, 23*, 61–68.

Jessor, R. (1981). The perceived environment in psychological theory and research. In D. Magnusson (Ed.), *Toward a psychology of situations: An interactional perspective* (pp. 297–311). Hillsdale, NJ: Lawrence Erlbaum.

Jessor, R. (1983). The stability of change: Psychosocial development from adolescence to young adulthood. In D. Magnusson & V. Allen (Eds.), *Human development: An interactional perspective* (pp. 321–341). New York: Academic Press.

Jessor, R., Carman, R. S., & Grossman, P. (1968). Expectations for need satisfaction and drinking patterns of college students. *Quarterly Journal of Studies on Alcohol, 29*, 101–116.

Jessor, R., Chase, J. A., & Donovan, J. E. (1980). Psychosocial correlates of marijuana use and problem drinking in a national sample of adolescents. *American Journal of Public Health, 70*, 604–613.

Jessor. R., Donovan, J. E., & Widmer, K. (1980). *Psychosocial factors in adolescent alcohol and drug use: The 1978 national sample study and the 1974–78 panel study.* Boulder: University of Colorado, Institute of Behavioral Science.

Jessor, R., Graves, T. D., Hanson, R. C., & Jessor, S. L. (1968). *Society, personality and deviant behavior: A study of a tri-ethnic community.* New York: Holt, Rinehart & Winston.

Jessor, R., & Jessor, S. L. (1975). Adolescent development and the onset of drinking: A longitudinal study. *Journal of Studies on Alcohol, 36*, 27–51.

Jessor, R., & Jessor, S. L. (1977). *Problem behavior and psychosocial development: A longitudinal study of youth.* New York: Academic Press.

Jessor, R., & Jessor, S. L. (1978). Theory testing in longitudinal research on marijuana use. In D. B. Kandel (Ed.), *Longitudinal research on drug use: Empirical findings and methodological issues* (pp. 41–71). Washington, DC: Hemisphere Publications

Jessor, R., Young, H. B., Young, E. B., & Tesi, G. (1970). Perceived opportunity, alientation and drinking behavior among Italian and American youth. *Journal of Personality and Social Psychology, 15*, 215–222.

Jones, M. C. (1968). Personality correlates and antecedents of drinking patterns in adult males. *Journal of Consulting and Clinical Psychology, 32*, 2–12.

Jones, M. C. (1971). Personality antecedents and correlates of drinking patterns in women. *Journal of Consulting and Clinical Psychology, 36*, 61–69.

Jöreskog, K. G., & Sörbom, D. (1978). *LISREL-IV: Analysis of linear structural relationships by the method of maximum likelihood.* Chicago: National Educational Resources.

Kandel, D. (1975). Stages in adolescent involvement in drug use. *Science, 190*, 912–914.

Kandel, D. B. (1978). Convergences in prospective longitudinal surveys of drug use in normal populations. In D. B. Kandel (Ed.), *Longitudinal research on drug use Empirical findings and methodological issues* (pp. 1–38). Washington, DC: Hemisphere Publications.

Kandel, D. B., Kessler, R. C., & Margulies, R. Z. (1978). Antecedents of adolescent initiation into stages of drug use: A developmental analysis. In D. B. Kandel (Ed.), *Longitudinal research on drug use: Empirical findings and methodological issues* (pp. 73–99). New York: Halsted.

Kaplan, H. B. (1982). Self-attitudes and deviant behavior. New directions for theory and research. *Youth and Society, 14*, 185–211.

Kellam, S. G., Brown, C. H., Rubin, B. R., & Emsminger, M. E. (1983). Paths leading to teenage psychiatric symptoms and substance use: Developmental epidemiological studies in Woodlawn. In S. B. Guze, F. J. Earls, & J. E. Barrett (Eds.), *Childhood psychopathology and development* (pp. 17–51) New York: Raven Press.

Knupfer, G. (1961). *Characteristics of abstainers; comparison of drinkers and non-drinkers in a large California city*/California Drinking Practices Study Report No. 3. Berkeley: CA: California State Department of Public Health.

Lettieri, D. J., Sayers, M., & Pearson, H. W. (Eds). (1980) *Theories on drug abuse. Selected contemporary perspectives*/National Institute of Drug Abuse Research Monograph 30. Washington, DC: Government Printing Office.

Levinson, D. J. (1978). *The seasons of a man's life.* New York: A. A. Knopf.

Lewin, K. (1951). *Field theory in social science.* New York: Harper.

Magnusson, D. (Ed.) (1981). *Toward a psychology of situations: An interactional perspective.*

Hillsdale, NJ: Lawrence Erlbaum.

Magnusson, D., & Allen, V. (Eds.). (1983). *Human development: An interactionist perspective.* New York: Academic Press.

Magnusson, D., & Endler, N. S. (Eds.). (1977). *Personality at the crossroads: Current issues in interactional psychology.* Hillsdale, NJ: Lawrence Erlbaum.

Martin, J. A. (1982). Application of structural modeling with latent variables to adolescent drug use: A reply to Huba, Wingard and Bentler. *Journal of Personality and Social Psychology, 43*, 598–603.

McCord, W., & McCord, J. (1962). A longitudinal study of the personality of alcoholics. In D. J. Pittman & C. R. Snyder (Eds.), *Society, culture and drinking patterns* (pp. 413–430). New York: John Wiley & Sons.

Merton, R. K. (1957). *Social theory and social structure.* New York: Free Press.

Midanik, L. (1982). Validity of self-reported alcohol consumption and alcohol problems: A literature review. *British Journal of Addiction, 77*, 357–382.

Mischel, W. (1968). *Personality and assessment.* New York: John Wiley & Sons.

Nathan, P. E., & Lansky, D. (1978). Common methodological problems in research on the addictions. *Journal of Consulting and Clinical Psychology, 46*, 713–726.

Newcomb, M.D., & Bentler, P.M. (1985). The impact of high school substance use on choice of young adult living environment and career directive. *Journal of Drug Education 15*, 253–261.

Newcomb, M. D., Huba, G. J., & Bentler, P. M. (1983). Mothers' influence on the drug use of their children: Confirmatory tests of direct modeling and mediational theories. *Developmental Psychology, 19*, 714–726.

Noll, R. B., & Zucker, R. A. (1983, August). *Developmental findings from an alcoholic vulnerability study: The preschool years.* Paper presented at the 91st Annual Convention of the American Psychological Association, Anaheim, CA.

O'Leary, D. E., & O'Leary, M. R. (1976). Social skill acquisition and psychological development of alcoholics: A review. *Addictive Behaviors, 1*, 111–120.

Pandina, R. J., Labouvie, E. W., & White, H. R. (1984). Potential contributions of the life span developmental approach to the study of adolescent alcohol and drug use: The Rutgers Health and Human Development Project, a working model. *Journal of Drug Issues, 14*, 253–268.

Pernanen, K. (1974). Validity of survey data on alcohol use. In R. J. Gibbens (Ed.), *Research advances in alcohol and drug problems* (Vol. 1, pp. 355–374). New York: John Wiley & Sons.

Perry, C. L., & Jessor, R. (1983, April). *Doing the cube: Preventing drug abuse through adolescent health promotion.* Paper presented at the Conference on Preventing Adolescent Drug Abuse: Intervention Strategies, sponsored by National Institute on Drug Abuse, Rockville, MD.

Pulkkinen, L. (1983). Youthful smoking and drinking in a longitudinal perspective. *Journal of Youth and Adolescence, 12*, 253–283.

Riegel, K. F. (1979). *Foundations of dialectical psychology.* New York: Academic Press.

Rooney, J. F., & Wright, T. L. (1982). An extension of Jessor and Jessor's Problem Behavior theory from marijuana to cigarette use. *International Journal of the Addictions, 17*, 1273–1287.

Rotter, (1954). *Social learning and clinical psychology.* Englewood Cliffs, N.J.: Prentice-Hall.

Rutter, M., Graham, P., Chadwick, O. F. D., & Yule, W. (1976). Adolescent turmoil: Fact or fiction? *Journal of Child Psychology and Psychiatry, 17*, 35–56.

Sadava, S. W. (1977): *A social psychology of non-medical drug use in working samples* (research report). Brock University, Department of Psychology, St. Catharines, Ontario, Canada.

Sadava, S. W. (1978). Etiology, personality and alcoholism. *Canadian Psychological Review, 19*, 198–214.

Sadava, S. W. (1980). Towards a molar interactional psychology. *Canadian Journal of Behavioral Science, 12*, 33–51.

Sadava, S. W. (1984). Concurrent multiple drug use. Review and implications. *Journal of Drug Issues, 14*, 623–636.

Sadava, S. W. (1985). Problem behavior theory and the consumption and consequences of alcohol use. *Journal of Studies on Alcohol 46*, 392–397.

Sadava, S. W., & Forsyth, R. (1977a). Person–environment interaction and college student drug use: A multivariate longitudinal study. *Genetic Psychology Monographs, 96*, 211–245.

Sadava, S. W., & Forsyth, R. (1977b). Turning on, turning off and relapse: Social psychological determinants of status change in cannabis use. *International Journal of Addictions, 12*, 509–528.

Sadava, S. W., Thistle, R., & Forsyth, R. (1978). Stress, escapism and the patterns of alcohol and drug use. *Journal of Studies on Alcohol, 39*, 725–735.

Schlegel, R., Crawford, C. A., & Sanborn, M. D. (1977). Correspondence and mediational properties of the Fishbein model: An application to adolescent alcohol use. *Journal of Experimental Social Psychology, 13*, 421–430.

Schlegel, R. P., d'Avernas, J. R., & Manske, S. R. (1984, September). *Longitudinal patterns of alcohol use: Psychosocial predictors of transition.* Presented in symposium, "Alcohol/drug use and the principle of interactionism" at the 23rd International Congress of Psychology, Acapulco, Mexico.

Southwood, K. E. (1978). Substantive theory and statistical interaction: Five models. *American Journal of Sociology, 83*, 1154–1203.

Stabenau, J. R. (1984). Implications of family history of alcoholism antisocial personality and sex differencs in alcohol dependence. *American Journal of Psychiatry, 141*, 1178–1182.

Tabachnick, B. G., & Fidell, L. S. (1983). *Using multivariate statistics.* New York: Harper & Row.

Vaillant, G. E. (1983). *The natural history of alcoholism* Cambridge, MA: Harvard University Press.

Verhofstadt-Denève, L. M. F. (1984, September). *Crises in adolescence amd psychosocial development in young adulthood: A seven-year follow-up study from a dialectical perspective.* Paper presented at the meeting of the 23rd International Congress of Psychology, Acapulco, Mexico.

Vicary, J. R., & Lerner, J. N. (1983). Longitudinal perspectives on drug use: Analyses from the New York longitudinal study. *Journal of Drug Education, 13*, 275–285.

Walizer, D. G. (1975). The need for standardized scientific criteria for describing drug-using behavior. *International Journal of the Addictions, 10*, 927–936.

Zucker, R. A. (1976). Parental influences upon drinking patterns of their children. In M. Greenblatt & M. A. Schuckit (Eds.), *Alcoholism problems in women and children* (pp. 211–238). New York: Grune & Stratton.

Zucker, R. A. (1979). Developmental aspects of drinking through the young adult years. In H. T. Blane & M. E. Chafetz (Eds.), *Youth, alcohol and social policy* (pp. 91–146). New York: Plenum Press.

Zucker, R. A., & Barron, F. H. (1973). Parental behaviors associated with problem drinking and antisocial behavior among adolescent males. In M. E. Chafetz (Ed.), *Research on alcoholism: 1. Clinical problems and special populations* (pp. 276–296). Washington, DC: Government Printing Office.

Zucker, R. A., & DeVoe, C. I. (1975). Life history characteristics associated with problem drinking and antisocial behavior in adolescent girls: A comparison with male findings. In R. D. Wirt, G. Winokur, & M. Roff (Edks.), *Life history research in psychopathology*, (Vol. 4, pp. 109–134). Minneapolis: University of Minnesota Press.

Zucker, R. A., & Noll, R. B. (1982). Precursors and developmental influences on drinking and alcoholism: Etiology from a longitudinal perspective. In *Alcohol Consumption and Related Problems* (Alcohol and Health Monograph 1, Department of Health and Human Services Publication No. ADM 82-1190, pp. 289–330). Washington, DC: Government Printing Office.

Zucker, R. A., Noll, R. B., Drazin, T. H., Braxter, J. A., Weil, C. M., Theads, D. P., Greenberg, G. S., Charlot, C., & Reider, E. (1984). *The ecology of alcoholic families: Conceptual framework for the Michigan State University Longitudinal Study.* Paper presented at the meeting of the National Council on Alcoholism, National Alcoholism Forum, Detroit.

# 5 Social Learning Theory

DAVID B. ABRAMS

RAYMOND S. NIAURA

## Basic Assumptions of Social Learning Theory

An introduction to social learning theory (SLT), as expressed by Bandura (1969, 1977b, 1978, 1982, 1985) is best begun by considering it, albeit briefly, in historical perspective, relative to earlier views on learning and the determinants of behavior. In the spirit of early behaviorism, SLT rejects the notion that behavior can be explained solely by a consideration of underlying motivational forces in the form of needs, drives, and impulses. Such explanations are thought to be inadequate by themselves since they are inferred usually by the behavior they supposedly caused, and do not lend themselves readily to empirical scrutiny. Partly for these reasons, general theories of behavior shifted the focus from internal determinants to an examination of external influences on action. Social learning theory, however, also rejects explanations of human behavior based solely on classical conditioning, strict stimulus–response learning theory, or operant conditioning descriptions. A radical behaviorism posture is unsatisfactory since, by implicitly ascribing causality for behavior solely to external events, one cannot explain adequately the apparent inconsistency of behaviors under similar circumstances. At this point interactionist theories of behavior were resurrected and a compromise of sorts was attained: Behavior results from the interaction of intrapersonal factors on dispositions and situations, the relative contribution of either factor being variable (see Bowers, 1973; Endler & Magnusson, 1976; Mischel, 1968, 1973, 1981).

Social learning theory can be considered an interactionist theory. However, in contrast with earlier views that assume that behavior is a product of the two-way interaction between personal dispositions and situations, SLT

DAVID B. ABRAMS and RAYMOND S. NIAURA. Division of Behavioral Medicine, The Miriam Hospital, Brown University, Providence, Rhode Island.

posits that personal factors, environment, and behavior are interlocking determinants of each other. Causality is, therefore, multidirectional among the factors. The relative influences exerted by these interdependent factors are assumed to differ in different settings and for different behaviors. This model of reciprocal causal function is termed *reciprocal determinism*. Behavior can be studied and explained adequately only by observing simultaneous variations among personal dispositions, environments, and behaviors over time.

Social learning theory moves beyond the assumption that learning occurs by experiencing the effects of behavior, or the repeated pairing of stimuli and responses. Social learning theory assigns prominence to cognitive–mediational—"person factors"—in explaining learning and behavior (Bandura, 1977b). An individual is both an agent and recipient of behavior patterns. Behaviors and environments are thought to interact with a number of basic individual cognitive capabilities: symbolizing capability, forethought capability, vicarious capabjlity, self-regulatory capability, and self-reflective capability.

Borrowing from Bandura (1985), *symbolizing capability* refers to the capacity of individuals to develop internal cognitive models of experience that serve as guides for decision making and future actions. *Symbolization* allows an individual to project courses of action and to generate and test alternatives. *Forethought capability* refers to the capacity to anticipate consequences of action and set goals. Thus, cognitive representations of future events are thought to have a strong causal impact on present actions. Symbolization and forethought play a major role in determining choices of behavior in a specific environmental context. An individual is an active agent, weighing pros and cons before taking action. Good decision making and effective behavior results from an ability to make an accurate appraisal of environmental demands, know the strengths and limits of one's repertoire of coping skills, and weigh both the long and short-term positive and negative consequences of projected outcomes.

The ability to optimize and integrate these various sources of information and to make use of previous experience will determine how effectively an individual copes with situational demands. Thus a general set of life style management skills results in a balanced life style, resilience in the face of unexpected life stressors, and a flexibility in the choice of behaviors that optimize both long-term outcomes and immediate consequences. Since immediate rewards exercise more powerful control over behavior than distant rewards, the individual must acquire the skills to exercise restraint (delay gratification). Cognitive factors play a strong role in *delay of gratification* situations in children (Mischel, 1974) and are also relevant for understanding substance abuse (Abrams & Wilson, 1983). The immediate tension reducing properties of alcohol must be weighed up against the longer-term negative consequences of drinking. Alternatives to drinking (but perhaps less immediately effective ways to cope with tension) must be considered. Individuals must exercise self-control to resist highly tempting immediate rewards that have devastating long-term consequences.

*Vicarious capability* assumes that learning occurs by observing other people's behavior and its consequences for them. In some ways, vicarious capability, or learning through modeling, is also at the root of the definition of SLT since social learning is fostered by observing others' behavior and its consequences. Modeling is a highly efficient way of learning about complex social behavior patterns and cultural norms of conduct. As we shall see, modeling also assumes a primary role in a SLT theory of alcohol use and misuse. Importantly, SLT distinguishes between acquisition and performance of modeled behavior. Individuals do not perform everything they learn. They must first attend to the modeled behavior and remember it. Symbolic processes must then be translated into action. Incentives to reproduce the behavior, either as a function of the situation, observed vicariously or self-produced, will finally determine whether the modeled behaviors will be produced.

*Self-regulatory capability* refers to the capacity to regulate behavior through internal standards and self-evaluative reactions. If there is a discrepancy between internal standards and behaviors, the individual will be motivated to change standards, behavior, or both. Finally, self-reflective capability refers to the distinctive human capacity to reflect upon one's thoughts or monitor one's ideas. All of the above cognitive factors assume a central role in SLT and help explain how individuals are active agents in their own destiny and exercise self-control over their behavior within the situational context.

*Reciprocal determinism* and the thesis that individuals are active agents in determining their own destiny are also central to a SLT model of alcohol use and abuse. As we shall see, SLT differs from traditional theories of addiction that focus on a medical disease model emphasizing the pharmacologic–physiologic properties of alcohol and its effects (Collins & Marlatt, 1983). The primary emphasis of the biological theories is on uncontrollable biochemical processes as the basis for addiction with the addicted individual as the helpless victim of the disease and chemical agents. Drug availability and exposure to even the smallest amount results in an inevitable "loss of control" over behavior with tolerance, dependency, and withdrawal as key variables in explaining alcoholism (Jellinek, 1960). While biological theories acknowledge the importance of individual differences (e.g., genetics and personality traits) their primary emphasis is on processes that are beyond volitional control in a "passive organism."

A social learning model also acknowledges biological factors as predisposing conditions that modulate learning and behavior. However, the underlying principles of SLT assume an adaptive orientation in a purposive rather than passive organism. Thus cognitive activities such as anticipation, expectancy, memory about history of use, and modeling play the primary role as determinants of behavior. An individual chooses to use alcohol to obtain specific outcomes and can choose to use other, more adaptive or less damaging behaviors to achieve his or her goals. Thus the underlying psychological principle of an SLT model of alcohol use and abuse differs markedly from a biological or medical model. This, in turn, results in major differences in prediction of behavior and in treatment of addictive disorders (Miller, 1980; Nathan, 1980; Marlatt, 1976; Marlatt & Gordon, 1985; Wilson, 1978).

The SLT perspective emphasizes a multidetermined interaction between biological, environmental, and other organismic variables (cognitive–emotional and psychophysiologic). Social learning theory stresses how biological–biochemical factors might influence an individual's cognitions (e.g., expectancies of stress reduction) and attempts to initiate alternative methods of coping to prevent relapse. Similar to biological variables, situational determinants of drinking behavior (e.g., modeling effects, reactivity to alcohol cues) are also modulated by cognitions thus providing an alternative to either traitlike dispositional constructs (personality) or fixed biochemical reactions under all situations.

Social learning theory assigns central importance to a self-efficacy mechanism in explaining how thought affects action and how behavior patterns are selected by the individual (Bandura, 1977a, 1982). Briefly, *self-efficacy* refers to a perception or judgment of one's capability to execute a particular course of action required to deal effectively with an impending situation. *Efficacy expectations* reflect an estimate that an individual has sufficient mastery of the skills required to cope with a specific situation. *Efficacy judgments* are thought to influence the choice of actions, the effort expended, perseverance in a course of action, attributions for success or failure, quality and strength of emotional reactions during anticipation of an event, and performance in the actual situation. Efficacy judgments influence directly preparatory learning skills, and influence one's ability to withstand failures.

Efficacy judgments are based upon, and altered by, four sources of information. Performance accomplishments or previous experience of action in a given situation are thought to exert the most powerful influences upon efficacy beliefs insofar as failure experiences will undermine, and success experiences will boost directly efficacy judgments. Efficacy expectations are also instigated vicariously through modeling influences. Observation of success or failure of others similar to oneself will be reflected in a corresponding increase or decrease in self-efficacy. Social persuasion can also act to influence efficacy judgments. Finally, individuals will rely on their physiologic state in judging their efficacy to perform a set task in a given situation. If someone is highly anxious or fatigued, for example, this will influence an estimate of their capability to perform adequately.

Efficacy judgments are thought to influence directly a person's coping efforts in threatening or aversive situations. For example, efficacy perceptions have been related to initiation and duration of coping actions in fear and anxiety-related disorders (Biran & Wilson, 1981), management of pain (Reese, 1983), tension headaches (Holroyd *et al.*, 1985), postcoronary rehabilitation (Ewart, Taylor, Reese, & DeBusk, 1983), and relapse in treated smokers (Condiotte & Lichtenstein, 1981). As we shall attempt to show, efficacy beliefs, by influencing directly coping efforts during aversive stimulation, will bear upon both the development and maintenance of alcohol abuse and dependence. They also will be related directly to predictions about recovery and prevention of relapse.

In the following sections we will attempt to show specifically how the central principles of SLT can be applied to understanding alcohol use and abuse. We will explore the origins of the SLT of alcohol use and abuse, the acquisition and initiation of drinking from a developmental perspective, the immediate determinants (proximal) of drinking behavior, alcohol abuse, and the process of recovery and of relapse.

## Early Formulations of a Social Learning Theory of Alcohol Abuse

Bandura (1969) states that "alcoholics are people who have acquired through differential reinforcement and modeling experiences alcohol consumption as a widely generalized dominant response to aversive stimulation" (p. 536). In support of this general statement, Bandura (1969) proposes that social learning variables, in several forms, influence the reinforcement contingencies associated with alcohol use. Included are concepts derived from learning theory in the form of classical and operant conditioning. These principles such as tension reduction theory are covered in detail elsewhere (see Cappell, 1975; Cappell & Greeley, Chapter 2, this volume). Variables other than those derived from strict learning theory were also included in SLT. Cultural norms and prescriptions for drinking and sobriety, for example, may explain the disparity in the incidence of alcoholism among cultures and subcultures. Implicit in cultural norms, Bandura (1969) argues, are the modeling behaviors of socializing agents, including family and peers. Patterns of drinking behaviors, including drinking under circumscribed conditions (e.g., mealtime or religious occasions) or drinking in a large variety of circumstances and in response to monotony or stress, are thought to be modeled by family members and peers. Thus from an early age, individuals learn how alcohol is used and in what situations, and what behaviors are "permitted" when one is intoxicated (MacAndrew & Edgerton, 1969).

Furthermore, Bandura (1969) states that, after initial exposure to alcohol use, the individual will experience directly the positive reinforcing effects of alcohol's stress-reducing properties. Consumption of alcohol, then, eventually will be elicited readily by, and generalized to, a growing array of aversive conditions and reinforced positively by tension reduction. Bandura (1969) also suggests that other operant learning factors (i.e., where alcohol use serves an instrumental function) may also act to sustain drinking behaviors. For example, drinkers may consume alcohol, in part "to obtain a variety of rewards deriving from social interactions with imbibing companions" (Bandura, 1969, p. 536). Eventually, with prolonged, excessive use of alcohol, physical dependence, and the fear and pain of alcohol withdrawal, is then thought to maintain consumption of alcohol independent of its original functional value. Thus, biological mechanisms can interact with psychosocial factors so that the maintenance of problem drinking is separate from its acquisition.

Bandura's (1969) theory differs in several important ways from other theories of alcohol abuse and misuse. The theory assumes, at least implicitly, that all drinking behavior, from abstinence to normal social drinking to alcohol abuse, is governed in varying degrees by similar principles of learning, cognition, and reinforcement. The theory also assumes that, since social learning determinants of drinking behaviors may vary as a function of settings and time, drinking behaviors may also vary concurrently. There is no necessary or inexorable progression through various stages of alcoholism, as suggested by some "disease" models (Jellinek, 1960). Similarly, a SLT of alcoholism rejects the consideration of fixed person-factors (e.g., personality predisposition, internal dynamics) as prepotent in the development of alcoholism. Indeed, longitudinal investigations have confirmed the extreme variability of the course of problem drinking and alcoholism both between and within individuals over time (Cahalan & Cisin, 1976; Jessor, 1984; Polich, Armor, & Braiker, 1981; Vaillant, 1983).

Social learning theory suggests that drinking, as a social behavior, is acquired and maintained by modeling, social reinforcement, the anticipated effects of alcohol, direct experience of alcohol's effects as rewarding or punishing, and physical dependence. Moos and his colleagues (e.g., Cronkite & Moos, 1980) likewise have drawn attention to various situational determinants of drinking variability such as stressful life events, work and family pressures, and the role played by social networks and social supports. As these biopsychosocial factors vary over time within individuals and from one individual to another, so too will drinking behaviors. Thus drinking patterns vary along a "continuum" beginning with experimentation in adolescence and progressing to normal social drinking and/or episodes of abuse, abstinence, or controlled use throughout the adult life cycle. It is possible to have episodic alcohol abuse without necessarily having alcoholism characterized by physical dependence. It has also been observed that some problem drinkers can and do drink moderately for significant periods of time despite their participation in abstinence-oriented treatments, and this observation has led to controversial new treatments such as "controlled drinking" (Heather & Robertson, 1983).

Social learning theory can account for variations in drinking patterns across individual and cultures as well as within individuals over time and across situations. In many ways, Bandura's (1969) earlier statements about alcohol use and abuse, building on previous learning theory approaches, have set the stage for more comprehensive cognitive–social learning formulations of alcoholism (see Marlatt & Gordon, 1985; Miller & Mastria, 1977; Miller, 1980; Nathan, 1976; Sobell & Sobell, 1978; Wilson, 1978, 1985), including the present chapter.

## Major Principles of Social Learning Theory of Alcohol Use and Abuse

Developments since 1969 have resulted in an enormous amount of research on alcohol use and abuse. A more elaborate and refined set of social learning principles has emerged. These principles are listed below and will then be addressed in detail, together with their empirical base, in the remainder of this chapter. As far as we know, this is the first time an attempt has been made to bring together the varying aspects of current theory and research. Included are developmental factors, experimentation in adolescence, determinants of normal drinking, alcohol abuse, relapse, and recovery. However, because of space limitations, not every principle is addressed in detail in subsequent sections and some principles are combined under a single subheading. The principles are arranged within a developmental framework but this is in no way to be construed as a "stage" theory as previously stated.

1. Learning to drink alcohol is an integral part of psychosocial development and socialization within a culture. Youthful drinking behaviors, beliefs, attitudes, and expectancies concerning alcohol are formed mainly through the social influences of culture, family, and peers. Much learning takes place before the child or young adolescent consumes any alcohol at all. This influence is exerted indirectly by attitudes, expectancies, and beliefs, and directly by modeling alcohol consumption, media portrayals of drinking, and social reinforcement for drinking. The influence of socializing agents may be necessary, but is not sufficient to explain the development of alcohol abuse and dependence.

2. Predisposing individual-difference factors may interact with the influence of socializing agents and situations to determine initial patterns of alcohol

consumption. These individual differences may be biological and/or psychological in nature, and may be inherited and/or acquired. Genetic and pharmacologic factors may increase the risk of alcohol abuse in vulnerable individuals. Psychosocial factors include skill deficits or excesses such as social incompetence or difficulty managing negative emotions. The absence of normal-drinking role models or the presence of abusive-drinking role models can also result in higher risk of alcohol abuse.

3. Direct experiences with alcohol become increasingly important as development and experimentation with alcohol continues. Continued alcohol use is thought to be reinforced negatively by factors such as its tension reducing/stress dampening effects and reinforced positively by factors such as its euphoric properties in enhancing social interaction. These effects are mediated strongly by socially learned expectations which may be the predominant determinant of the effects, especially at lower doses.

4. To the extent that any predisposing individual difference factor (or a combination of factors) interacts with a current situational demand to overwhelm an individual's capacity to cope effectively, the person's perception of efficacy will be undermined and alcohol abuse rather than normal use may occur. To the extent that an individual has learned (positive outcome expectations) that consumption of alcohol provides at least a short-term method of coping with the demands of a situation, or results in relief from aversive consequences, it will be selected. The probability of continued alcohol use is high if an individual is unable to learn to develop alternative, more adaptive coping skills. Thus, a deficit in psychosocial coping skills (predisposition) in the face of an external challenge may tax efficacy percepts, leading to a decrease in the strength and duration of alternative coping efforts. And if, through learned expectations or direct experience (or both), the individual expects alcohol to produce a desired outcome, alcohol use will tend to continue. In essence, the major proximal determinant of drinking is characterized by a high degree of strain because (a) environmental stressors exceed coping capacity, (b) low self-efficacy for alternative coping behaviors, and (c) high-outcome expectations that alcohol will produce the desired results while, (d) minimizing the long-term negative consequences. Depending on the severity of environmental demands, the availability of alcohol, and the repertoire of alternative coping skills, episodes of abusive drinking could occur. In normal drinking, the individual is assumed to have adequate self-control and delay of gratification capacity so that alternative forms of coping can be easily chosen despite the fact that they are less immediate, less powerful, and do not produce as good a "quick fix" as alcohol does.

5. If alcohol use is sustained, acquired tolerance to its direct, reinforcing properties (e.g., stress dampening effects) will act to promote the ingestion

of greater quantities in order to achieve the same effects that were previously attained with smaller quantities. Thus, acquired tolerance to alcohol's direct reinforcing effects may act as a secondary mediator of further alcohol consumption and may, in part, also be determined by biologically inherited factors.

6. If the level of alcohol consumption increases, and consumption is sustained over time, the risk for developing physical and/or psychological dependence increases. At this point, alcohol consumption may be reinforced negatively by avoidance of withdrawal symptoms associated with acute periods of abstinence from alcohol. Psychological dependence can also motivate alcohol abuse. The individual relies increasingly on alcohol as the sole method of coping with psychosocial problems such as severe mood swings, social anxiety, and social skills deficits. Environmental cues such as the sight and smell of alcohol can themselves produce "environmental demands" (i.e., become stimuli that result in a form of cognitive craving experienced as a strong desire or urge to drink).

7. The abuse of alcohol, however, will not only result from biological, proximal environmental, and psychological variables (listed under points 4, 5, and 6, above). Any episode of alcohol abuse has reciprocal individual and social consequences that can exacerbate further drinking by placing increasing stress and strain on subsequent person–environment interactions. On the one hand, the individual becomes increasingly dependent on alcohol to achieve short-term positive outcomes (euphoria, better social interaction, tension relief). On the other hand, the individual's behavior has increasingly devastating long-term personal and environmental consequences. Repeated drunken behavior often results in undesirable social consequences such as aggressive acting out, mood swings, loss of job, divorce, and a downward spiral toward isolation from the mainstream of society and its alternative reinforcers. The severe problem drinker or alcoholic is left either alone or with poor role models (other alcoholic drinking buddies) and with a very limited and inflexible set of alternative methods of coping. Thus reciprocal determinism predicts that the reactions of others in the environment (to avoid the alcoholic) will also result in increased stress, loss of social support, and a further decrease in self-efficacy and coping capacity. Thus, loss of social support leads to increased difficulty coping with environmental stressors which, in turn, results in further drinking which results in short-term relief but further loss of social support, and so on. A vicious circle of negative person–environment interactions is produced. The negative consequences are reciprocally maintained until a crisis point is reached such as when the alcoholism is severe enough for societal agencies to intervene (police, medical system, rehabilitation). It is important to note that reciprocal determinism can explain the powerful

"loss of control" process without necessarily resorting to an underlying biological disease process and the assumption of an individual who is "allergic" to alcohol.

8. The influence of these various social, situational, and intraindividual factors on alcohol consumption will vary both between individuals and within individuals over time. The influence of any factor or combination of factors is also thought to apply across the range of alcohol consumption, from abstinence to controlled social drinking, through to episodic problem drinking and alcohol dependence. Thus, it is assumed that there is no necessary combination of factors required to produce a problem drinker or alcoholism (i.e., no alcoholic personality, single genetic marker, or environmental stressor) and no inexorable progression through clearly defined "stages" of alcoholism. Put another way, it is assumed that there are multiple biopsychosocial pathways to alcohol use, abuse, and recovery, subject to the same principles of social learning.

9. Recovery will depend on the individual's ability to choose to explore alternative ways of coping. Both general coping skills required for everyday life, and the specific self-control skills necessary to manage drinking are needed. Through direct practice, verbal persuasion, modeling, and physiologic pathways, the individual must acquire successfully and practice alternative intrapersonal and interpersonal skills to develop high enough levels of self-efficacy to resist demanding situations. The individual must be more self-reflective so as to identify potentially risky environmental (e.g., at a party) or personal (e.g., negative moods) antecedents of drinking. The individual must acquire the self-regulatory, and delay of gratification skills that will allow for better decision making around alcohol use. Overly positive expectations about the consequences of alcohol use must be replaced by a more balanced set of expectations including the long-term negative consequences. Those with particularly severe drinking problems and predisposing risk factors are probably best served by making a decision to totally abstain. Other individuals may "grow out" of their problem or experience only brief episodes of problem drinking. Some may be able to resort to controlled drinking but the specific individual profiles and behaviors to be mastered must be established clearly for this subgroup (Heather & Robertson, 1983). Ultimately, the central thesis of SLT of alcohol use is that responsible alcohol use depends on cognitive self-regulation in a stressful world where many "quick fixes" are readily available.

Taken together, the nine principles outlined above reveal an increasingly complex SLT model from that proposed by Bandura and others. In essence, SLT makes broad contributions to our understanding of alcohol use patterns across cultures and over the life span. Alcohol use is a method of coping with the demands of everyday life that can be maladaptive if excessively used. In its most severe form, it is a serious disorder with life threatening personal, and devastating social consequences.

## Initiation of Alcohol Use

### Family and Peer Influences within a Developmental Context

A SLT approach to alcohol use and abuse must consider early, direct, and vicarious experiences with alcohol within a developmental and social context. Indeed, despite the fact that the legal age for purchase and consumption of alcoholic beverages in the United States is 18 years or older, most teenagers have experienced the effects of alcohol, and a significant proportion have established a stable pattern of consumption, prior to this age (Blane & Hewitt, 1977; Harford, 1982; Rachal et al., 1975). Moreover, alcohol is the most widely used drug among youth aged 12 to 17; more young people are having their first drink and starting to drink regularly at progressively younger ages; and the rate of problem drinking among youth continues to rise, and now stands at about the 20% level (see Braucht, 1980, 1981, for reviews). Thus we can conclude that alcohol use is endemic to American youth and that, perhaps, problem drinking among youth is reaching epidemic proportions. By necessity, early experiences with alcohol-socializing agents—family and peers—must play a role in the initiation and maintenance of alcohol use among youth.

Drinking patterns are learned within the context of the general process of socialization such that, at different life stages, beliefs and alcohol use change in conjunction with changes in socializing forces (Barnes, 1977; Cellucci, 1982; Plant, 1979; Zucker, 1979). Alcohol use among youth is not an isolated activity but is part of the overall process of psychosocial development (Jessor & Jessor, 1977). Social learning theory assumes that family and peers can influence both the onset and maintenance of drinking behaviors among youth by affecting generally attitudes, standards, and values toward alcohol, and also by modeling drinking behaviors within social contexts. A thorough consideration of family and peer influences upon youthful drinking behaviors and attitudes toward drinking, however, is beyond the scope of this chapter. By necessity, some general statements culled from reviews by Biddle et al. (1980), Margulies, Kessler, and Kandel (1977), and Harford (1982) are offered.

Consistently, one of the best single predictors of adolescent drug habits including alcohol use and abuse, appears to be the attitudes and behaviors of parents regarding alcohol (Barnes, 1977; McDermott, 1984; O'Leary, O'Leary, & Donovan, 1976; Wechsler & McFadden, 1979). But although the overall relationships between parental attitudes and behavior toward alcohol and adolescent alcohol use is a strong one, the relationship is not necessarily linear (Davies & Stacey, 1972). For example, conflicting parental attitudes toward alcohol are related to excessive drinking among youth (Jackson & Connor, 1953), and children of abstainers who hold extreme, temperant attitudes, may also be at risk for developing alcohol problems (Wittman, 1939).

Age also moderates the relationship between parental attitudes toward alcohol and adolescent alcohol use. Generally, as age increases, peer influences assume gradually greater importance. Harford (1982) has shown that this shift in influence is, at least in part, related to changes in the setting and control of alcohol consumption. For example, for younger adolescents, drinking at home is more frequent, but is characterized by decreased levels of consumption (Davies & Stacey, 1972). Frequency of drinking in the home, however, decreases with age, while frequency of drinking in non-adult-supervised drinking contexts concurrently increases. Changes in drinking contexts occur as a concommitant of increased socialization. It is here in non-supervised contexts, not surprisingly, that levels of alcohol consumption also increase. These changes, importantly, seem to be modified both by actual and perceived availability of alcohol, lending indirect support to distribution-of-consumption models of alcohol consumption (Harford, Parker, & Light, 1980). Thus, the disengagment of the adolescent from parents is reflected in changes in the settings in which alcohol is consumed (Harford, 1982). And, although parental drinking behavior may be related to onset of drinking, adolescents are more likely to drink, and to consume larger quantities of alcohol, in peer settings (Harford & Spiegler, 1982; Maddox & McCall, 1964).

Biddle et al. (1980) studied the effects of four social determinants (parental and peer modeling, and parent and peer norms) on adolescents' perceived drinking norms, preferences for alcoholic beverages, and reported drinking behavior, as a function of age, sex, and social class. Generally, parents were found to influence drinking through norms (McDermott, 1984) while peers tended to influence drinking through behaviors, confirming earlier reports by Jessor and Jessor (1975) and Kandel et al. (1976). This relationship was also modified by age. Young adolescents responded to parental norms instrumentally, while middle-adolescents were most strongly influenced by peer behaviors, confirming Harford's (1982) general conclusions that alcohol consumption is related to the process of disengagement from parents' social influence. Interestingly, young adults tended to internalize parental and peer norms, and it was only at this stage of developmental that parental drinking was related directly to the drinking behaviors of young adults. Thus, parental modeling influences may only be expressed in later years, while early in adolescence it is peer drinking behaviors that are prepotent. Social class and race also modified the observed relationships, with white, middle-class youths more likely to be influenced by peers in midadolescence, while blacks and working-class youths were affected (most strongly) by parental norms.

*Modeling Influences*

While the research reviewed above suggests that peers exert their influence on alcohol consumption directly through modeling, experimental studies have confirmed the phenomenon and elucidated some of the mechanisms of this social influence process (see Collins & Marlatt, 1981; Collins, Parks, & Marlatt, 1985).

Modeling factors exert important influences on drinking patterns and expectations before the initiation of drinking per se. However, these factors have not as yet been subjected to rigorous research scrutiny. The powerful effects of modeling are assumed from other work in SLT (e.g., aggression in children; see Bandura, 1973) or research on modeling in college-age social drinkers. In college-age populations, modeling is a proximal determinant of drinking (see Proximal Determinants of Drinking, below). Caudill and Marlatt (1975) first reported that, among heavy social-drinking college students, subjects who were exposed to a heavy-drinking model consumed significantly more than subjects exposed to a light-drinking model or no model, in a bogus alcoholic beverage taste-rating task. Hendricks, Sobell, and Cooper (1978) extended these results by varying the presence or absence of a confederate model. They found that the modeling effect was facilitated when the subject and confederate participated together in another task prior to the alcohol taste-rating task. The modeling effect did not occur when the subject and the model did not perform the tasks in synchrony, but still observed each other's behavior. Thus, prior coaction formed a social bond between the subject and model. Social blending among adolescents, therefore, may facilitate direct modeling of alcohol consumption.

Other studies have shown that modeling effects are also influenced by settings (Strickler, Dobbs, & Maxwell, 1979), gender (Cooper, Waterhouse, & Sobell, 1979; Lied & Marlatt, 1979), drinking history (Lied & Marlatt, 1979), and the nature of the interaction between drinking partners (Collins, Parks, & Marlatt, 1985). While both males and females will drink more when exposed to a heavy-drinking model of either sex, males tend to drink more when exposed to a heavy- as opposed to a light-drinking male partner. Drinking history mediates the modeling effect insofar as the phenomenon is most significant for heavy, as opposed to light drinkers. Thus, heavy-drinking males may be at particular risk for overconsumption if they drink in the presence of other heavy-drinking males (Harford, Wechsler, & Rohman, 1981).

Overall, the results of the experimental studies suggest that the modeling phenomenon is robust. Importantly, the process of social bonding, and the perception of the model as a peer, increases the significance of the modeling effect. This phenomenon is influenced by drinking history and gender such that heavy-drinking males are most likely to escalate alcohol consumption in the presence of other heavy-drinking males. Modeling effects have been studied primarily in college students rather than in the earlier years prior to the onset of actual drinking behavior. While modeling factors are an obvious source of acquired expectancies, the acquisition process has not been researched in depth prior to onset of drinking. Modeling factors could receive more attention in future research, for example, with respect to "resilience" in high-risk groups such as some children of alcoholics who go on to develop "healthy" alcohol use skills, despite exposure to inappropriate role-models in early childhood.

### Development of Alcohol-Related Expectancies

Biddle *et al.* (1980) have suggested that parental norms and peer modeling of drinking behaviors also influence the development of internalized expectancies for alcohol effects. In fact, they suppose that modeled behaviors get translated into expectancies (e.g., preferences for alcohol), and that expectancies are more important, direct determinants of alcohol consumption than modeling per se. Thus, internalized expectancies for drinking may be important, direct determinants of drinking behaviors, and these expectancies, in turn, may be shaped initially by socializing agents. The important influence of cognitive–mediational factors on adolescent and adult drinking behavior is highlighted by the results of several recent studies that have examined the development of alcohol-related expectancies, and their relation to subsequent drinking behavior.

In a preliminary study, Brown, Goldman, Inn and Anderson (1980) factor-analyzed the responses of college students to a questionnaire that explored expectations of the positively reinforcing effects of moderate alcohol consumption in adults with differing drinking habits. Six distinct factors described the domain of expected reinforcing alcohol effects: Alcohol positively transforms experiences, alcohol enhances social and physical pleasure, alcohol enhances sexual performance and experience, alcohol increases power and aggression, alcohol increases social assertiveness, and alcohol reduces tension. Pattern of drinking modified these results somewhat, with lighter drinkers having more expectancies for positive experiences and enhancing social pleasure, and heavier drinkers expecting alcohol to increase sexual and aggressive behavior and reduce stress or tension.

In a follow-up study, Christiansen, Goldman, and Inn (1982) examined alcohol-related expectancies as a function of age and prior experience with alcohol. The results showed that, among mixed-sex 12- to 14-year olds, well-developed alcohol-related expectancies (essentially identical to Brown *et al.*'s preliminary study) exist prior to the establishment of stable drinking patterns. Taken together, these studies suggest that expectancies must be conveyed early on in development, and that they are modified as a function of age and drinking practices.

Indeed, Spiegler (1983) has shown that, by age 6, children already have clearly established perceptions of social drinking norms for men, women, and children. We suggest that these expectancies, established prior to direct experiences with alcohol, are transmitted primarily through parental and, to a lesser extent, peer influences. However, it should also be noted that other agents of acculturation (e.g., media) may also serve to transmit and/or reinforce these general expectancies for alcohol effects (Cafisco, Goodstadt, Garlington, & Sheppard, 1982; Lowery, 1980). Lowery (1980), for example, has shown that television programs tend to portray alcohol use as a means of enhancing the enjoyment of social interaction and the reduction of social tension, crisis management, and escape from chronic stress, with a majority of portrayals involving social facilitation. Alcohol use on television is also usually reinforced socially and has few negative consequences.

Given the existence of well-developed alcohol-related expectancies in predrinking youth, and given that these expectancies are largely positive ones, the question arises as to their relation to actual drinking behaviors, and to the etiology of problem drinking. Christiansen and Goldman (1983) attempted to answer this question by testing the predictive relation of eight alcohol-related expectancy factors to self-reported drinking behaviors in a group of 12- to 19-year-old adolescents. In addition, they compared the predictive power of these expectancies to demographic/background variables (i.e., parental drinking and attitudes, presence of an alcoholic in the family, ethnic–religious influences, socioeconomic differences, age, and sex of adolescent) that have been shown previously to be related to adolescent drinking.

As expected, the results showed the background/demographic variables to be related significantly to drinking behaviors. However, two expectancy factors—positive and negative alterations in social behavior and enhanced cognitive and motor functioning—were in fact superior predictors of frequent and problem drinking. Moreover, the expectancy factors added significant predictive power beyond what the background and demographic variables offered. Brown (1985) replicated and extended Christiansen and Goldman's (1983) findings in a college-age sample. Again, the results showed that, overall, the expectancy variables predicted drinking patterns at least as well as background/demographic variables. Additionally, while expectations of enhanced social and physical pleasure were related significantly to frequent heavy drinking, expectations of tension reduction predicted frequent heavy drinking combined with other alcohol problems. Thus, expectations of tension reduction differentiated between heavy drinkers who were and were not experiencing social complications secondary to their alcohol use (i.e., alcohol abuse).

These studies suggest that alcohol-related expectancies are inculcated early in life, prior to the establishment of stable drinking patterns, and are probably the result of influence from primary and secondary socializing agents. Alcohol-related expectancies then interact with direct experiences with alcohol and determine, in part, acute intoxication experiences (see Proximal Determinants of Drinking, below). Thus, the actual pharmacologic influence of alcohol may be less important in determining its psychological impact, at least at lower doses. Furthermore, negative experiences with initial alcohol use may not modify well-developed positive expectancies. Continued contact with socializing agents may also reinforce further already held expectancies, or override disconfirmatory, acute experiences with alcohol. Importantly, positive expectancies for alcohol use seem to be related to increased levels of drinking. In addition, expectancies for tension reduction seem to be related strongly to development of abusive drinking in young adulthood. It is also conceivable that a subset of youth with a balance of positive and negative alcohol-related expectation may go on to develop a moderate pattern of social drinking. However, data on this question are presently unavailable.

In summary, parents and peers influence alcohol consumption by affecting attitudes toward alcohol, engendering certain alcohol-related expectancies for positive and negative reinforcement, modeling directly appropriate or inappropriate consumption, and socially rewarding alcohol use. Parents' initial influence on alcohol consumption seems to be superceded by peers' influence (modeling) during the normal process of socialization and disengagement from parental controls. However, parents' attitudes and behaviors toward alcohol may place the individual at risk for development of alcohol problems in young adulthood—a kind of "sleeper" phenomenon. For example, a youth with heavy-drinking or alcoholic parents may not fall into an abusive pattern of drinking during adolescence, if peers' drinking behaviors are moderate. However, this individual may be at risk for abusive drinking as a young adult, for reasons that are, as yet, unclear. Conversely, a youth with parents who consume alcohol moderately and appropriately may, nevertheless, fall into an abusive drinking pattern during adolescence, based upon heavy-drinking peers' influence. However, this youth's drinking habits may again stabilize to a nonabusive pattern in young adulthood (Jessor, 1984). These developmental processes may be modified by other social factors, including race, gender, and socioeconomic status.

Importantly, positive outcome expectations for alcohol effects, developed prior to drinking, may override or otherwise interact with direct, pharmacologic experiences with alcohol, and may be an important factor in the development of abusive drinking styles in later years. These alcohol-related expectations are most probably influenced directly by family and peers, and secondarily through other cultural agents. For example, an individual may, on the basis of early parental modeling experiences and media portrayals, hold strong expectations that alcohol enhances social/physical pleasure and reduces tension. And despite some early aversive experiences, this individual may continue to expect these effects from alcohol. In adolescence, peers may reinforce further the expectation that alcohol is a tension reducing agent, and also reinforce the notion that alcohol is to be used to relieve tension and enhance social pleasure (e.g., peers may consume alcohol prior to a high school gathering to relieve the tension that is associated with interactions with opposite-sex peers). As the individual matures, he or she may never learn to modulate this anxiety without alcohol and he or she will come to rely increasingly upon alcohol to relieve tension in a growing array of aversive situations, thus increasing the risk for alcohol abuse. Finally, it should be noted that, while a person's social learning history may be related strongly to the development of abusive drinking practices, we assume that these preconditions are not necessarily sufficient, by themselves, to explain sustained consumption (see Proximal Determinants of Drinking, below).

### Predisposing Individual Differences

In our theoretical model, we propose that certain individual difference factors, interacting with situational or environmental demands, may overwhelm an individual's ability to cope effectively and may lead to a decreased sense of efficacy. If the individual has learned that alcohol can help to cope with the immediate situation, the probability of alcohol consumption is increased. We believe that these predispositions can be learned and/or inherited, and are biological and/or psychological in nature.

There are more predisposing factors than we are able to enumerate here, but important examples include the following. Individuals may inherit biological differences that make them more tolerant to the intoxicating and reinforcing effects of alcohol (Begleiter, Porgesz, Bihari, & Kissin, 1984; Schuckit, 1980). Individuals may inherit or acquire cognitive or neuropsychological deficits that may predispose them to problem drinking (Schaeffer, Parsons, & Yohman, 1984). Inherited or acquired affective disorders (i.e., depression, anxiety) appear to predispose certain individuals to alcoholism, perhaps in an attempt to "self-medicate" their symptoms (Schuckit, 1983). Furthermore, deficits in socialization skills are also related to risk for alcoholism (O'Leary, O'Leary, & Donovan, 1976).

Furthermore, we propose that there is no set combination of predisposing individual differences that increase the risk of problem drinking relative to other combinations of differences. In this sense, we agree with Nathan and Harris (1980) that there are multiple pathways to substance abuse and, in particular, alcohol abuse. Bry, McKeon, and Pandina (1982), for example, presented data suggesting that the extent of drug abuse among adolescents was more a function of the number of risk factors (i.e., predisposing individual differences) than any particular factor alone or combination of factors. Thus, we may conceptualize alcohol as a general coping mechanism, whose use is a function of the number of diverse etiologic variables, rather than particular sets of these variables.

This section will focus on a discussion of socialization deficits as they relate to the development of abusive and dependent drinking. Mindful of the caveat issued above, we feel that such a focus is justified, given our theoretical orientation. Moreover, as we shall attempt to show, socialization deficits are related both to the development and maintenance of abusive drinking, as well as to recovery and the process of relapse.

The thesis of this section is that social skills deficits restrict alternatives of action within a social context, minimize the control exerted over activities and environment, and decrease accessibility to desired resources (Bandura, 1969). Social skills are thought to be reinforced and maintained, in part, by their ability to decrease the level of anxiety experienced in social and interpersonal situation (O'Leary, O'Leary, & Donovan, 1976). Social skills deficits may, therefore, produce increased anxiety or tension in interpersonal situations that require such adaptive responding. This can be conceptualized as a high-risk-for-drinking situation if the individual does not possess adequate, alternative skills for coping with the situation at hand, and if the individual has learned that alcohol ingestion can provide at least short-term relief. If such deficits are chronic over the course of psychosocial development, the potential for abusive drinking is thought to increase (see Monti, Abrams, Binkoff, & Zwick, in press).

### Socialization Deficits

In an extensive review, O'Leary et al. (1976) examined the evidence supporting the view that prealcoholics can be considered generally deficient in social skills. They cited studies demonstrating that, during high school, prealcoholic boys were judged to be less productive, less socially perceptive, less calm, and more sensitive to criticism (Jones, 1968). Similarly, Braucht et al. (1973) found adolescent problem drinkers to be overly aggressive, impulsive, and lacking generally in personal controls. Other researchers have also indicated that symptoms characteristic of an antisocial personality—delinquent activities including running away, theft, and assault—were related to development of later alcoholism (Cadoret et al., 1985; Robins et al., 1962). Jessor (1984) has suggested that problem drinking in adolescents co-occurs with other problem behaviors that may be considered antisocial (e.g., delinquency, precocious sexuality) and that problem-drinking students valued achievement less, and had greater attitudinal tolerance for and engaged in more deviant behaviors (Jessor & Jessor, 1972).

Problem drinking in adolescence and adulthood also seems to co-occur with difficulties in peer relationships. Lentz (1941) found that heavy-drinking young adults participated in fewer extracurricular activities, and reported more interpersonal maladjustment. Kalin (1972) found that college-age problem drinkers were more antisocially assertive and they were less involved in long-term relationships. Other data cited by O'Leary et al. (1976) included the findings that alcoholics were more often single, separated, or divorced (Koller & Castanos, 1969; C.M. Rosenberg, 1969), and showed decreased levels of social competence (Levine & Zigler, 1973). However, Monti, Corriveau, and Zwick (1981) note that alcoholics may not be as socially incompetent as psychiatric patients.

These data are suggestive and provide support for the view that socialization deficits may, in some ways, predispose an individual to abusive drinking. These deficits may be modeled by parents (O'Leary et al., 1976) or may be biologically inherited to some degree (Cadoret, O'Gorman, Troughton, & Heywood, 1985). However, it should also be noted that alcohol use may serve to maintain preexisting socialization deficits or may prevent the learning of appropriate social skills as development continues.

### Selected Assessment Studies

In a study of the relationships between assertiveness and problem drinking, Sturgis, Calhoun, and Best (1979) found that, among problem drinkers, two general groups could be identified. For example, passive, less-assertive individuals reported that they consumed alcohol in order to facilitate social interactions. However, a subgroup of problem individuals who were highly assertive reported drinking more often to change their sensations and to reduce boredom. (This result underscores our assertion that no one predisposing individual-difference factor can be considered as prepotent.)

Miller and Eisler (1977) studied problem drinking and non-problem-drinking psychiatric patients on self-report and role-play measures of assertiveness, and operant drinking. Overall, both patient groups showed equal deficits on the role-play measure of assertiveness, but the problem drinkers perceived themselves as being more assertive. As a group, the problem drinkers also tended to consume more alcohol as their role-play assertiveness scores decreased. Hamilton and Maisto (1979) reported similar findings in a group of problem drinkers compared to matched nonproblem drinkers. Overall, the groups did not differ on self-report and behavioral tests of assertiveness, however, the problem drinkers reported more discomfort in assertion-required situations.

In addition to the assessment studies noted above, several experimental studies have suggested that, as social stress is increased, alcohol consumption increases. This is a general finding in social drinking populations (Higgins & Marlatt, 1975), and problem drinkers tend to consume more alcohol than social drinkers in a similar experimental paradigm (Miller, Hersen, Eisler, & Hilsman, 1974). Moreover, subjects who are given the means to cope effectively with the anxiety-provoking situation tend to consume less alcohol compared to subjects for whom there is no alternative means of coping (Marlatt, Kosturn, & Lang, 1975). Taken together, these studies suggest that a combination of a negative emotional state secondary to social or interpersonal conflict, plus an inability to express oneself effectively, can lead to an increase in alcohol consumption.

The process of alcoholic relapse also is related significantly to social factors, possibly socialization deficits. Marlatt and Gordon (1980) reported that two social situations tend to precede between 39 and 50% of alcohol relapses. In half the cases, interpersonal conflict preceeded the relapse, in the other half, social pressure to drink was the precipitant. H. Rosenberg (1983), in a retrospective study, showed that nonrelapsing alcoholics responded to problem situations in a more assertive and drink-refusing manner compared to those alcoholics who relapsed. Rist and Watzl (1983) found that, among women alcoholics, those who relapsed 3 months after treatment evaluated various situations involving social pressure to drink alcohol as more difficult to deal with and as creating more discomfort than did abstainers. But the groups did not differ in their self-rated assertiveness in non-alcohol-related situations, suggesting that drink-refusal skills deficits may be related particularly to relapse.

Although the data are by no means unequivocal, taken together, the studies reviewed above point out the importance of considering socialization deficits as factors predisposing toward alcohol consumption/abuse. Early developmental learning and/or biological differences may be directly responsible for these deficits. Or social skills deficits may be secondary to social anxiety (i.e., the individual may possess the requisite skills but is unable to bring them to bear due to debilitating anxiety; see Trower, Yardley, Bryant, & Shaw 1978). Whatever their origin, skills deficits may prevent desired outcomes from being obtained, especially in the context of a demanding social interaction. Alcohol may act to actually facilitate social interactions (or influence perception of the quality of social interactions) or to decrease the anxiety associated with such interactions, thus reinforcing continued use. Interestingly, the data imply that, if an alternative coping strategy is available, the probability of alcohol consumption decreases. However, continued skills deficits may be reinforced by association with other individuals who abuse alcohol, and alcohol use itself may preclude the development of adequate skills.

It should be pointed out again that a social-skills deficit is one hypothesized predisposition toward alcohol consumption. And even this conceptual category may be too broad in itself to be of much value in predicting alcohol use. From this selective review it is evident that types of skill deficits need to be specified more clearly (e.g., deficits in skills per se, or self-perception of skills), and the etiology of these deficits needs to be better delineated. Socialization deficits may be important for a particular subset, and drink refusal skills may be related to alcohol consumption in another problem drinking sample. Also, other predispositions may co-occur and interact with each other (i.e., in an additive fashion) to influence risk for drinking.

### Proximal Determinants of Drinking

Developmental factors including cultural norms, modeling, peer influences, and experimentation with alcohol form the "social learning history" of variables that moderate current drinking behavior. These past experiences may be modulated to some degree by inherent genetic/biological and predisposing psychological factors. They are constantly revised by current experiences and specific person–environment interactions. The combination of social learning history and current experiential factors contribute to individual differences in patterns of alcohol use and the risk of alcohol abuse. The present section focuses on the immediate cognitive and environmental determinants of drinking behavior (proximal determinants). Prior to drinking and during actual drinking, individuals are constantly using cognitive processes such as symbolization to project courses of action and guide decision making; forethought and expectation to set goals and anticipate likely consequences of action; and self-regulation using performance feedback, internal standards, and self-reflection to modify behavior and exercise self-control.

In terms of frequency and severity of occurrence of alcohol use, there is a continuum of alcohol use patterns. All points along this continuum, from no use at all to infrequent use to normal drinking to abuse, are governed by similar SLT principles. This is in sharp contrast to other models that suggest discrete categories (total abstinence—in control) or (drinking—total loss of control) to characterize those with drinking problems (see Marlatt & Gordon, 1985; Abrams, Niaura, Carey, Binkoff, & Monti, in press).

Important proximal determinants of drinking behavior include antecedents such as environmental settings, beliefs and expectations, the person's repertoire of general and drinking specific coping skills, and the current cognitive–emotional–physiologic state of the person at the time of drinking (Abrams, 1983). Equally important are the consequences of drinking behavior including both short-term and long-term reinforcing and punishing effects. The depth and breadth of the studies in this area make it possible to add substantially to Bandura's (1969) original contribution to a SLT of alcohol use and abuse.

According to SLT, cognitive factors modulate all person–environment interactions. The decision to drink or exercise restraint (self-control) is ultimately determined by self-efficacy and outcome expectations formulated around a current situational context. For example, a person who is socially phobic at a Christmas party may feel more confident in his or her ability to socialize (efficacy expectations) with a drink in hand. If the consumption of alcohol actually helps the person to achieve the desired effects, then further drinking is reinforced (by the outcome), and the probability of habitually using alcohol in similar situations is increased via outcome expectations. Given a specific situational demand, an individual's confidence at coping with the demand and his or her perceptions of achieving a desired outcome will determine which coping behaviors will be selected. Through direct practice, modeling experiences, verbal persuasion, and physiologic feedback, self-efficacy is strengthened by past behavior in the direction of either drinking or using alternative coping behaviors (see below). Thus the antecedents and consequences of drinking, together with the current state of the person, all combine to provide crucial information that can modify self-efficacy and outcome expectations for the self-regulation of each drinking decision and episode. Space does not allow a detailed exploration of all the mechanisms involved. Rather, some key mechanisms will be selectively reviewed to illustrate the central role cognitive factors may play.

A variety of specific cognitive–behavioral mechanisms are assumed to be crucial to the exercise of adequate self-regulation and delay of gratification capacity in normal drinkers. In order not to abuse alcohol an individual must (1) be able to judge in which settings drinking is appropriate; (2) have a rich enough and flexible repertoire of general and alcohol-specific coping skills to achieve desired goals without drinking at all or without drinking to excess; and (3) have a full awareness of the long-term negative consequences of alcohol abuse to offset the short-term powerful reinforcing effects of alcohol use (e.g., pleasure or reduction of aversive states). For example, an individual may be in a high state of stress due to a busy day at work plus a recent fight with his or her spouse. This individual has to go to a party where alcohol is available and the demands of the situation are to relax and enjoy oneself. Coping behavior will be determined by the person's current state and the extent to which the individual has adequate general and specific coping skills and high enough self-efficacy expectations to achieve desired outcomes without excessive drinking. Beliefs and expectations about the short- and long-term effects of drinking on behavior will also enter into the decision-making process. Self-efficacy for not drinking (or for moderate drinking) will be undermined by excessive strain on the person (physiologic pathway), a limited repertoire of alternative coping skills (direct practice), observation of others' use of drinking to cope (modeling and verbal persuasion), and overly positive outcome expectations of alcohol's effects.

If drinking is initiated, several additional self-regulation mechanisms must then operate to regulate both consumption and behavior when the individual is intoxicated. These include: (1) internal cues and use of social feedback about levels of intoxication to appropriately regulate further consumption and to stop abusive drinking; (2) internalized standards of conduct derived from appropriate role models and cultural norms so that intoxication does not serve as either a cognitive or a pharmacologic "excuse" for "loss of control" over sexual, aggressive, or further drinking behavior; (3) the biphasic effects of alcohol (i.e., pleasant, euphoric, arousing properties, and central nervous system depressant, relaxing properties) which can powerfully perpetuate distorted expectations regarding the short-term reinforcing effects of consumption.

Drinking behavior becomes maladaptive when individuals' "choices" to achieve desired goals are limited to alcohol use and they engage in frequent, repetitive use while minimizing or denying actual negative consequences. Thus episodes of alcohol abuse can be characterized by expectations for immediate gratification and/or relief from stressful antecedents that result from situational demands that exceed current coping capacity (cognitive, behavioral, and biological). Behavior is moderated by expectations or anticipation of desired outcomes and low self-efficacy for alternative methods of achieving short-term goals in specific situations. Prolonged drinking results in additional biobehavioral dependency where additional factors can play a strong role in maintaining drinking independent of the original etiologic determinants (see General and Alcohol-Specific Coping Skills, below).

Before presenting selected studies that illustrate the mechanisms outlined above, a caveat is necessary. A SLT model of alcohol abuse appears to place full responsibility on the individual for their condition and this has been equated with "blaming the victim" (Sontag, 1978). In other words, individuals "choose" to be self-destructive and deserve what they get. However, this is based on a false assumption since individuals are not entirely responsible for their social learning history, their current behavioral skill deficits or excesses, their biological capacity to tolerate stress, and their problems in exercising self-control based on distorted beliefs and expectations obtained from culture, poor role models, and the media. As Marlatt (1985) points out:

> Behavioral theorists define addiction as a powerful habit pattern, an acquired vicious cycle of self-destructive behavior that is locked in by the collective effects of classical conditioning (acquired tolerance mediated in part by classically conditioned compensatory responses to the deleterious effects of the addictive substance), and operant reinforcement (both the positive reinforcement of the high of the drug rush and the negative reinforcement associated with drug use as a means of escaping or avoiding dysphoric physical and/or mental states—including those associated with the negative aftereffects of prior drug use). In terms of conditioning factors alone, an individual who acquires an addictive habit is no more to be held "responsible" for this behavior than one of Pavlov's dogs would be held responsible for salivating at the sound of a ringing bell. In addition to classical and operant conditioning factors, human drug use is also determined to a large extent by acquired expectancies and beliefs about drugs as an antidote to stress and anxiety. Social learning and modeling factors (observational learning) also exert a strong influence (e.g., drug use in the family and peer environment, along with the pervasive portrayal of drug use in advertising and the media). Just because a behavioral problem can be described as a learned habit pattern does not imply that the person is to be held responsible for the acquisition of the habit, nor that the individual is capable of exercising voluntary control over the behavior. (p. 11)

But it is important to note that treatment of alcohol abuse within an SLT model does require that an individual accept personal responsibility for learning self-regulatory skills and using them as alternatives in future settings where drinking is highly likely. Any one or a combination of excesses or deficits in the key self-regulation mechanisms (outlined above) interacting with social learning history, predisposing biological and other individual differences, and the situational context can result in alcohol abuse. In order to truly exercise self-control over drinking behavior an individual must have a rich and flexible repertoire of cognitive–behavioral skills so as to make a truly informed decision about whether to drink at all, how much to drink, and how to behave when drinking. The following section examines selected studies illustrating how situational and cognitive–behavioral factors play a crucial role in alcohol use and abuse.

### Situational Factors

The situational context (e.g., business lunch, Alcoholics Anonymous Meeting, wedding, party) and the presence of drinking role models can influence drinking behavior. Studies have demonstrated that subjects who are tested in convivial social atmospheres are more likely to experience the positive effects of alcohol consumption as compared with subjects tested in more formal settings (Williams, 1966). Further evidence for the importance of social context comes from cross-cultural studies of drinking behavior (MacAndrew & Edgerton, 1969). These authors note that there are cultures where drinking to the point of intoxication and even coma are controlled highly by cultural norms and ritual. Heavy drinking in some of these contexts is not associated with the "loss of control" over sexual or aggressive impulses as is traditionally assumed in American culture according to a pharmacologic "disinhibition" model (Rada, 1975). Individuals' appraisal of what society will or will not "allow" in terms of deviant behavior when intoxicated can determine their drinking pattern and, most important, their behavior under the influence of alcohol.

The social context and related determinants of alcohol consumption have been investigated in a series of studies by Marlatt and his colleagues (Caudill & Marlatt, 1975; Collins & Marlatt, 1981; Collins, Parks, & Marlatt, 1985). The general paradigm has been to investigate the influence of heavy-drinking versus light-drinking role-models, and the nature of these models' social interaction (unsociable versus sociable) on an individual's drinking behavior. Thus, modeling factors are important proximal determinants of adult drinking behavior; in addition, they play a role in the early acquisition of drinking-related expectations during adolescence (as described above in Family and Peer Influences within a Developmental Context). The main findings to date suggest that the drinking rate of a role model (light vs. heavy drinking) influences significantly the drinking rate of the subject observing the role model. These findings have also been replicated in laboratory taste-rating tasks (Cooper et al., 1979) as well as in seminaturalistic and natural bar settings (Reid, 1978; Caudill & Lipscomb, 1980). In a significant extension of these findings, Reid (1978) studied the relationship between heavy versus light drinking and social versus unsociable interactions. He found a highly significant modeling effect but only in the warm-sociable condition. The alcohol consumption of subjects exposed to a cold and unsociable model did not differ significantly as a function of the model's drinking rate.

In a 1985 study, Collins et al. once again found that a subject's alcohol consumption rate was dependent on both the consumption rate of the role model and on the model's level of sociability. However, in their study, heavier drinking in the subject was produced by exposure to either a sociable heavy-drinking model, an unsociable heavy-drinking model, or an unsociable light drinking model. The authors speculate that an unsociable model may be aversive for subjects and they tend to respond by drinking more heavily. This may provide an analogue to the negative reinforcement pattern of drinking to alleviate negative emotional states, in this case social anxiety (see Abrams,

1983; Abrams & Wilson, 1979). These studies demonstrate that the social consequences of behavior can be changed when alcohol is present and that alcohol consumption can be influenced by proximal social consequences.

Wilson (1977) points out that the presence of alcohol defines a set of social role conditions that can influence behavior such as the facilitation or disinhibition of otherwise constricted social behaviors as in shyness, social phobia, or the expression of sexual or aggressive behaviors. In one study designed to investigate the effects of alcohol on social anxiety, Wilson et al. (1981) led male subjects to believe that they were consuming an alcoholic or a nonalcoholic beverage. The subjects were also told that a female confederate, with whom they were to interact, had also been given an alcoholic or a nonalcoholic beverage in a balanced 2 × 2 factorial design. No alcohol was actually consumed. Subjects who were led to believe that their partners were intoxicated, were less anxious, more attractive, and more likeable, as rated by self-report and by observers kept blind to the conditions. Thus, the male subject's expectation that a female confederate had been drinking, produced favorable psychological and interpersonal consequences, even when no alcohol was actually administered. The study is important because it illustrates that expectations about others' drinking can also influence behavior.

Drinking practices are strongly influenced by modeling and by differential reinforcement patterns within social subgroups such as in national, ethnic, or religious normative practices (Abrams & Wilson, 1986). Positive consequences reliably increase drinking, and negative consequences decrease drinking (Wilson, 1985). Together with modeling, these patterns of differential reinforcement can account for differing rates of alcoholism among national and ethnic groups (MacAndrew & Edgerton, 1969). For example, groups that model and reward appropriate drinking in some situations (e.g., as part of a Jewish Sabbath ritual) but disapprove of heavy abusive drinking and out-of-control behavior in other circumstances, tend to have lower rates of alcohol problems than groups that do not differentiate appropriate from inappropriate situations and behaviors when intoxicated. In a longitudinal study of per-morbid differences between alcoholics and normal drinkers, Vaillant (1983) reported that alcoholics were more likely to come from ethnic groups that discourage adolescents from learning appropriate drinking behavior and tolerate excessive drinking in adulthood. Alcoholics were also more likely to have a history of antisocial behavior and to have relatives who were alcoholic.

The above studies are limited in that the majority are confined to laboratory analogue settings with the exception of some of the studies of the influence on drinking of heavy- versus light-drinking role models. Studies have also been conducted primarily on college students or nonproblem drinkers and the majority have used male subjects. Thus, the strength and generalizability of the findings are restricted, especially with respect to implications for treatment. However, taken together the studies on the relationship between environment/social context and drinking suggest that these factors can play an important role as immediate determinants of drinking, the quantity of alcohol consumed, and individuals' behavior under the influence of alcohol.

### Cognitive Factors

There are several critical points where deficits or excesses in cognitive information processing could interfere with the ability to make appropriate decisions about whether to drink, how much to drink, and how to behave when intoxicated: (1) Individuals' expectations could be influenced by a "problematic" social learning history such as the absence of normal-drinking role models, the presence of poor role models (e.g., an alcoholic parent), or the absence of well-defined cultural norms for drinking, (2) Individuals may overemphasize the immediate, positive consequences of drinking and ignore or minimize the long-term, negative results, thereby leading to faulty or biased outcome expectations that result in excessive drinking, (3) Individuals may believe that alcohol is a powerful mood manipulator or modulator of physiologic arousal; (4) Individuals may not have the general coping skills to negotiate life stressors and accomplish goals without the aid of alcohol, (5) Individuals may not have specific coping skills to regulate adequately their actual drinking behavior, (6) Individuals may not attend to critical psychophysiologic and behavioral information providing feedback about the effects of alcohol on their biology and its impact on their behavior (e.g., impaired performance, ataxia, level of intoxication).

The crux of the social learning model is that alcohol use and abuse involves persons with particular social learning histories, placed in specific situations, in a certain current state, and with personal needs and expectations (cognitive–emotional and biological/physiologic) so that alcohol is chosen as an "optimal" method of coping (Abrams, 1983; Marlatt & Gordon, 1985; Wills & Shiffman, 1985). Cognitive factors play a crucial role in determining when drinking will take place, how much will be consumed and what behaviors will be displayed. Among the cognitive variables, expectations have received the majority of research attention over the last 10 years.

### Expectancy Set

Social learning theory has generated a large body of research on the role expectations play as mediating variables in explaining drinking and behavior when intoxicated. *Expectancy* refers to the beliefs about the effects of alcohol that are held by an individual or group resulting from learning history. As already described in Family and Peer Influences within a Developmental Context, above, beliefs about drinking and behavior when intoxicated are formed very early in life, prior to actual experiences with alcohol. However, in this section, we focus on the more proximal antecedents and consequences that may govern alcohol use and abuse.

Expectancy effects and their interaction with setting may help to explain inconsistencies in both pharmacologic theories and early learning theories based solely on classical or operant principles. For example, the tension reduction hypothesis, although enjoying much clinical support and intuitive appeal, has been fraught with equivocal research findings over the years (see Cappell & Greeley, Chapter 2, this volume; Wilson, 1978, 1985; Marlatt & Rohsenow, 1980). Failure to control for expectancy and setting variables may in part explain the equivocal results. The available evidence reveals that there is no simple relationship between alcohol and its behavioral consequences, whether based on pharmacologic theory or learning theory. Depending on the current state of the person, his or her expectations, and the context, alcohol can produce a variety of effects.

The literature on expectancy set has been extensively reviewed and critiqued (see Marlatt & Rohsenow, 1980). The general research paradigm employs a 2 × 2 factorial design that controls for both expectancy set and pharmacologic action—the "balanced placebo design" (BPD). Subjects are told that their drinks either contain an alcoholic (vodka) or a nonalcoholic (tonic) beverage and the beverage itself either contains alcohol or it does not. This results in four conditions: (1) told alcohol, given alcohol; (2) told alcohol, given tonic; (3) told tonic, given alcohol; and (4) told tonic, given tonic. At low to moderate doses of ethanol (0.5–1.0 g/kg) subjects cannot discriminate correctly the placebo and reverse placebo conditions, and the procedure has stood the test of time and replication in several laboratories since the early 1970s (see Marlatt & Rohsenow, 1980). Generally the studies conducted using the BPD have tested specific hypotheses related to alcohol use and abuse such as whether expectancy or pharmacology is the primary mechanism in loss of control over drinking, "disinhibition" of sexual or aggressive behavior, mood changes, tension reduction, and cognitive and psychomotor performance.

Engle and Williams (1972) investigated subjective craving in 40 inpatient alcoholics using the BPD. They measured subjective craving before and 40 min after the administration to subjects of either a mixture of 1 ounce of vodka in a vitamin drink or the vitamin drink alone. Half of the subjects in each of these two conditions were told that their drinks contained alcohol and half were told that the drinks contained only fruit juice. The only main effect was for expectancy set: Those subjects who were told that they were receiving alcohol regardless of drink content, reported significantly more craving than those subjects who believed they were only receiving fruit juice. Marlatt, Demming, and Reid (1973) used a similar design but measured drinking consumption directly. Both alcoholics and social drinkers were randomly assigned to one of the four cells of the BPD and were then led to believe that they were sampling drinks in a "taste-rating task." Though subjects believed that the primary goal of the study was to rate the beverages according to taste, the major dependent variable of interest was the quantity of alcohol that they consumed during the task. The results of this study were in the same direction as the previous study on craving. Those subjects who believed that they were sampling an alcoholic beverage drank significantly more in the taste-rating task than subjects who believed that they were consuming a nonalcoholic beverage. Thus there was a main effect for expectancy set, regardless of drink content.

Subsequent research using the BPD has replicated and extended the results of the above studies implicating expectancy set as a powerful proximal determinant of both drinking and behavior when intoxicated. The BPD has also been employed to investigate the effects of alcohol on mood states. Using the BPD, Lang, Goeckner, Adesso, and Marlatt (1975) investigated the relative contributions of the cognitive and pharmacologic determinants of aggressive behavior in heavy-drinking male subjects. The results indicated that subjects who had believed that they had consumed alcohol were significantly more aggressive than subjects who believed that they had consumed a nonalcoholic beverage. There was no main effect for actual drink content. In a related study, Marlatt, Kosturn, and Lang (1975) investigated provocation to anger and the opportunity for retaliation on subsequent alcohol consumption using the taste-rating task previously described. They found that subjects who were provoked to anger drank significantly more alcohol than subjects who were given the opportunity to retaliate. The results of these studies suggest that individuals provoked to anger who failed to assert themselves may consume more alcohol, and that drinking may be followed by aggressive acts because people believe that such acts are "justified" when intoxicated.

Attempts to investigate the tension reduction hypothesis using the BPD have resulted in a series of studies with mixed results. (For a critical review for this area, see Cappell and Greeley, Chapter 2, this volume.) For example, Wilson and Abrams (1977) reported that the belief that alcohol was consumed, regardless of beverage content, resulted in decreased social anxiety in males, whereas it resulted in increased social anxiety in females (Abrams & Wilson, 1979). However, while these studies show that alcohol can increase or decrease social anxiety, it is interesting to note that in both cases the effect was again based on expectancy set and not on drink content. Interestingly, in another study investigating the fear of interpersonal evaluation, Higgins and Marlatt

(1975) also showed that subjects tended to drink more after fear of interpersonal evaluation. This suggests that social anxiety may play a role in alcohol use and abuse in those who have problems with self-confidence and/or their social competence (Monti, Abrams, Binkoff, & Zwick, in press). For a more extensive examination of the stress dampening hypothesis, also see Sher, Chapter 7, this volume.

In studies using the BPD to investigate the effects of alcohol on sexual arousal, some sex differences have also been noted. Wilson and Lawson (1976b) reported that male subjects who believed they had consumed alcohol showed significantly greater levels of sexual arousal as measured by penile tumescence, regardless of drink content. However, Wilson and Lawson (1976a) reported that women who received alcohol, regardless of expectancy set, showed significantly reduced sexual arousal. The doses of alcohol in both of these studies were relatively low (blood alcohol concentration of 40 mg/100 ml). In other studies using both low and moderately high doses (blood alcohol concentration of 80 mg/100 ml), it has been shown that increased levels of intoxication are related negatively to sexual arousal (Wilson, Lawson, & Abrams, 1978). In this study, male alcoholics showed decreased penile tumenscence with increasing doses of alcohol even though they reported that alcohol would either have no effect on their arousal or would increase it.

It is interesting to note that in the context of sexual arousal, expectancy set and drink content appear to work in opposite directions, and that at low doses expectancy set may override pharmacologic effects for male subjects but not for females. Despite the fact that increasing doses of alcohol decreases sexual arousal, most individuals continue to believe that it enhances sexual arousal. Thus beliefs about the short-term and low-dosage effects of alcohol are maintained by the majority of individuals despite the fact that alcohol impairs sexual performance at higher doses.

In term of generalizability, the studies of expectancy set have included alcoholics or heavy social drinkers, although the majority have used college students. Many of the studies are limited in that they consist of laboratory analogues of clinical phenomena (Abrams, 1983). The studies have also been criticized because of the low doses of alcohol employed. It is difficult or impossible to protect the internal validity of the BPD with doses that are extremely high, thus dose may interact with expectancy set in ways that have not yet been empirically tested. Few studies have been conducted on women subjects, and gender differences may lead to important findings with implications for treatment. However, taken together, the overwhelming majority of the studies indicate that expectancy set cannot be ignored in explanations of drinking and behavior when intoxicated. Expectancy set may be the dominant factor in initiation of drinking, especially where low doses are consumed, or prior to the full absorption of higher doses. The short-term immediate consequences of drinking may be in line with prior expectations regardless of pharmacologic action or more delayed consequences.

### General and Alcohol-Specific Coping Skills

The domain of coping skills is a critical determinant in the decision to drink or not to drink and whether the drinking is "normal" or "maladaptive." It is useful to discriminate between generalized coping skills that are required to deal with a variety of life situations (e.g., personal mental and physical health, interpersonal relationships, work) and specific coping skills that are relevant to alcohol regulation per se (e.g., awareness of cues related to intoxication, assertiveness skills to refuse drinks under peer pressure). This is an important distinction because it may, in part, predict the severity and length of alcohol abuse and what individuals are at greater risk for progressing from normal social drinking to alcohol dependence. For example, Marlatt and Gordon (1985) suggest that a "lifestyle balance" is an important goal for recovering alcoholics so that the individual has an adequate reserve capacity in order to cope with life stressors as they come up. This prevents the accumulation of stressors over time and the subsequent taxing of coping responses with each new everyday "hassle" (Abrams, 1983; Lazarus & Folkman, 1985).

Deficits in generalized coping ability are reflected in epidemiologic studies of developmental factors that predict substance abuse in young persons, such as poor academic performance, social marginality, family conflict, and low self-esteem (Jessor & Jessor, 1977). These factors were extensively reviewed in predisposing Individual Differences, and Major Principles of Social Learning Theory of Alcohol Use and Abuse, above. Briefly, generalized skill deficits appear to increase the probability that alcohol experimentation will lead to heavy use and ultimately to dependency. There is the perception and expectation that alcohol will enhance the user's self-esteem and social image, reduce his or her tension, and help the individual gain access to desirable peer groups by making him or her appear more "adultlike" (Chassin, Presson, Sherman, Corty, & Olshavsky, 1981). Not only will these young adults be more likely to experiment with alcohol but they are also more likely to become dependent on alcohol (Wills & Warshawsky, 1983).

An important but underemphasized implication of a general coping model for alcohol use is the reciprocal changes in social interaction predicted by SLT. According to SLT, individuals who have general coping deficits would progressively isolate themselves, and would in turn be isolated by those peers who have adequate coping abilities. Opposed to those with coping deficits would be those individuals who have high self-esteem, adequate efficacy and outcome expectations, a good repertoire of intrapersonal and interpersonal competence, greater awareness of the negative rather than positive consequence of substance use, and an attachment to peer groups with values that model appropriate alcohol use and discourage habitual use of alcohol as a coping method. These groups have the ability to exercise self-control over drinking, are self-selected into a "healthy" peer subculture, and for the most part become "normal social drinkers." By contrast, those individuals who eventually become alcohol abusers will find themselves in a reciprocally determined downward spiral. They are self-selected into a different kind of subculture, with other peers who have similar skill deficits, engage in similar "delinquent" behavior, and have distorted, overly positive expectations of drug effects. Their life style of alcohol use is reciprocally reinforced and maintained within their subculture.

The reciprocal interaction between members of each subculture both reinforces the skills and myths within that culture and isolates them from other subcultures. In particular, it deprives the skill-deficit groups of the healthy role modeling and other learning experiences that would counteract their distorted expectations and decision making. Thus the skill-deficit group must rely increasingly on other alcohol abusers for social and emotional support. It is interesting to note that Moos and his colleagues (e.g., Moos & Finney, 1983; Cronkite & Moos, 1980) point out that alcoholics who have impoverished social networks, a poor work history, and are divorced also have a poorer prognosis for recovery than less socially isolated alcoholics. This may not be the result of a "powerful disease process" or "genetic predisposition" but rather may be due to a powerful reciprocally determined social selection process, governed by the principles of SLT. For a detailed explanation of how SLT factors are implicated in healthful versus unhealthful life styles, see Abrams, Elder, Lasater, Carleton, and Artz (1986).

In order to avoid problem drinking, individuals must possess specific skills enabling them to cope with drinking situations (e.g., assertive drink refusal), in addition to general coping skills to achieve life style balance. Once one or two drinks are consumed, self-regulation of drinking is needed, based on internal feedback (cognitive–physiologic) and external behavior cues (e.g., ataxia, comments from significant others). For example, Nathan and his colleagues have suggested that excessive drinking can result from inattention to blood alcohol cues, or deficits in feedback mechanisms conveying internal cues of intoxication to the brain (Lansky, Nathan, & Lawson, 1978; Lipscomb & Nathan, 1980; Huber, Karlin, & Nathan, 1976). Nathan and colleagues advocated blood alcohol level discrimination training to increase awareness of these feedback systems and to teach better self-control.

Alcohol is frequently available in social situations where adults are faced with both subtle and more direct pressures to drink. An adequate repertoire of drink refusal skills must include the ability to refuse to drink and/or to stop drinking before the risks of negative consequences are too great. Recent research suggests that cues such as the sight and smell of a favorite alcoholic beverage may impair an individual's social skills to refuse an offer of a drink (Binkoff *et al.*, 1984; Binkoff, 1985; Monti *et al.*, in press). Thus, self-regulation of drinking requires attention to feedback systems such as physiologic cues within the human organism, in addition to the individual cognitive and social skills required to regulate drinking in social contexts. The repertoire of coping skills, both general and specific, are important factors in determining an individual's risk of alcohol use and abuse.

Use of alcohol in a particular situation is also determined by other cognitive self-regulatory mechanisms. Basically, conditions requiring coping responses can be divided into intrapersonal and interpersonal dimensions. Intrapersonal dimensions can be further subdivided into cognitive–emotional factors and psychophysiologic–biochemical factors. Individuals who have inadequate methods of coping with intrapersonal factors (i.e., who have responses such as fatigue, boredom, stress, tension, depression, anger) may resort to alcohol use or abuse. Alcohol can also be viewed as a drug to potentiate or enhance positive affect such as pleasure, increased arousal, or sensation seeking. In intrapersonal situations, there may be coping skill deficits (e.g., difficulty achieving a state of relaxation), and low self-efficacy expectations for achieving desired intrapersonal goals without use of alcohol.

Alcohol can be used as a coping mechanism because it can reduce negative affect or increase positive affect. This assumption expands on the more narrow tension reduction theory that has dominated learning theory and has been implicitly accepted within SLT (see Bandura, 1969; Cappell and Greeley, Chapter 2, this volume). It is possible that both positive and negative mood manipulation may be accomplished either during one episode over time or on different occasions. That alcohol is a powerful mood manipulator may derive both from the individual's expectancy and from the biphasic effects of alcohol over time.

The biphasic effects of alcohol may in part explain how alcohol can be chosen both for the relief of negative affect and the enhancement of positive affect (i.e., arousal reduction or arousal induction). In this case, biochemical factors can interact with psychosocial factors to produce specific outcomes. Mello (1968) points out that alcohol acts as a stimulant early in the absorption curve, when there is a rising blood alcohol level. This is associated with mild euphoria and a pleasant feeling of arousal. Alcohol also increases heart rate by 10–12 beats/min. Later, as higher blood concentrations of alcohol are reached and during the period marked by a falling blood alcohol level curve, the depressing effects become more dominant, possibly resulting in tension reduction, sedation, and decreased aversiveness of negative mood states.

McCollam, Burish, Maisto, and Sobell (1978) studied 60 male social drinkers and reported that sensations were rated higher during the ascending compared with the descending limb of the blood alcohol curve. Thus it is possible that pharmacologic factors may interact with psychosocial variables over time. Since the potency of reinforcers is in part determined by the length of time between the reward and the behavior, the more immediate pharmacological effects (pleasant euphoria) may become more powerful stimuli for future usage.

Russell and Mehrabian (1975) suggest that the biphasic effects of alcohol result in different drinking patterns in anticipation of the desired outcomes required at the time. In individuals who seek heightened arousal and euphoria, drinking is prolonged and small sips are taken to lengthen the time of the rising blood alcohol level and delay the onset of the CNS depressing effect. By contrast, the tendency of individuals who are already hyperaroused, stressed, or tense would be to drink large amounts of alcohol as rapidly as possible so as to shorten the time of the rising blood alcohol level, and quickly reach and prolong the desired CNS depression effects during the falling limb of the blood alcohol curve (tension reduction). Thus it is possible, according to SLT, for different individuals, or the same individual at different times, to alter their drinking patterns to produce arousing or relaxing effects. In essence, individuals use alcohol both as a mood enhancer for pleasant emotions, to increase arousal, and to attenuate negative moods such as anxiety or tension. Alcohol can "assist" individuals in coping with a wide variety of intrapersonal and physiological states (Abrams, 1983).

To summarize, alcohol use and abuse is moderated by a variety of situational and personal proximal determinants. Alcohol abuse can be seen as a maladaptive method of coping when self-efficacy and outcome expectations are such that alcohol is chosen as the best or only currently available method of obtaining a desired result. Situational context and modeling effects influence drinking behavior. Alcohol consumption has also been shown to be influenced by operant factors such as reinforcing or punishing consequences. Important factors in drinking include both the biphasic effects of alcohol and the powerful role played by expectancy set in determining drinking. In problem drinkers, expectations about the short-term benefits of alcohol use outweigh the long-term negative consequences. Alcohol can also serve as a mood manipulator to enhance positive affect or to attenuate negative affect. Both the repertoire of general coping skills and alcohol-specific coping skills play a central role in determining drinking patterns. Once drinking has begun, feedback about one's level of intoxication and specific drink refusal skills must be available and utilized to regulate further drinking. Various combinations of situational stressors, cognitive (person) variables, and the current biological state of the person at the time of drinking can result in a taxing of existing coping mechanisms and a tendency to become overly reliant on alcohol to accomplish short-term solutions to life problems. Once drinking is used as a frequent and habitual coping mechanism the risk of abuse is increased. Self-regulation of alcohol consumption and issues of tolerance and withdrawal become additional factors that can account for the transition from normal use to problem drinking, and especially the escalation to alcoholism or alcohol dependence (Abrams & Wilson 1986).

## Tolerance, Withdrawal and Loss-of-Control

In both Bandura's (1969) and our SLT model, tolerance and physical dependence upon alcohol are viewed as important determinants of sustained consumption. Tolerance is thought to promote increased consumption by decreasing the positive reinforcing aspects of alcohol use. Individuals will then consume greater amounts of the substance in order to achieve the desired effect. Physical dependence is thought to result in increased alcohol consumption as a means of avoiding the painful effects of alcohol withdrawal bought about by acute periods of abstinence (Hershon, 1977). However, in our model, we reject the notion that tolerance and withdrawal are static influences acquired only through the process of repeated ingestion of alcohol. While recognizing that direct pharmacologic influences are important in the development of tolerance and dependence, it is important to consider how these factors may interact with cognitive and social learning variables to moderate drinking behavior.

Human tolerance to alcohol has been found to be influenced by variables that affect other kinds of learning. For example, tolerance to alcohol's effects is related to the context in which it is ingested. If the context of administration changes, tolerance may decrease (Shapiro, 1984; Dafters & Anderson, 1982). This may be related to a conditioning phenomenon, in which a previously neutral stimulus (the drinking context) is repeatedly paired with the unconditioned effects of the drug. Eventually the neutral (or unconditioned stimulus) may come to elicit a compensatory response, opposite in direction to the effects of the drug, designed to maintain organismic homeostasis (see Solomon & Corbit, 1974; Siegal, 1979). Tolerance to alcohol's interfering effects on psychomotor skills in humans can also be enhanced by positive reinforcement for good performance (Mann & Vogel-Sprott, 1984). Thus, it is conceivable that tolerance is influenced by both drinking contexts (including social contexts) and operant learning factors. And, as these factors vary, so too may alcohol consumption.

Tolerance, however, should not necessarily be considered as a unitary phenomenon (Niaura & Nathan, 1984). It may be that tolerance to only certain alcohol effects may lead to increased alcohol consumption. Wilson, Lipscomb, Nathan, and Abrams (1980) reported an interaction between tolerance and dose of alcohol to produce stress-reducing effects. Individuals were measured for tolerance using a standing steadiness test after an alcohol preload. They were then exposed to a stressful interaction, and triple response mode measures were recorded (i.e., heart rate and skin conductance, behavioral skills and anxiety, self-reported anxiety). Subjects were given a placebo, or a low dose or high dose of alcohol and were divided into high- and low-tolerance groups on the basis of the standing steadiness measure. A significant interaction effect was reported in that high-tolerance subjects, as compared with low-tolerance subjects, displayed less change in heart rate arousal during stress in the high-dose but not in the low-dose condition. Thus, tolerance, however it is acquired, has implications for pattern of drinking, so that some subjects may tend to drink more heavily to achieve stress dampening effects in social situations.

Physical dependence and withdrawal phenomena can also be interpreted through classical, operant, and cognitive learning models. In the classical conditioning paradigm, a neutral stimulus is paired with an unconditioned stimulus that naturally elicits an unconditioned response. After repeated trials, the neutral stimulus becomes a conditioned stimulus and is capable of eliciting a conditioned response in the absence of the unconditioned stimulus. Dependence or "craving" for alcohol can be explained using this paradigm. Initially, craving occurs during withdrawal and becomes associated with certain stimuli (environmental cues and bodily sensations) that are present during withdrawal. If at some future time the abstinent alcoholic is exposed to stimuli that were previously associated with withdrawal (e.g., physiologic arousal, the sight or smell of alcohol), a conditioned response, or craving, will result (Ludwig & Wikler, 1974). The conditioned craving will now cause the individual to seek relief through further substance abuse, which may eventuate in a loss-of-control phenomenon (Pomerleau, Fertig, Baker, & Cooney, 1983). Thus, reactivity to internal or environmental cues can set the stage for heavy drinking; the first drink is assumed to act to produce additional craving in much the same way as an "appetizer." Other learning-based models suggest that cues previously associated not only with withdrawal but also with alcohol consumption or termination of drinking, may come to elicit withdrawal and subjective craving (Siegal, 1979; Hodgson, Rankin, & Stockwell, 1979).

There is accumulating empirical research showing that alcoholics differ from nonalcoholics in their salivation or digastric muscle responses to the sight and smell of alcohol (Pomerleau et al., 1983; Cooney, Baker, & Pomerleau, 1983; Binkoff et al., 1984). For example, alcoholics were found to salivate significantly more as a reaction to the sight and smell of their favorite alcoholic beverage when compared with nonalcoholics. Binkoff (1985) has shown that drinking cues can impair drink refusal skills in a laboratory analogue study with alcoholics. However, whether these differences predict relapse or heavy drinking in the natural environment, is yet to be demonstrated. The notion that cues can elicit craving long after physiologic withdrawal has ceased, has important ramifications for research and practice. This area of SLT is likely to attract much attention in the future.

Early definitions defined loss-of-control as a unidimensional construct in which minimum amounts of alcohol resulted in a pharmacologic process leading to craving and loss-of-control over subsequent drinking. A multidimensional model was later proposed including situational, psychological, and cultural factors that could trigger craving and loss-of-control drinking (Jellinek, 1960). Although research on loss-of-control drinking has been beset by definitional problems (Maisto & Schefft, 1977), attempts to examine the social learning mechanisms of this phenomenon have provided additional insights into a social learning model of alcohol use and abuse (see Development of Alcohol-Related Expectancies, above). Engle and Williams (1972) and Marlatt et al. (1973) using the BPD, have shown that psychological (expectancy) and environmental factors may be more important influences in initiating loss-of-control drinking than pharmacology.

Since many of these studies used low to moderate doses of alcohol, it is possible that higher doses do result in a strong pharmacologic action that triggers loss-of-control drinking. For example, Glatt (1976) proposed a multifactorial model that includes psychosocial and pharmacologic factors. Glatt proposed that an as-yet-unspecified "critical threshold" exists such that loss-of-control drinking is pharmacologically based when the blood alcohol level is above the threshold, and psychosocially mediated when the blood alcohol level is below the threshold.

Thus, withdrawal and craving for alcohol may be associated to a significant degree with the situational, cognitive, and physiologic cues associated with previous drinking, termination of drinking, and previous episodes of withdrawal associated with acute abstinence from alcohol. Cooney et al. (1982) have proposed that among alcoholics, responses to these cues may not only result in increased physiologic and subjective responsiveness (withdrawal symptoms and craving) but also will be paralleled by subsequent increases in positive outcome expectations regarding the effects of alcohol and decreases in perceived efficacy to cope in the situation without resorting to alcohol consumption. These speculations, however, await confirmation by further research.

To summarize, a variety of learning-based models have been proposed to explain the influence of psychosocial variables on alcohol craving, withdrawal, and loss-of-control drinking. Although many questions remain, the finding that expectancy set mediates drinking and that one drink does not inevitably lead to loss-of-control has been replicated. This finding has significant treatment implications that have led to the notion of controlled drinking as an alternative treatment for some problem drinkers (Miller & Caddy, 1977; Marlatt, 1984; Nathan & Niaura, 1985; Sobell & Sobell, 1978; Wilson, 1985). Reactivity to alcohol cues as a precipitant of drinking is also likely to generate much interest in the coming years.

## Relapse Prevention and Recovery

Marlatt and Gordon's (1985) social learning model of relapse provides additional insights into episodes of problem drinking and the road back to either normal drinking or total abstinence in those who have had drinking problems. However, it also provides insights into the etiology and integration of many of the variables mentioned in the previous sections of this chapter. Thus, in some respects, Marlatt and Gordon's model of relapse can be conceived as a comprehensive summary of a SLT of alcohol use and abuse. Although of relatively recent origin and as yet not thoroughly tested, the Marlatt and Gordon (1985) model of relapse is the most well articulated and comprehensive statement of a SLT of alcohol abuse. It will doubtless produce a wealth of research and has the potential to make one of the largest new contributions to treatment of addictive disorders in this century.

Marlatt (1979) summarizes the key factors that may precipitate the reoccurrence of excessive drinking as follows: (1) the degree to which the drinker feels controlled by or helpless relative to the influence of others; (2) the individual's view of the self in relation to the environmental events that are perceived as beyond personal control (i.e., low self-efficacy) in the face of the demands of everyday life, including feelings of powerlessness, fatalism, and learned helplessness; (3) the availability of alcohol and the constraints placed on drinking in a particular situational context; (4) the availability of adequate alternative coping responses to drinking, both general and specific; (5) the drinker's expectations about the effects of alcohol as a method of coping. Those with positive expectations of outcome will be more likely to drink.

In order to study how person variables and environmental factors come together to create a drinking situation, Marlatt and Gordon (1985) examined relapse episodes in 70 male alcoholics, as well as smokers and heroin addicts. Information concerning the circumstances surrounding initial use of these substances following a period of abstinence was analyzed. It was found that 61% of the relapse situations fell into categories involving stressful personal or environmental determinants. The major subcategories included negative emotional states such as frustration, anger, anxiety, and fear which accounted for 38% of the relapse situations; urges and temptations such as craving and exposure to cues which accounted for 16% of relapse situations; and social and interpersonal context such as conflict and pressure which accounted for 20% of relapse situations. Other important but less frequently reported categories included using drugs to achieve positive emotional states and as a means of creating feelings of pleasantness or euphoria (3% of situations). It is not surprising to note that these factors are in agreement with the developmental, early drinking experiences, and proximal determinants (e.g., expectations) of alcohol use, described earlier in this chapter. For the recovering problem drinker or alcoholic these factors have come to be known as "high-risk-for-relapse" situations.

The central assumption in Marlatt and Gordon's (1985) SLT model of relapse is that the individual has voluntarily made a choice to abstain or to control alcohol consumption. An individual must develop general and specific coping skills as alternatives to drinking. The choice of abstaining or limiting intake leads to a sense of personal control over drinking and a growing mastery over those situations that may precipitate relapse (i.e., "high-risk-for-relapse" situations). The presence of adequate alternative coping skills and the belief that one has sufficient mastery over these skills (self-efficacy expectations) to achieve the desired goals (outcome expectations) will determine whether alcohol or an alternative behavior is chosen. Relapse will occur if the perception of control and self-efficacy diminishes when an individual is confronted with a particularly difficult situation. If the individual is indeed able to cope with a high-risk situation without drinking then a sense of self-efficacy is enhanced. This results in a higher probability that an individual will resist drinking in future situations.

According to self-efficacy theory, there are four methods for enhancing self-efficacy expectations (Bandura, 1977a). In the early phases of treatment and recovery, role-modeling of appropriate coping responses (e.g., social skill training around drink refusal and verbal persuasion) are probably useful, especially when the problem drinker is in a controlled rehabilitation setting where the risk of relapse is strongly diminished. Later on, as new coping skills are acquired and self-efficacy begins to increase, graduated exposure to more and more difficult situations would be recommended. Ultimately, the most powerful sources of maintaining high self-efficacy expectations (direct practice with successful feedback) must become operative. Actual participation in successful coping (without alcohol) in the natural environment is essential to enhance self-efficacy. The individual must begin extinction of physiologic cues that in the past undermined self-efficacy via physiologic pathways such as conditioned reactivity to cues, anxiety, panic, or a sense of loss of control. With repeated trials, self-efficacy is enhanced and the individual is able to cope with a variety of intrapersonal (e.g., management of mood states) and interpersonal (e.g., at a social gathering) situations. Each success experience contributes to a heightened sense of self-control and leads to better resistance to temptation in the face of adversity.

By contrast, a lack of alternative coping skills, or low efficacy expectations, will result in a negative, vicious circle in which loss of confidence leads to alcohol use and then subsequent abuse. This is even more likely to occur if the individual has retained positive outcome expectations and not learned about the negative consequences of drinking. After consuming a small amount of alcohol following a period of abstinence, the individual can experience a variety of cognitive reactions which Marlatt and Gordon (1985) have termed the abstinence violation effect (AVE). The AVE is made up of two components: cognitive dissonance and a personal attribution effect. Cognitive dissonance involves a conflict between the self-image as an abstainer and behavior that has violated self-imposed limits. The violation of the self-imposed limits is then attributed to personal weakness and failure such as a lack of willpower. Thus, self-efficacy expectations are strongly undermined, the individual is convinced that failing once suggests continued failure, and that they may as well give up and drink themselves into oblivion. The initial stimulating effects of alcohol are experienced as very pleasant and add even more to the likelihood of continued use. Once drinking has progressed, the usual factors of acquired tolerance, craving and, expected loss-of-control once again become operative in a vicious and self-destructive cycle. To counteract the effect, a cognitive restructuring is required so that the individual sees a "relapse" as a learning experience, in essence as another form of feedback on how to do better the next time. The aim is to stop drinking very early on so that the behavior is viewed as a "slip" or minor transgression rather than as an excuse for loss of control. The term "lapse" has been suggested, rather than "relapse" (see Abrams et al., 1986).

### Summary and Conclusion

The implications of the social learning model of alcohol use, abuse, and recovery are widespread. It suggests that individuals' beliefs about alcohol and their ability to cope with the demands of everyday life are crucial determinants of how psychologically dependent on alcohol they become. Cultural norms, role models, and learned expectations have a powerful effect on drinking behavior and play a central role in determining drinking patterns. Individuals with behavioral excesses or deficits in general coping skills, such as inability to manage everyday stress, may be particularly vulnerable to using chemicals as an artificial method of modulating their functioning. Certain biological factors may also interact with psychosocial variables and result in abusive drinking.

Unfortunately, alcohol use has short-term beneficial effects, but generally creates devastating long-term results that themselves become additional stressors. Prolonged alcohol use damages the body, changes social interaction and supports, and perpetuates faulty cognitive information processing, creating a downward spiral toward social isolation and neglect. These factors, in turn, produce increased stress in the form of divorce, loss of employment, and lack of social support. Moos and his colleagues (Cronkite & Moos, 1980) have illustrated how sociocultural factors can also mediate treatment and recovery.

Thus, a social learning model of alcohol use and abuse suggests that nothing short of a total life style change should be contemplated as part of rehabilitating the problem drinker. Individuals must acquire general and specific coping skills so as to regulate stress in their lives to cope with major life stress events and everyday hassles in a balanced manner. Alternative forms of relaxation, work patterns, and social life must all be attended to, and individuals must develop adequate forethought and self-regulation capacity to successfully negotiate the demands of everyday life without resorting necessarily to artificial substances. Alternative reinforcers that are as powerful and immediately effective as alcohol are difficult to find and use, especially for problem drinkers who must learn to delay gratification and exercise self-control.

Social learning theory has made significant advance since early formulations based on learning theory and Bandura's initial formulations of the late 1960s. Contributions to understanding alcohol use and abuse have been made in several areas to date. Promising areas for future research include the use of SLT findings to develop prevention programs in adolescents or younger-age children. More work in this area may ultimately lead to primary prevention of alcohol abuse, an area sorely in need of research (Abrams et al., 1986; Nathan, 1983). Another area that is likely to have a major impact on the field of alcohol treatment is the seminal work of Marlatt and Gordon (1985) and others on relapse prevention. Research on understanding the interaction between biological (biochemical, endocrine, and psychophysiologic) factors and psychosocial variables is also likely to lead to major advances in the field. Already the contribution of SLT to the study of drug relationships (e.g., the BPD) has resulted in significant advances. Pomerleau (1981) and Pomerleau et al. (1983) and others represent examples of advancing the interface between biological and behavioral mechanisms.

In the past SLT has been criticized as being a mere collection of isolated observations rather than a comprehensive theory. It is easy to see why this is so, since SLT of alcohol use and abuse is anchored in the experimental method and demands empirical testing of specific hypotheses. Furthermore, diverse aspects of SLT have rarely been integrated (e.g., expectancies, modeling, relapse, adolescent applications, and cross-cultural aspects). It is hoped that the present chapter, although broad in nature, integrates key research studies across the life span and from micro (individual) to macro (cultural) perspectives. It is critical for a theory that posits a complex interaction between person and environment to be empirically based and rooted in specific research studies of component processes and mediating mechanisms. It is this research base that makes SLT an ever-growing model with the capacity for self correction of faulty hypotheses and with the ability to generate new ideas that are testable and subject to disconfirmation. The strength of SLT is its solid research base and its ability to be heuristic.

## References

Abrams, D. B. (1983). Psychosocial assessment of alcohol-stress interactions: Bridging the gap between laboratory and treatment outcome research. In L. Pohorecky & J. Brick, (Eds.), *Stress and Alcohol Use* (pp. 61–86). New York: Elsevier.

Abrams, D. B., Elder, J., Lasater, T., Carlton, R., & Artz, L. (1986). A comprehensive framework for conceptualizing and planning organizational health promotion programs. In M. Cataldo & T. Coates (Eds.), *Behavioral medicine in industry*. New York: John Wiley & Sons.

Abrams, D. B., Niaura, R. S., Carey, K. B., Binkoff, J. A., & Monti, P. M. (in press). Understanding relapse and recovery in alcohol abuse. *Annals of Behavioral Medicine, 8.*

Abrams, D. B., & Wilson, G. T. (1979). Effects of alcohol on social anxiety in women: Cognitive versus physiological processes. *Journal of Abnormal Psychology, 88,* 161–173.

Abrams, D. B., & Wilson, G. T. (1983). Alcohol, sexual arousal, and self-control. *Journal of Personality and Social Psychology, 45,* 188–198.

Abrams, D. B., & Wilson, G. T. (1986). Habit disorders: Alcohol and tobacco dependence. In A. Frances and R. Hales (Eds.), *American Psychiatric Association: Annual review* (Vol. 5). Washington, DC: American Psychiatric Press.

Bandura, A. (1969). *Principles of behavior modification.* New York: Holt, Rinehart & Winston.

Bandura, A. (1973). *Aggression: A social learning analysis.* Englewood Cliff, NJ, Prentice-Hall.

Bandura, A. (1977a). Self-efficacy: Toward a unifying theory of behavioral change. *Psychological Review, 84,* 191–215.

Bandura, A. (1977b). *Social learning theory.* Englewood Cliffs, NJ: Prentice-Hall.

Bandura, A. (1978). The self-system in reciprocal determinism. *American Psychologist, 33,* 344–358.

Bandura, A. (1982). Self-efficacy mechanism in human agency. *American Psychologist, 37,* 122–147.

Bandura, A. (1985). *Social foundations of thought and action.* Englewood Cliffs, NJ: Prentice-Hall.

Barnes, G. M. (1977). The development of adolescent drinking behavior: An evaluative review of the impact of the socialization process within the family. *Adolescence, 12,* 571–591.

Begleiter, H., Porgesz, B., Bihari, B., & Kissin, B. (1984). Event-related brain potentials in boys at risk for alcoholism. *Science, 225,* 1493–1496.

Biddle, B. J., Bank, B. J., & Marlin, M. M. (1980). Social determinants of adolescent drinking: What they think, what they do and what I think they do. *Journal of Studies on Alcohol, 41,* 215–241.

Binkoff, J. (1985). *Cue exposure and drink refusal.* Unpublished doctoral dissertation, State University of New York at Stony Brook.

Binkoff, J., Abrams, D., Collins, L., Monti, P., Nirenberg, T., Liepman, M., & Zwick, W. (1984, August). *Cue-exposure and drink refusal skills in alcoholics.* Paper presented at the 92nd Annual Convention of the American Psychological Association, Toronto, Ontario, Canada.

Biran, M., & Wilson, G. T. (1981). Treatment of phobic disorders using cognitive and exposure methods: A self-efficacy analysis. *Journal of Consulting and Clinical Psychology*, *49*, 886–899.

Blane, H. T., & Hewitt, L. E. (1977). *Alcohol and youth: An analysis of the literature* (Report No. PB-268-698). Rockville, MD: National Institute on Alcohol Abuse and Alcoholism.

Bowers, K. (1973). Situationism in psychology: An analysis and critique. *Psychological Review*, *80*, 307–336.

Braucht, G. N. (1980). Psychosocial research on teenage drinking: Past and future. In F. R. Scarpitti and S. K. Datesman (Eds.), *Drugs and the youth culture: Sage annual reviews of drug and alcohol abuse* (Vol. 4). Beverly Hills, CA: Sage.

Braucht, G. N. (1981). Problem drinking among adolescents: A review and analysis of psychosocial research. In *Special Population Issues* (Alcohol and Health Monograph 4, Department of Health and Human Services Publication No. ADM 82-1193, pp. 143–164). Washington, DC: Government Printing Office.

Braucht, G. N., Follingstad, D., Brakarsh, D., & Berry, K. L. (1973). Drug education: A review of goals, approaches, and effectiveness, and a paradigm for evaluation. *Quarterly Journal of Studies on Alcohol*, *34*, 1279–1292.

Brown, S. A. (1985). Expectancies versus background in the prediction of college drinking patterns. *Journal of Consulting and Clinical Psychology*, *53*, 123–130.

Brown, S. A., Goldman, M. S., Inn, A., & Anderson, L. R. (1980). Expectations of reinforcement from alcohol: Their domain and relation to drinking patterns. *Journal of Consulting and Clinical Psychology*, *48*, 419–426.

Bry, B. H., McKeon, P., & Pandina, R. J. (1982). Extent of drug use as a function of number of risk factors. *Journal of Abnormal Psychology*, *91*, 273–279.

Cadoret, R. J., O'Gorman, T. W., Troughton, E. & Heywood, E. (1985). Alcoholism and antisocial personality: Interrelationships, genetic, and environmental factors. *Archives of General Psychiatry*, *42*, 161–167.

Cafiso, J., Goodstadt, M. S., Garlington, W. K., & Sheppard, M. A. (1982). Television portrayal of alcohol and other beverages. *Journal of Studies on Alcohol*, *43*, 1232–1243.

Cahalan, D., & Cisin, I. (1976). Epidemiological and social factors associated with drinking problems. In R. E. Tarter & A. A. Sugerman (Eds.), *Alcoholism: interdisciplinary approaches to an enduring problem* (pp. 523–572). Reading, MA: Addison-Wesley.

Cappell, H. (1975). An evaluation of tension models of alcohol consumption. In R. J. Gibbins, Y. Israel, H. Galant, R. E. Popham, W. Schmidt, & R. G. Smart (Eds.), *Research advances in alcohol and drug problems* (Vol. 2, pp. 177–209). New York: John Wiley & Sons.

Caudill, B. D., & Lipscomb, T. R. (1980). Modeling influences on alcoholics' rates of alcohol consumption. *Journal of Applied Behavior Analysis*, *13*, 355–365.

Caudill, B. D., & Marlatt, G. A. (1975). Modeling influences in social drinking: An experimental analogue. *Journal of Consulting and Clinical Psychology*, *43*, 405–415.

Cellucci, T. (1982). The prevention of alcohol problems: Conceptual and methodological issues. In P. M. Miller & T. D. Nirenberg (Eds.), *Prevention of alcohol abuse* (pp. 15–33). New York: Plenum Press.

Chassin, L., Presson, C., Sherman, S., Corty, E., & Olshavsky, R. (1981). Self-images and cigarette smoking in adolescence. *Personality and Social Psychology Bulletin*, *7*, 670–676.

Christiansen, B. A., & Goldman, M. S. (1983). Alcohol-related expectancies versus demographic/background variables in the prediction of adolescent drinking. *Journal of Consulting and Clinical Psychology*, *51*, 249–257.

Christiansen, B. A., Goldman, M. S., & Inn, A. (1982). Development of alcohol-related expectancies in adolescents: Separating pharmacological from social-learning influences. *Journal of Consulting and Clinical Psychology*, *30*, 336–344.

Collins, R. L., & Marlatt, G. A. (1981). Social modeling as a determinant of drinking behavior: Implications for prevention and treatment. *Addictive Behaviors*, *6*, 233–239.

Collins, R. L., & Marlatt, G. A. (1983). Psychological correlates and explanations of alcohol use and abuse. In B. Tabakoff, P. Sutker, & C. Randall (Eds.), *Medical and social aspects of alcohol abuse* (pp. 273–308). New York: Plenum Press.

Collins, R., Parks, G., & Marlatt, G. (1985). Social determinants of alcohol consumption: The effects of social interaction and model status on the self-administration of alcohol. *Journal of Consulting and Clinical Psychology, 53*, 189–200.

Condiotte, M. M., & Lichtenstein, E. (1981). Self-efficacy and relapse in smoking cessation programs. *Journal of Consulting and Clinical Psychology, 49*, 648–658.

Cooney, N. L., Baker, L., & Pomerleau, O. F. (1983). Cue-exposure for relapse prevention in alcohol treatment. In K. D. Craig & R. J. McMahon (Eds.), *Advances in clinical behavior therapy* pp. 194–210. New York: Brunner/Mazel.

Cooper, A. M., Waterhouse, G. J., & Sobell, M. B. (1979). Influence of gender on drinking in a modeling situation. *Journal on Studies on Alcohol, 40*, 562–570.

Cronkite, R., & Moos, R. (1980). The determinants of posttreatment functioning of alcoholic patients: A conceptual framework. *Journal of Consulting and Clinical Psychology, 48*, 305–316.

Dafters, R., & Anderson, G. (1982). Conditioned tolerance to the tachycardia effect of ethanol in humans. *Psychopharmacology, 78*, 365–367.

Davies, J., & Stacey, B. (1972). *Teenagers and alcohol* (Vol. 2). London: Her Majesty's Stationery Office.

Endler, N. S., & Magnusson, D. (1976). *Interactional psychology and personality*. New York: John Wiley & Sons.

Engle, K. B., & Williams, T. K. (1972). Effects of an ounce of vodka on alcoholics' desire for alcohol. *Quarterly Journal of Studies on Alcohol, 33*, 1099–1105.

Ewart, C. K., Taylor, C. B., Reese, L. B., & DeBusk, R. F. (1983). Effects of early post-myocardial infarction exercise testing on self-perception and subsequent physical activity. *American Journal of Cardiology, 51*, 1076–1080.

Glatt, M. M. (1976). Alcoholism disease concept and loss of control revisited. *British Journal of the Addictions, 71*, 135–144.

Hamilton, F., & Maisto, S. A. (1979). Assertive behavior and perceived discomfort of alcoholics in assertion-required situations. *Journal of Consulting and Clinical Psychology, 47*, 196–197.

Harford, T. C. (1982). Situational factors in drinking context. In P. M. Miller and T. D. Nirenberg (Eds.), *Prevention of Alcohol Abuse*, (pp. 119–156). New York: Plenum Press.

Harford, T. C., Parker, D. A., & Light, L. (1980). *Normative approaches to the prevention of alcoholism* (Department of Health, Education and Welfare Publication No. 79-847). Washington, DC. Government Printing Office.

Harford, T. C., & Spiegler, D. L. (1982). Environmental influences in adolescent drinking. In *Special Population Issues* (Alcohol and Health Monogram 4, Department of Health and Human Services No. ADM 82-1193, pp. 167–193). Washington, DC: Government Printing Office.

Harford, T. C., Wechsler, H., & Rohman, N. (1981). Contextual drinking patterns of college students: The relationship between typical companion status and consumption level. In M. Galanter (Ed.), *Currents in Alcoholism* (Vol. 8, pp. 327–338). New York: Grune & Stratton.

Heather, N., & Robertson, I. (1983). *Controlled drinking*. New York: Methuen.

Hendricks, R. D., Sobell, M. B., & Cooper, A. M. (1978). Social influences on human ethanol consumption in an analogue situation. *Addictive Behaviors, 3*, 253–259.

Hershon, H. I. (1977). Alcohol withdrawal symptoms and drinking behavior. *Journal of Studies on Alcohol, 38*, 953–971.

Higgins, R. L., & Marlatt, G. A. (1975). Fear of interpersonal evaluation as a determinant of alcohol consumption in male drinkers. *Journal of Abnormal Psychology, 84*, 644–651.

Hodgson, R. J., Rankin, H. J., & Stockwell, T. R. (1979). Can alcohol reduce tension? *Behaviour Research and Therapy, 17*, 459–466.

Holroyd, K. A., Penzien, D. B., Hursey, K. G., Tobin, D. L., Rogers, L., Holm, J. E., Marcille, P. J., Hall, J. R., & Chila, A. G. (1985). Change mechanisms in EMG biofeedback training: Cognitive changes underlying improvement in tension headache. *Journal of Consulting and Clinical Psychology, 52*, 1039–1053.

Huber, H., Karlin, R., & Nathan, P. E. (1976). Blood alcohol level discrimination by nonalcoholics: The role of internal and external cues. *Journal of Studies on Alcohol, 37,* 27–39.

Jackson, J. K., & Connor, R. (1953). Attitudes of the parents of alcoholics, moderate drinkers, and nondrinkers toward drinking. *Quarterly Journal of Studies on Alcohol, 14,* 596–613.

Jellinek, E. M. (1960). *The disease concept of alcoholism.* New Brunswick, NJ: Hillhouse Press.

Jessor, R. (1984, November). *Adolescent problem drinking: Psychosocial aspects and developmental outcomes.* Paper presented at the Carnegie Conference on Unhealthful Risk-Taking Behavior among Adolescents, Stanford, CA.

Jessor, R., & Jessor, S. L. (1972). Problem drinking in youth: Personality, social and behavioral antecedents and correlates. In M. E. Chafetz (Ed.), *Proceedings of the Second Annual Alcoholism Conference* (Department of Health, Education and Welfare Publication No. HSM 73-9083, pp. 3–23). Washington, DC: Government Printing Office.

Jessor, R., & Jessor, S. L. (1975). Adolescent development and the onset of drinking. A longitudinal study. *Journal of Studies on Alcohol, 36,* 27–51.

Jessor, R., & Jessor, S. L. (1977). *Problem behavior and psychosocial development: A longitudinal study of youth.* New York: Academic Press.

Jones, M. C. (1968). Personality correlates and antecedents of drinking patterns in adult males. *Journal of Consulting and Clinical Psychology, 32,* 2–12.

Kalin, R. (1972). Self-descriptions of college problem drinkers. In D. C. McClelland, W. N. Davis, R. Kalin, & E. Wanner. (Eds.), *The drinking man* (pp. 217–231). New York: Free Press.

Kandel, D., Single, E., & Kessler, R. C. (1976). The epidemiology of drug use among New York State high school students: Distributions, trends and change in rates of use. *American Journal of Public Health, 66,* 43–53.

Koller, K. M. & Castanos, T. N. (1969). Family background and life situation in alcoholics. *Archives of General Psychiatry, 21,* 602–610.

Kraft, T. (1971). Social anxiety model of alcoholism. *Perceptual and Motor Skills, 33,* 797–798.

Lang, A. R., Goeckner, D. J., Addesso, V. J., & Marlatt, G. A. (1975). The effects of alcohol and aggression in male social drinkers. *Journal of Abnormal Psychology, 85,* 508–518.

Lansky, D., Nathan, P. E., & Lawson, D. M. (1978). Blood alcohol level discrimination by alcoholics: The role of internal and external cues. *Journal of Consulting and Clinical Psychology, 46,* 953–960.

Lazarus, R., & Folkman, S. (1985). *Stress, appraisal and coping.* New York: Springer.

Lentz, T. F. (1941). Personality correlates of alcohol beverage consumption. *Psychological Bulletin, 38,* 600.

Levine, J., & Zigler, E. (1973). The essential-reactive distinction in alcoholism: A developmental approach. *Journal of Abnormal Psychology, 81,* 242-249.

Lied, E. R., & Marlatt, G. A. (1979). Modeling as a determinant of alcohol consumption: Effect of subject sex and prior drinking history. *Addictive Behavior, 4,* 47–54.

Lipscomb, T. H., & Nathan, P. E. (1980). The effects of family history of alcoholism, drinking pattern, and tolerance (blood alcohol level discrimination). *Archives of General Psychiatry, 37,* 571–582.

Lowery, S. A. (1980). Soap and booze in the afternoon. *Journal of Studies on Alcohol, 41,* 829–838.

Ludwig, A. M., & Wikler, A. (1974). A "craving" and relapse to drink. *Quarterly Journal of Studies on Alcohol, 35,* 108–130.

MacAndrew, C., & Edgerton, R. B. (1969). *Drunken comportment.* Chicago: Aldine.

Maddox, G. L., & McCall, B. C. (1964). *Drinking among teenagers: A sociological interpretation of alcohol use by high school students.* New Brunswick, NJ: Rutgers Center for Alcohol Studies.

Maisto, S. A., & Schefft, B. K. (1977). The constructs of craving for alcohol and loss of control drinking: Help or hindrance to research. *Addictive Behavior, 2,* 207–217.

Mann, R. E., & Vogel-Sprott, M. (1984). Control of alcohol tolerance by reinforcement in nonalcoholics. *Psychopharmacology, 75,* 315–320.

Margulies, R. Z., Kessler, R. C., & Kandel, D. B. (1977). A longitudinal study of drinking among high-school students. *Journal of Studies on Alcohol, 38,* 897–912.

Marlatt, G. A. (1976). Alcohol, stress, and cognitive control. In J. G. Sarason and C. D. Spielberger (Eds.), *Stress and anxiety* (Vol. 3, pp. 271–296). Washington, DC: Hemisphere Publishing.

Marlatt, G. A. (1979). Alcohol use and problem drinking: A cognitive–behavioral analysis. In P. C. Kendall, S.D. Hollon (Eds.), *Cognitive behavioral intervention: Theory, research, and procedure* (pp. 319–355). New York: Academic Press.

Marlatt, G. A. (1983). The controlled-drinking controversy: A commentary. *American Psychologist, 38,* 1097-1110.

Marlatt, G. A. (1985). Relapse prevention: Theoretical rationale and overview of the model. In G. A. Marlatt & J. R. Gordon (Eds.), *Relapse prevention: Maintenance strategies in the treatment of addictive behaviors* (pp. 3–70). New York: Guilford Press.

Marlatt, G. A., Demming, B., & Reid, J. B. (1973). Loss of control drinking in alcoholics: An experimental analogue. *Journal of Abnormal Psychology, 81,* 223–241.

Marlatt, G. A., & Gordon, J. R. (1980). Determinants of relapse: Implications for the maintenance of behavior change. In P. O. Davidson & S. M. Davidson (Eds.), *Behavioral medicine: Changing health lifestyles* (pp. 410–452) New York: Brunner/Mazel.

Marlatt, G. A., & Gordon, J. R. (1985). *Relapse prevention: Maintenance strategies in the treatment of addictive behaviors.* New York: Guilford Press.

Marlatt, G. A., Kosturn, C. F., & Lang, A. R. (1975). Provocation to anger and opportunity for retaliation as determinants of alcohol consumption in social drinkers. *Journal of Abnormal Psychology, 84,* 652–659.

Marlatt, G. A., & Rohsenow, D. J. (1980). Cognitive process in alcohol use: Expectancy and the balanced placebo design. In N. K. Mello (Ed.), *Advances in substance abuse* (Vol. 1, pp. 159–199). Greenwich, CT: JAI Press.

McCollam, J. B., Burish, S., Maisto, S., & Sobell, L. (1978). *Affect, arousal, and alcohol: An alternative to tension reduction.* Paper presented at the 86th Annual Convention of the American Psychological Association, Toronto, Ontario, Canada.

McDermott, D. (1984). The relationship of parental drug use and parents' attitude concerning adolescent drug use to adolescent drug use. *Adolescence, 19,* 89–97.

Mello, N. K. (1968). Some aspects of the behavioral pharmacology of alcohol. In D. H. Efrow (Ed.), *Psychopharmacology: A review of progress, 1957-1967* (Public Health Service Publication No. 1836, pp. 787–809). Washington, DC: Government Printing Office.

Merry, J. (1966). The "loss of control" myth. *Lancet, 1,* 1267–1268.

Miller, W. R. (1980). *The addictive behaviors: Treatment of alcoholism, drug abuse, smoking, and obesity.* New York: Pergamon Press.

Miller, W. R., & Caddy, G. R. (1977). Abstinence and controlled drinking in the treatment of problem drinkers. *Journal of Studies on Alcohol, 38,* 986–1003.

Miller, P. M., & Eisler, R. M. (1977). Assertive behavior of alcoholics: A descriptive analysis. *Behavior Therapy, 8,* 146–149.

Miller, P. M., Hersen, M., Eisler, R. M., & Hilsman, G. (1974). Effects of social stress on operant drinking of alcoholics and social drinkers. *Behaviour Research and Therapy, 12,* 67–72.

Miller, P. M., & Mastria, M. (1977). *Alternatives to alcohol abuse.* Champaign, IL: Research Press.

Mischel, W. (1968). *Personality and assessment.* New York: John Wiley & Sons.

Mischel, W. (1973). Toward a cognitive social learning reconceptualization of personality. *Psychological Review, 80,* 252–283.

Mischel, W. (1974). Processes in delay of gratification. In L. Berkowitz (Ed.), *Advances in experimental social psychology* (Vol. 7, pp. 249–292). New York: Academic Press.

Mischel, W. (1981). A cognitive-social learning approach to assessment. In T. Merluzzi, C. Glass, & M. Genest (Eds.), *Cognitive Assessment* (pp. 479–502). New York: Guilford Press.

Monti, P., Abrams D., Binkoff, J. & Zwick, W. (in press). The relevance of social skills training for alcohol and drug abuse problems. In C. Hollin and P. Trower (Eds.), *Handbook of social skills training.* New York: Pergamon Press.

Monti, P. M., Corriveau, D. P., & Zwick, W. (1981). Assessment of social skills among alcoholics versus other psychiatric patients. *Journal of Studies on Alcohol, 42,* 527–530.

Moos, R., & Finney, J. (1983). The expanding scope of alcoholism treatment evaluation. *American Psychologist, 38*, 1036–1044.

Nathan, P. E. (1976). Alcoholism. In H. Leitenberg (Ed.), *Handbook of behavior modification and behavior therapy* (pp. 3–44). New York: Appleton-Century-Crofts.

Nathan, P. E. (1980). Etiology and process in the addictive behaviors. In W. R. Miller (Ed.), *The addictive behaviors: Treatment of alcoholism, drug abuse, smoking, and obesity* (pp. 241–263). New York: Pergamon Press.

Nathan, P. E. (1983). Failures in prevention. *American Psychologist, 38*, 459–467.

Nathan, P. E., & Harris, S. L. (1980). *Psychopathology and society* (2nd ed.). New York: McGraw-Hill.

Nathan, P. E., & Niaura, R. S. (1985). Behavioral assessment and treatment of alcoholism. In J. H. Mendelson & N. K. Mello (Eds.), *The diagnosis and treatment of alcoholism* (2nd ed., pp. 391–455). New York: McGraw-Hill.

Niaura, R. S., & Nathan, P. E. (1984, August). *Development of tolerance to alcohol: Time course and effects of drinking history*. Paper presented at the 92nd Annual Convention of the American Psychological Association, Toronto, Ontario, Canada.

O'Leary D. E., O'Leary, M. R., & Donovan, D. M. (1976). Social skill acquisition and psychosocial development of alcoholics: A review. *Addictive Behaviors, 1*, 111–120.

Plant, M. A. (1979). Learning to drink. In M. Grant & P. Gwinner (Eds.), *Alcoholism in perspective*. Baltimore: University Park Press.

Polich, J. M., Armor, D. J., & Braiker, N. B. (1981). *The course of alcoholism: Four years after treatment*. New York: John Wiley & Sons.

Pomerleau, O. F. (1981). Underlying mechanisms in substance abuse: Examples of research on smoking. *Addictive Behaviors, 6*, 187–196.

Pomerleau, O., Fertig, J., Baker, L., & Cooney, N. (1983). Reactivity to alcohol cues in alcoholics and non-alcoholics: Implications for a stimulus control analysis of drinking. *Addictive Behaviors, 8*, 1–10.

Rachal, J. V., Williams, J. R., Brehem, M. L., Cavanaugh, B., Moore, R. P., & Eckerman, W. C. (1975). *A national study of adolescent drinking behavior, attitudes, and correlates* (Contract No. ADM 281-76-0019). Research Triangle Park, NC: Research Triangle Institute.

Rada, R. T. (1975). Alcohol and rape. *Medical Aspect of Human Sexuality, 9*, 48–65.

Reese, L. (1983). *Coping with pain: The role of perceived self-efficacy*. Unpublished doctoral dissertation, Stanford University, Palo Alto, CA.

Reid, J. B. (1978). Study of drinking in natural settings. In G. A. Marlatt & P. E. Nathan (Eds.), *Behavioral approaches to alcoholism* (pp. 58–74). New Brunswick, NJ: Rutgers Center for Alcohol Studies.

Rist, F., & Watzl, H. (1983). Self-assessment of social competence in situations with and without alcohol by female alcoholics in treatment. *Drug and Alcohol Dependence, 11*, 367–371.

Robins, L. N., Bates, W. M., & O'Neal, P. (1962). Adult drinking patterns of former problem children. In D. J. Pittman & C.R. Snyder (Eds.), *Society, culture, and drinking patterns* (pp. 395–412). New York: John Wiley & Sons.

Rosenberg, C. M. (1969). Determinants of psychiatric illness in young people. *British Journal of Psychiatry, 115*, 907–915.

Rosenberg, H. (1983). Relapsed versus non-relapsed alcohol abusers: Coping skills, life events, and social support. *Addictive Behaviors, 8*, 183–186.

Russell, J. A., & Mehrabian, A. (1975). The mediating role of emotions in alcohol use. *Journal of Studies on Alcohol, 36*, 1508–1536.

Schaeffer, K. M., Parsons, O.A., & Yohman, J. R. (1984). Neuropsychological differences between male familial and nonfamilial alcoholics and nonalcoholics. *Alcoholism: Clinical and Experimental Research, 8*, 347–351.

Schuckit, M. A. (1980). Self-rating of alcohol intoxication by young men with and without family histories of alcoholism. *Journal of Studies on Alcohol, 41*, 242–249.

Schuckit, M. A. (1983). Alcoholism and other psychiatric disorders. *Hospital and Community Psychiatry, 34* 1022–1030.

Shapiro, A. P. (1984). *Human tolerance to alcohol: The role of Pavlovian conditioning processes*. Unpublished doctoral dissertation, Rutgers University, New Brunswick, NJ.

Siegal, S. (1979). The role of conditioning in drug tolerance and addiction. In J. D. Keehn (Ed.), *Psychopathology in animals: Research and clinical application* (pp. 143–168). New York: Academic Press.

Sobell, M., & Sobell, L. (1978). *Behavioral treatment of alcohol problems*. New York: Plenum Press.

Solomon, R. L., & Corbit, J. (1974). An opponent-process theory of motivation: I. Temporal dynamics of affect. *Psychological Review, 81*, 119–145.

Sontag, S. (1978). *Illness as a metaphor*. New York: Farrar, Strauss & Giroux.

Spiegler, D. L. (1983). Children's attitudes toward alcohol. *Journal of Studies on Alcohol, 44*, 545–548.

Strickler, D. P., Dobbs, S. O., & Maxwell, W. A. (1979). The influence of setting on drinking behavior: The laboratory versus the barroom. *Addictive Behaviors, 4*, 339–344.

Sturgis, E. T., Calhoun, K. S., & Best, C. L. (1979). Correlates of assertive behavior in alcoholics. *Addictive Behaviors, 4*, 193–197.

Trower, P., Yardley, K., Bryant, B. M., & Shaw, P. (1978). The treatment of social failure. *Behavior Modification, 2*, 41–60.

Vaillant, G. (1983). *The natural history of alcoholism: Causes, patterns, and paths to recovery*. Cambridge, MA: Harvard University Press.

Wechsler, H., & McFadden, M. (1979). Drinking among college students in New England: Extent, social correlates and consequences of alcohol use. *Journal of Studies on Alcohol, 40*, 969–996.

Williams, A. F. (1966). Social drinking, anxiety, and depression. *Journal of Personality and Social Psychology, 3*, 689–693.

Wills, T., & Shiffman, S. (in press). Stress, coping, and substance use: A conceptual framework. In S. Shiffman, T. Wills (Eds.), *Stress, coping and substance use*. New York: Academic Press.

Wills, T. A., & Warshawsky, A. (1983, August). Stressful events, coping patterns and substance use in middle adolescence. In S. Shiffman (chairperson), *Stress and Smoking*. Symposium conducted at the 91st Annual Convention of the American Psychological Association, Anaheim, CA.

Wilson, G. T. (1977). Alcohol and human sexual behavior. *Behaviour Research and Therapy, 15*, 239–252.

Wilson, G. T. (1978). Booze, beliefs and behavior: Cognitive factors in alcohol use and abuse. In P. Nathan, G. Marlatt, & T. Loberg (Eds.), *Alcoholism: New directions in behavioral research and treatment* (pp. 315–339). New York: Plenum Press.

Wilson, G. T. (1985). Alcohol use and abuse: A social learning analysis. In A. Wilkinson and D. Chaudron (Eds.), *Theories of Alcoholism*. Toronto, Canada: Addiction Research Foundation.

Wilson, G. T., & Lawson, D. M. (1976a). The effects of alcohol on sexual arousal in women. *Journal of Abnormal Psychology, 85*, 489–497.

Wilson, G. T., & Lawson, D. M. (1976b). Expectancies, alcohol, and sexual arousal in male social drinkers. *Journal of Abnormal Psychology, 85*, 587–594.

Wilson, G. T., & Abrams, D. B. (1977). Effects of alcohol on social anxiety and physiological arousal: Cognitive versus pharmacological processes. *Cognitive Therapy and Research, 1*, 195–210.

Wilson, G. T., Lawson, D. M., & Abrams, D. B. (1978). Effects of alcohol on sexual arousal in male alcoholics. *Journal of Abnormal Psychology, 87*, 609–616.

Wilson, G. T., Lipscomb, T. R., Nathan, P. E., & Abrams, D. B. (1980). Effects of tolerance on the anxiety reducing function of ethanol. *Archives of General Psychiatry, 37*, 577–582.

Wilson, G. T., Perold, E., & Abrams, D. (1981). The influence of attribution of alcohol intoxication on interpersonal interaction patterns. *Cognitive Therapy and Research, 5*, 215–264.

Wittman, M. P. (1939). Developmental characteristics and personalities of chronic alcoholics. *Journal of Abnormal Psychology, 34*, 361–377.

Zucker, R. A. (1979). Developmental aspects of drinking through the young adult years. In H. T. Blane and M. E. Chafetz (Eds.), *Youth, alcohol, and social policy*. New York: Plenum.

# II RECENT THEORETICAL MODELS

# 6 Expectancy Theory: Thinking about Drinking

MARK S. GOLDMAN

SANDRA A. BROWN

BRUCE A. CHRISTIANSEN

> The approach distinguishes between these relatively stable competencies which underlie the capacity to construct behaviors and social cognitions, and the encodings, *expectations*, [italics added] goals and values, and self-regulatory systems and plans that guide the individual's choices. Collectively, such a set of person variables allows one to describe discriminative, adaptive, contextually responsive functioning at the level of specific behavior from situation to situation.
>
> Drinking makes the future seem brighter.
>
> Alcohol seems like magic.

The above excerpts from a recent paper on new approaches to personality theory by Walter Mischel (1984, p. 353) and from Factor 1 of the Alcohol Expectancy Questionnaire (AEQ) (Brown, Goldman, Inn, & Anderson, (1980) highlight the central role that cognitive variables have come to play in our understanding of general behavior, and more specifically, behavior related to alcohol consumption. The increasing convergence between the emphasis on cognitive factors in the alcohol literature and in the general psychological literature is a logical occurrence. It has been recognized for decades that adequate research on drug effects requires the use of a placebo control; a

MARK S. GOLDMAN. Department of Psychology, University of South Florida, Tampa, Florida.

SANDRA A. BROWN. Veterans Administration Medical Center and Department of Psychiatry, University of California, San Diego, San Diego, California.

BRUCE A. CHRISTIANSEN. Mt. Sinai Medical Center, Milwaukee, Wisconsin.

placebo control involves (at least in part) direct manipulation of cognitive variables.

In relation to alcohol and other substance abuse, systematic attention to the cognitive realm has been in evidence only over the last 10–15 years, however. During this time there has been increasing recognition that cognitive variables are not merely potential confounds to be controlled, but instead may play an integral role in determining drug effects and in an individual's choice to use or not use a drug. This chapter will review the evidence that has accrued over the past 10–15 years that implicates cognitive factors in the production of psychopharmacologic effects and will discuss our current understanding of the role of these variables. Emphasis will be placed on the cognitive variable known as "expectancy," although in practice it becomes very difficult at times to separate precisely this variable from attributions, attitudes, values, and so on.

It must be emphasized, however, that expectancy theorizing in the alcohol realm has not yet evolved into formal theory. Hence, specific and distinctive predictions are sometimes difficult to state and to test against predictions from other theories. With all due respect to the recent cognitive "revolution" in psychology, we must also be mindful of the intense controversies that have taken place over the years with regard to the use of cognitive mediators as explanatory variables. There was (and still is) good reason for these controversies. Cognitive variables are sometimes loosely stated, difficult to measure, and poorly tied to their antecedent and consequent observable behaviors. Just because they make intuitive sense, and appear to have descriptive explanatory power, does not mean that they will always satisfy the ultimate criteria for success in science: namely, satisfactory prediction and possible control of behavior (see Staddon, 1984). On the other hand, we must also understand that multiple levels of explanation are not only possible, but even necessary when explaining a complex phenomenon such as the behavioral effects of alcohol and continued alcohol usage. Molecular analyses of specific stimuli–responses and neurophysiologic activities must be carried on in parallel with a molar level of analysis which may include cognitions as intervening variables.

One further note: It is possible using expectancy concepts to come very close to the point at which all alcohol-related behavior can be explained without reference to any pharmacological effects of alcohol as a drug. While this line of thinking serves as an interesting and challenging counterpoint to the more typical approach in the drug field of explaining everything with biological variables, one should never be so naive as to disregard pharmacology. Instead, an adequate balance between behavioral and pharmacologic mechanisms is the ultimate goal.

## The Expectancy Concept

The psychological literature is replete with divergent uses of the term "expectancy." Shapiro and Morris (1978) refer to expectancies as "specific attitudes" in their discussion of the genesis of placebo effects. In psychotherapy research, expectancies have been viewed as attitudes formed and modified by previous experience that have an important, nonspecific impact on the process and outcome of psychotherapy (Nash, Frank, Imber, & Stone, 1964). In drug studies investigating placebo effects, and in particular, in those studies utilizing the balanced placebo design (Marlatt & Rohsenow, 1980; Ross, Krugman, Lyerly, & Clyde, 1962), expectancy has been equated with instructional set. That is, when subjects are told that they are to consume alcohol (whether or not alcohol is actually administered), they are spoken of as having been given an "expectancy." In the social psychological literature, the terms attitudes, beliefs, attributions, and expectancies have often been used interchangeably.

Since there is no clearly agreed upon usage for the term expectancy, researchers are obligated to specify the particular usage they intend. However, significant commonalities among these divergent uses should be recognized. The term *expectancy* typically refers to an intervening variable of a cognitive nature. Whether explicit or implied, this cognitive variable is understood to be knowledge (information, encodings, schema, scripts, and so on) about relationships between events or objects in the real world. The term expectancy, rather than attitude or belief, is usually invoked when the author refers to the anticipation of a systematic relationship between events or objects in some upcoming situation. The relationship is understood to be of an if–then variety; *if* a certain event or object is registered *then* a certain event is expected to follow (although the *if* condition may be correlated with, rather than causal of, the *then* event). Expectancies can be inferred to have causal status in that an individual, with his or her own actions, may actually produce a certain consequence upon noting that an *if* condition is fulfilled. Researchers usually intend a close linkage between the cognitive expectancy and antecedent stimuli and consequent behaviors in the real world, although the relationship is too often not clearly specified.

### Development of the Expectancy Concept

In *Purposive Behavior in Animals and Man* (1932), Tolman began the systematic explication of the term expectancy in his Gestalt-significate or expectancy theory. Tolman argues that a full appreciation of human behavior required concepts such as knowledge, thinking, planning, inference, and purpose, as intervening variables between stimuli and responses. However, he remained a behaviorist in that he strongly believed in the linkage of all intervening variables to observables. MacCorquodale and Meehl (1954) further systematized Tolman's expectancy theory by defining expectancy as the learning of a relationship between an initial stimulus (the elicitor), a response, and the expectandum of the response (outcome) in the presence of the elicitor. In this line of thinking, the organism may learn an expectancy linkage without behaving in accord with it. Other factors, including the valence of the consequence, determine whether the expectancy sequence is performed in any specific situation. Within Tolman's framework it is possible for an organism to learn an expectancy without ever performing the behavior or achieving the intended goal (i.e., vicarious learning).

In 1954, Rotter incorporated Lewin's (1951) notion of subjective probability into his definition of expectancy as the "probability held by the individual that a particular reinforcement will occur as a function of a specific behavior on his (her) part in a specific situation or situations." An individual's internal probability estimates are based both on the actual frequency of occurrence of objective past events and by factors specific to an individual. Rotter also conceived of expectancies as generalizing from other similar behavior-reinforcement sequences. Empirical studies reported by Rotter demonstrated the generalization of expectancies along a gradient that could be predicted from "common sense" or cultural knowledge of situational similarities.

Rotter (1981) emphasized that expectancies could increase in stability; that is, as one's experiences in a given stimulus situation become repetitive, the probability held of a particular situation–behavior–reinforcement relationship increases toward an asymptote. Hence, it becomes less likely that an alteration in the real-world contingencies will alter expectancies, and consequently behavior, in a specific situation. This possibility has important implications for any efforts to alter behavior by modifying expectancies. With behaviors such as alcohol or drug taking, the importance of altering expectancies is obvious and will be addressed later in this paper.

In 1972, in a very careful analysis of learning mechanisms, Bolles argued for the replacement of the associative concept of reinforcement with the concept of expectancy. He proposed that what subjects learn is not an associative link between a stimulus and response followed by reinforcement, but rather two kinds of expectancies. In one kind of expectancy, S–S* (the asterisk denotes a stimulus functioning as a biologically important *consequence* rather than as a *cue*), the organism acquires knowledge of the contingencies between a specific stimulus environment and specific outcomes. In the second, R–S*, the organism acquires knowledge of the relationship between its own responses and environmental outcomes. Thus, Bolles elevates the concept of expectancy to a central position in our understanding of learning and agrees that a behavior–outcome expectancy may be held without the organism behaving in accord with it. In this view, the term "expectancy" is simply a name for stored information about contingencies relating environmental cues and organismic responses to biologically important consequences. Mischel (1973) went on to employ Bolles's concepts specifically to human learning.

### Relationship of Expectancies to Observable Behavior

Consider the following quote from Bolles (1972, p. 404): "The point was raised perhaps most dramatically by Guthrie when he made his famous remark that Tolman's rat is so immersed in thought at the choice point that it is quite unable to move a muscle. Guthrie, acting here as a spokesman for all S-R theorists, seems unable to comprehend how having an expectancy can produce movement. An expectancy is merely a hypothetical construct; it is postulated to be an unobservable central event. How can it generate behavior?" Bolles points out, however, that the hypothesized association (bond) between S and R in classical learning theory, and the "hypothesized expectancy," are both constructs, are both unobservable, and are therefore, from a theoretical viewpoint, indistinguishable. It is likely, of course, that Gurthrie and other associationists included an implicit physiologic component in their concept of association. That is, they likely conceived of a complex neural pathway leading from the proximal stimulus to the efferent output that was responsible for movement. In the absence of explicit verification of such a pathway, Bolles correctly points out that neither the concept of association nor the concept of expectancy has a preeminent claim to explaining the increasing correlation between a stimulus and a response with increasing experience. Rather than a complex reflex pathway, the cognitive psychologist (Bolles, 1972, p. 404) likens the nature of the intervening process to map-reading (Tolman) or to "coding, storing, and retrieving information, or making a decision (Irvin, 1971)." Thus, while it is clearly appropriate to advance the concept of expectancy as an important explanatory variable, it must never be forgotten that expectancy research is always an implicit or explicit test of the theoretical utility of expectancy as an intervening variable, which cannot be taken for granted in advance.

If one allows for the moment the replacement of the term expectancy with that of attitude (as is often done in the social psychology literature), then the literature is filled with attempts to determine the correspondence between attitudes and behavior (see review by Ajzen & Fishbein, 1973). While historically the prediction of overt behavior from attitude measures has not been entirely successful (Wicker, 1969), recent work has emphasized situational specificity to improve prediction. That is, the more closely the measures of an attitude correspond to specific features of the situation in which a behavior will be performed, the better the predictability of the behavior. Ajzen and Fishbein (1977) add three elements to the specific behavior to be performed (action) as bearing upon the likelihood of performance: The target toward which the behavior is directed, the context (situation) in which the behavior is to be performed, and the time at which the behavior is to be performed.

In 1977, Bandura offered a categorization of expectancies into two types, outcome and efficacy expectancies, also to increase their utility in the prediction of behavior. He wished to distinguish between expectancies relating particular behaviors to desired outcomes, and an individual's higher-order expectancies that he or she could execute these critical behaviors. The ability to execute particular behaviors was seen by Bandura as limited either by a lack of (social) skills, or performance inhibitions due to fear of failure. As George and Marlatt (1983) have suggested, the response of alcohol consumption may easily become tied to an individual's estimation of their likelihood of being able to execute a desired behavior so that they come to anticipate a performance inability in the absence of alcohol (as we shall see subsequently).

Another conceptual advance made in recent years is the prototype concept. In this view, a decision to apply an expectancy to a stimulus situation is made, not by using the myriad of available cues, but instead based upon a few key features which most characterize that stimulus category (Mischel & Peake, 1982). An example may clarify this concept. Assume we were policemen in charge of monitoring a road where only private passenger cars, but no commercial vehicles, were allowed. How would we decide whether a particular vehicle was a passenger car or a commercial vehicle? Passenger cars may vary widely along dimensions of size and shape, and may include some vans that look very much like trucks. Instead of trying to employ every stimulus characteristic of the vehicle in question, we base our decision on a few stimulus characteristics which are highly prototypic of the category. Therefore, we might begin our job by separating cars from trucks based upon size and shape, and then look further for external lettering as a means of distinguishing between commercial vehicles and passenger cars. Similarly, expectancies about stimulus–outcome relationships may be employed when a particular stimulus complex meets the criteria for a prototype. In this way, particular expectancies can generalize to situations with which the individual has no prior experience, or may be inappropriately applied in a situation in which the prototypic cues are misleading; that is, a situation in which the relationship between stimulus and outcome does not hold. The concept of prototypes modifies the classic notion of stimulus generalization.

In sum, expectancy concepts are not theoretically deficient in their potential ability to predict overt behavior relative to any classical learning theory. The addition of the above refinements may actually offer some advantages in terms of ultimate predictive power. The nuts-and-bolts work to formalize the theory and conduct empirical tests remains, however.

## Origins of Expectancies

Having discussed major theorists (Tolman and Bolles) who have elevated expectancy to a central position in the learning process, it may appear redundant to ask how expectancies originate. From their perspective, expectancies are what is learned in any learning situation; when situational cues or a particular organismic response, and a particular environmental outcome, are correlated and repetitive, an expectancy is acquired by the organism. The registration, encoding, and storage of a high correlation between cues and outcome *is* the expectancy.

However, in relation to alcohol and other drug use, such a conceptualization deemphasizes important considerations. Alcohol consumption potentially has many intraorganismic effects that may alter the perceptual system and provide interoceptive cues (thus altering the overall stimulus context), and may even alter the motor response (efferent) system. Hence, the boundaries between the stimulus–response and the hypothetical (intervening) variable become difficult to establish. The problem becomes compounded when we realize that we are no longer ignorant about the site of action of alcohol and other drugs even at the cellular level within the nervous system (see Goldstein, 1983). How should our knowledge of the effect of alcohol and other drugs on membranes, synaptic transmission, receptor sites, and so forth, be included in our understanding of the nature of an intervening variable such as expectancy?

Unfortunately, refined theorizing which addresses these issues has yet to be undertaken. We shall elaborate on this topic shortly, but first let us address some other approaches to the origin of expectancies that have particular relevance to pharmacologic issues. Some of these approaches may overlap general expectancy theories. They are dealt with separately because each highlights an important aspect of the alcohol-expectancy process.

### Causal Attributions

Concepts under the heading "attribution theory" are closely linked to those of expectancy (Harvey & Weary, 1984) and the concept of attribution is implicit in the expectancy theories reviewed above. In one sense, expectancy and attribution may be viewed as reciprocal; that is, when one holds an expectancy one must have previously attributed a causal (inferred from high observed correlations) relationship to the events in question, and when one attributes a relationship, one ends up holding an expectancy.

One reason for the distinction between attribution and expectancy is historical in that attribution theory derived from social psychology rather than experimental psychology. However, attribution theory emphasizes that humans do not just passively observe correlations between events, but instead deliberately search for causal relationships. Therefore, the linkage of a consequence to an antecedent event could happen very quickly (perhaps with only one occurrence) if circumstances are favorable. Attribution theory also emphasizes the commonsensical theorizing of the everyday individual to explain behaviors that they observe. Thus, attribution theory does not just relate observables, but might also relate an individual's implicit theory of behavior to an observable outcome; for example, a person's "aggressiveness"causes a physical attack. Heider (1958) called this "naive psychology" or the cause–effect analysis of behavior made by the "man in the street." These attributed causes may then determine subsequent responses (Nisbett & Wilson, 1977; Shomer, 1966; Storms & Nisbett, 1970; Valins & Nisbett, 1972). For example, one person may hit another because the first person provoked him, because he or she is aggressive in nature, or because the alcohol made him or her do it.

Attributions may be internal or external (Heider, 1958; Jones & Nisbett, 1971; Kelly, 1967). In internal attributions, causes lie within the person; that is, a specified behavior is considered a consequence of personality, dispositions, preferences, abilities, and so forth. Inferences that a behavior is due to environmental or situational factor(s) are external attributions. Research indicates that individuals tend to attribute their own actions to situational determinants, whereas the same actions by others are more likely attributed to stable personal dispositions (Jones & Nisbett, 1971; Quattrone, 1982). Society-at-large and an individual's cultural background may also pull for particular attributions through cultural theories and stereotypes (Kruglinski, 1979; Nisbett & Wilson, 1977; Ross, 1977).

## Observational (Vicarious) Learning

The possibility of learning by observing others' actions and their effects, rather than by direct experience with stimulus and response contingencies oneself, has been a part of expectancy formulations from the beginning (Tolman, 1932). If what one is learning is a relationship between environmental stimuli, organismic response, and environmental outcomes, then knowledge of these relationships can be acquired indirectly through observations of others as well as directly through one's own experience. Therefore, the reason for highlighting this mechanism is not novelty, but rather because the acquisition of information about alcohol use through vicarious learning seems to play such a central role in alcohol-related behavior. This sort of observational learning may also come via the mass media. Bandura has provided the most extensive empirical demonstrations of vicarious learning beginning in 1962 (Bandura, Ross, & Ross, 1963) and vicarious learning has now been demonstrated across a number of species (e.g., Adler & Adler, 1977) and classes of behavior (Bandura, 1984).

## Classical Conditioning

The potential importance of expectancies as explanatory variables in relation to alcohol-induced behavior was indicated by the observation of apparent alcohol effects in the absence of actual drug administration [that is, in a placebo situation (Marlatt & Rohsenow, 1980; Shapiro & Morris, 1978)]. Equally plausible as an explanation of these effects, however, is classical conditioning. Responses observed following administration of an alcohol placebo are often highly affective or emotional. The autonomic component of such responses could be conditioned classically. Those cues normally paired with alcohol consumption (glass, smell, whiskey bottle, bar, and so forth) may come to elicit a conditioned response similar to that which follows alcohol consumption. Hence, classical conditioning might be viewed either as a source of expectancies, or as a concept that could render expectancies epiphenomenal in explaining the induction of drug effects in the absence of the drug. Classically conditioned alcohol-related responses also could be regarded as cues for alcohol seeking and consumption. Note that theorists such as Bolles (1972) explain classical conditioning via expectancy theorizing.

## Actual Drug Effects

It might appear redundant at this point to note that actual pharmacologic effects could be the source of alcohol-related expectancies. The role of pharmacology in producing expectancies will be elaborated in subsequent sections. Interestingly, however, none of the aforementioned mechanisms require any pharmacologic effects. If alcohol consumption is highly correlated with a particular behavioral outcome, an expectancy can develop *even though alcohol may not produce that effect*. Valins (1966) recognized this possibility in his modification of Schacter's well-known two-factor theory of emotion (Schacter, 1964; Schacter & Singer, 1962). Schacter had theorized that specific emotion derives from generalized physiologic arousal (which might come from a drug such as alcohol) combined with a subsequent cognitive-labeling process. Valins's research indicated that labeling could influence emotional responding even without the presence of biological arousal, although Zajonc (1980) has more recently argued that labeling is not a necessary precursor to emotional reactivity. Such thinking has been recently elaborated by Ross and Olson (1981) in their expectancy-attribution analysis of placebo effects.

### Expectancies and Alcohol Use and Abuse

Any comprehensive attempt to explain alcohol use, and the development of problem drinking and alcoholism, must provide answers to four basic questions. First, how is drinking initiated in a person's lifetime? Alcohol is not a basic foodstuff, and individuals survive very nicely without ever having used alcohol. What are the processes or mechanisms that do induce drinking in those who use alcohol?

Second, what maintains further drinking once drinking has been initiated? It is well known that without some manipulation, animals will not spontaneously consume more than the smallest amounts of alcohol. Combine this observation with anecdotal evidence with which we are all familiar, namely, the reaction of a young child to the first taste of a strong alcoholic beverage (in low alcohol concentration beverages, other olfactory and gustatory cues may mask the alcohol taste, rendering the beverage more palatable), and we must wonder why anyone would continue to drink after their first experience with this drug.

Third, how does alcohol consumption accelerate in some individuals? That is, why do some individuals drink more than others at levels below problem drinking or alcoholism? The answer to this question may overlap with the answer to Question Two, but should be attended to separately.

Last, how do some individuals come to use alcohol at levels that become physically and behaviorally damaging? This question highlights a fundamental paradox in alcohol use: How does behavior persist even in the face of mounting aversive consequences? It has been most common for workers in the alcohol field to address this question using biological mechanisms. Although such mechanisms may play a role, they are not the only means of answering this question.

In the following sections of this chapter we will elaborate upon expectancy formulations which can be proposed to answer each of these questions. At the same time we will review the empiricial data that are consistent with such formulations.

Rather than begin at the beginning, we will begin by answering Question Two, How is alcohol maintained after initial contact? Answering this question provides the best opportunity for a comprehensive explication of expectancy formulations. Once the reader is familiar with these formulations, it will be easy to return to Question One and then proceed onward with Questions Three and Four.

### Maintenance—Why Do People Drink?

Whether the underlying motivating factors are biological or psychological, alcohol use is, at least in part, an acquired (learned) behavior. Alcohol is certainly not an immediate need for infants and children, and once alcohol use is begun in adolescence or adulthood, its pattern tends to accommodate to external contingencies in terms of frequency and amount of drinking, and appropriate time and context for drinking. It has long been recognized that individuals within different societies use alcohol in different ways and may show different effects (MacAndrews & Edgerton, 1969).

In classical associationist learning theory, behavior is learned and maintained by its consequences (outcomes). That is, the consequences of a behavior (reinforcement) are viewed as strengthening an associational link or bond between the stimulus and response. If we cast alcohol use into this line of thinking, the simplest level of analysis would suggest that alcohol use serves as a reinforcer (either positive or negative) that strengthens the associational link between a particular stimulus context and the response of alcohol consumption. This reasoning is the basis for the tension reduction (negative reinforcement) formulation, as originally explicated by Conger (1956). Other types of associationist analysis usually treat alcohol-related behavior as a set of instrumental responses that are reinforced by other environmental outcomes. It is not our purpose, however, to provide a more fine-grained analysis of an associationist view. Instead, this reasoning is noted as a contrast to an expectancy view of alcohol consumption. From an expectancy viewpoint, it is information about the relationship between alcohol consumption and certain outcomes that is learned, and an individual drinks because drinking is anticipated to result in the attainment of desired outcomes.

A moment of reflection, however, indicates that we cannot stop with such a simplistic analysis. The act of alcohol consumption is both a response (putting the glass to your lips and drinking) and a stimulus (taste, the sensations of swallowing, and so on). Once alcohol is absorbed into the bloodstream and begins to impact on neurophysiologic systems, it may also produce interoceptive stimuli (e.g., dizziness) and, as it affects the efferent or motor system, it may result in molecular as well as molar motoric changes (e.g., postural alterations). An individual may also hold expectancies of the relationship between these internal stimuli and responses and external outcomes. At the same time, these internal stimuli and proprioceptive feedback from efferent changes may also serve as sought-after outcomes expected as a consequence of initial alcohol consumption. Furthermore, possible changes in the sensory and motor systems due to alcohol consumption may produce environmental outcomes that would not be achievable without the presence of the drug. That is, looking at the world through "alcohol-colored glasses" may be a far different experience than the world in the absence of the drug. Finally, most drinking takes place in particular contexts (a bar, a party, and so on). Alcohol-related expectancies may pertain to these contexts, in addition to those deriving from alcohol consumption itself. For example, appropriate behavior at a party is not the same as at a faculty meeting; however, since alcohol is often consumed at a party, to the drinker the distinction between alcohol-induced behavior and party-induced behavior may get lost. Thereafter, they may come to expect all such behavior from alcohol consumption.

To help with these concepts, Figure 6.1 offers a simplified schematic representation of the possible expectancy relationships. To the left of the figure we find the environmental stimuli that are common in the usual environmental contexts for drinking, such as a bar, dim lights, people milling about, and so forth. The individual comes to expect that particular environmental outcomes are possible in this stimulus context. Part of this expectancy may be, however, that these environmental consequences are possible only if the alcohol is consumed in that context. Note that in expectancy theorizing the context does not push or force the occurrence of alcohol consumption because the notion of an associative bond between the stimuli and responses is not included. However, the individual may perform the responses of alcohol consumption because this response is expected in this context to result in certain sought-after environmental outcomes. The response of drug taking is

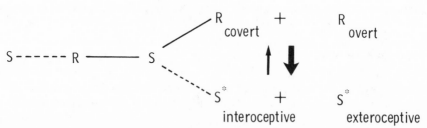

FIGURE 6.1. Diagram of complex expectancy which includes psychopharmacologic effects. S-S* and R-S* expectancies are overlapped. The *S*timulus to the left refers to a drinking context; the *R*esponse to the left refers to alcohol consumption; the *S*timuli before the fork are gustatory; the *R*esponses to the top of the figure are covert and overt motor activities; the *S*timuli to the bottom of the figure are sought-after interoceptive pharmacologic stimuli and sought-after environmental outcomes.

the second element in Figure 6.1. The next element in the figure is the $S$ representing the stimuli that derive from the odor of alcohol, alcohol in the mouth, and the swallowing of alcohol. If we trace the lower pathway in the figure, we will then see, following by some time lag, interoceptive stimuli resulting from the effect of alcohol on the nervous system, and exteroceptive stimuli resulting from alterations in the perceptual system. These intero- and exteroceptive stimuli may, of course, change with the rise and fall of the blood alcohol level (BAL). The intero- and exteroceptive stimuli may also derive from covert and overt motor responses (depicted as the upper pathway in Figure 6.1), which the individual emits in the context of the prior stimuli connected with a drinking setting and alcohol consumption itself. These two types of stimuli and responses may cycle to augment each other (hence, the vertical arrows); the motor responses produce stimuli and the stimuli serve as a context in which motor responses are carried out (which are then expected to result in desired stimulus outcomes). Because specific alcohol-related expectancies may include both the external situational context and internal cues in a varying ratio, it is possible for some alcohol expectancies to be less situationally bound than others. That is, some expectancies may be primarily based on internal alcohol cues and therefore could readily occur in many contexts. Most expectations, however, have developed in specific situations and include these situational cues as part of the expectancy.

So far we have discussed this model with the understanding that some of the stimulus outcomes and the alcohol-related responses are the direct result of psychopharmacologic effects. What is intriguing about this model, however, is that it is quite applicable even if we do not assume that alcohol has any relevant psychopharmacologic effect. That is, the same behavioral and stimulus outcomes could be produced in the absence of a true drug effect. All this model requires is a belief in a relationship between stimuli and outcomes or between behaviors and outcomes. The model operates even if these beliefs are not based on reality. For example, if a person in a typical drinking environment believed they had consumed alcohol, they might produce covert and overt alcohol-related responses (which appear to observers as pharmacologic effects), not because the drug action of alcohol made them do it, but instead because they believed desired outcomes were available if they behaved in this way in this context. The covert and overt responses produced in this situation might even result in interoceptive cues which, to the drinker, mimic psychopharmacologic effects of alcohol. It is essential to note that such an explanation is relevant even if a drug has an actual psychopharmacologic action, as long as the use of the drug ever results in a behavior that is not a direct consequence of its pharmacology. For example, the drug may just produce discriminable interoceptive cues without significant behavioral consequences, which then trigger the operation of expectancies, thereby resulting in overt behaviors that are not directly due to pharmacologic drug actions. Such an effect could also occur in an active drug at doses at which the drug is not behaviorally potent. Thus, the potential occurrence of expectancy effects always complicates the interpretation of pure psychopharmacologic effects. Without careful analysis we can never be sure which drug effects are directly the result of pharmacologic/physiologic mechanisms and which may be expectancy effects.

Later we will explore possible sources of alcohol-related expectancies, but one source is embedded in the explanatory process noted above. Consider a person who is introduced to alcohol use in a festive, partying context. Prior expectancies of appropriate behavior in such a situation might result in the individual's feeling euphoric and acting in an upbeat, party-type manner even without the use of alcohol. However, since alcohol use is included as part of the festive context, the person may leave that situation with expectancies of a party context plus alcohol use resulting in valued outcomes such as rewarding social interaction. At the time of the next party, this person may expect that alcohol use will once again achieve these desired outcomes.

Note that in the analysis outlined above no attribution concepts have been employed. The behaviors to be predicted are entirely a function of the expectancies held by the individual. Attribution concepts would be necessary only if it were found that an individual had a bias toward outcome expectancies from situational cues or from their own behavior independent of pharmacologic effects. Even here, attributional analysis is unnecessary if it can be shown that some stimuli are more salient. For example, drug taking may be a more salient cue than background stimuli, and thus individuals might tend to expect outcomes as a function of drug taking rather than as a function of their own behavior. Therefore, it remains to be seen whether including attributional concepts offers an advantage over pure expectancy formulations.

## Empirical Studies—Maintenance

General expectancy formulations can be applied to any study on the behavioral effect of alcohol, as well as to sociological, anthropological, personality, or epidemiologic literature on alcohol use. In order to apply boundaries to the literature that might be reviewed, we will confine ourselves to those studies that most directly address the issue of expectancies.

***Placebo and Balanced Placebo Studies.*** For many years, the use of the placebo condition in alcohol investigations was largely a control formality, following common practice in pharmacology research. It was not anticipated (or hoped) that the placebo condition would produce effects of the same magnitude and type as actual alcohol administration, and therefore few steps were taken to convince subjects that they were being given alcohol (even though they were not). Increasing appreciation in recent years for nonpharmacologic factors has led to methodological additions to tease out these factors.

Reviews of the conceptual issues and methodologies attendant to adequate study of placebo effects can be found elsewhere (Marlatt & Rohsenow, 1980; Shapiro, 1978), but a few pitfalls should be noted to help the reader evaluate placebo studies. First, the "double-blind" strategy for the control of placebo effects is difficult in alcohol studies where the preparation of drinks immediately prior to consumption is preferable. But, of course, in the absence of the double-blind strategy, experimenter bias can occur. Second, if the interoceptive cues associated with alcohol consumption are perceived as absent or incomplete, the placebo condition may be rendered ineffective, particularly if subjects are told as part of an informed consent procedure that they may receive alcohol. Such incongruities may undermine expectancy effects that otherwise would have been operative. Shapiro (1978) recommends an "active" placebo that mimics relevant internal cues, but such cues are difficult to mimic for alcohol without the administration of another behaviorally active drug. In the same vein, the common use of mouthwash to help disguise the taste of alcohol may at the same time alter cues important to the operation of expectancy effects. Finally, if the behavioral effects of actual alcohol administration are found to be significantly greater than those of placebo administration, it is not necessarily true that the placebo condition produced no effect.

Researchers have begun recently to include "antiplacebo" conditions (Carpenter, 1968), in which the subjects are lead to believe that they are not receiving the active drug when in fact they are given the active drug. This condition assesses drug effects in the absence of any instructional set. The addition of this cell has resulted in the "balanced placebo design" (Marlatt & Rohsenow, 1980), which includes four cells: told drug, given drug; told no drug, given no drug; told drug, given no drug; and told no drug, given drug. It offers advantages over the single placebo design, but does not solve all problems attendant to investigating expectancy effects. It is difficult in light of interoceptive cues to give people alcohol and keep them convinced that they have not received alcohol. Subjects should therefore be distracted from their internal cues by inducing them to focus on some external source of stimulation, but gauging the effectiveness of such strategies is difficult. For the same reason, one is restricted to dosages that provide minimal interoceptive cues, for above 100 mg% subjects would likely become very aware of having consumed alcohol. Given that this design requires four cells for the investigation of even a single dose, the addition of other dosage levels for determination of dose-response curves renders studies increasingly unwieldy, Subjects' confusion between interoceptive drug cues and contradictory instructional sets may produce some misleading results.

*Craving and loss of control.* The first traditional beliefs approached from this new perspective were the associated concepts of craving and loss of control in alcoholics. Craving was understood to be an intense, probably physiologically induced, desire for continued alcohol consumption once any alcohol was consumed, that would lead to a loss of control over the amount of one's drinking. In an attempt to distinguish pharmacologic from nonpharmacologic sources of craving, Merry (1966) administered alcohol to inpatient alcoholics without their knowledge. Each morning for approximately 2 weeks each patient was given a fruit-flavored beverage. On alternate days the beverage was either completely nonalcoholic or included one ounce of vodka (which would not be readily detected). Patients were then asked to rate their level of alcohol craving later each day, apparently as part of the routine treatment program. These ratings were not affected by the beverage consumed, and therefore a nonpharmacologic basis for craving was indicated.

Engle and Williams (1972) followed with a similar study that used both the antiplacebo condition employed by Merry and the customary direct placebo condition (the full balanced placebo design). Subjects rated their degree of craving for alcohol the day before, 40 minutes after, and 5 hours after receiving an administered beverage. Subjects were told they were receiving either alcohol or a vitamin drink, and were actually given alcohol or a vitamin drink independently of what they were told. Once again, craving ratings were a function of the instructional manipulation; subjects told they were getting alcohol reported more craving.

Going beyond mere ratings of craving, Marlatt, Demming, and Reid (1973) assessed actual alcohol consumption using the balanced placebo design in conjunction with a "taste-rating task." Nonabstinent alcoholic subjects were primed with a beverage 15 minutes prior to the taste-rating task. As they were given to understand it, their job was to drink from marked flasks containing the beverage and rate the taste qualities of that beverage. The actual dependent measure was how much ad libitum drinking they actually did. The results were clear; alcoholics who believed they were administered an alcoholic beverage consumed more than those subjects who believed they were given only tonic, regardless of whether or not they actually had been administered alcohol.

Of course, it is possible that had higher doses of alcohol been used in these studies, the results might have shown a pharmacologically induced craving or loss of control. Whether or not that is the case, however, the results strongly support nonpharmacologic factors (perhaps expectancies) as crucial to one of the most traditionally held beliefs about the effects of alcohol on alcoholics. Even Ludwig, Wikler, and Stark (1974), who averred that craving is a real, rather than subjective phenomenon, have argued that a classically conditioned subclinical alcohol withdrawal syndrome rather than a pharmacologically induced mechanism is responsible.

*Disinhibition—Sex and Aggression.* Among the effects that folklore commonly attributes to the pharmacology of alcohol are that alcohol increases sexual arousal and functioning, and that alcohol increases aggressivity. "Disinhibition theory," or the belief that alcohol suppresses inhibitory constraints on "instinctual" impulses, serves as an umbrella for these more specific beliefs. Carpenter and Armenti (1972) pointed out that disinhibition theory was severely flawed from the outset because of a lack of evidence that any of these behaviors is normally pressing for expression but is held in check by inhibitions. Moreover, MacAndrew and Edgerton (1969) in their cross-cultural analysis of the effects of alcohol on sexual and aggressive behavior concluded that "the presence of alcohol in the body does not necessarily even conduce to disinhibition, much less inevitably produce such an effect" (p. 88). Instead, these behaviors seem to occur within culturally sanctioned limits that may vary among cultures.

Recent laboratory studies have focused on cognitive factors as an underlying source of these beliefs. In relation to human sexual functioning, this research was aided by the introduction of the penile and vaginal plethysmograph to measure actual physiologic sexual arousal. These devices made possible research previously undertaken only with animals. Prior work with humans had primarily used projective tests as dependent measures and was primitive by comparison.

Studies on male sexual response uniformly revealed that increasing alcohol dose was related to decreases in penile tumescence (Briddell & Wilson, 1976; Farkas & Rosen, 1976; Wilson, Lawson, & Abrams, 1978). Complicating the picture, however, were balanced placebo design studies that showed that if males believed they had consumed alcohol, both penile tumescence and self-reported arousal increased (as long as the alcohol dose in the expected alcohol-received alcohol cell was not so high as to counteract the expectancy effect) (Briddell *et al.*, 1978; Lansky & Wilson, 1981; Wilson & Lawson, 1976). The study by Briddell *et al.* even showed that the instructional set for alcohol could increase other physiologic measures of arousal, including heart rate and skin temperature.

Two other studies in this sequence further revealed that instructional set interacted with individual differences. Lang, Searles, Lauerman, and Adesso (1980) found that all subjects increased their viewing time of erotic slides as a function of the pornography ratings of the slides, including those subjects initially high in guilt about sex. However, high-sex-guilt subjects who believed they received only tonic did not show this relationship. Hence, the belief that alcohol was consumed permitted high-sex-guilt subjects to exercise their sexual curiosity in the same manner as low-sex-guilt subjects. Lansky and Wilson (1981) then reported that high-sex-guilt subjects showed increased penile tumescence when they believed they had consumed alcohol. In an attempt to discover the medicating mechanism, these authors assessed selective attention and recognition memory for erotic stimuli in both the visual and auditory modalities. Unfortunately, their findings only narrowed the field of possible mechanisms; the effect of alcohol expectations on sexual responsivenss was apparently not mediated through its influence on selective attention and memory processes.

In women the picture has been somewhat less clear, partly due to the paucity of studies with human females using the more advanced methodology. Wilson and Lawson (1976) showed that for women, as in men, a direct physiologic index of sexual arousal (vaginal engorgement) decreased with alcohol dose. Remarkably, women's self-reports of arousal increased with increasing intoxication even as their physiologic sexual response declined. This increase in subjective arousal might be ascribed to expectancy effects. In a follow-up balanced placebo study, Wilson and Lawson (1978) found that the expectancy manipulation did not produce increased physiologic (vaginal) arousal to sexual stimuli as it had in men. However, once again women's self-reported arousal increased as they subjectively felt more intoxicated despite decreasing physical arousal.

In sum, we remain far from a complete understanding of the interaction between alcohol, expectations, and sexual behavior, although some advances have been made. It seems clear that increasing alcohol dose has a negative effect on penile tumescence and vaginal engorgement. Remarkably, however, at doses at which alcohol has little effect on physical arousal in males, the belief that one has consumed alcohol can increase self-reported arousal, penile tumescence, and other physical measures of arousal. This surely demonstrates the profound effects of instructional set (an perhaps expectancy). In women, belief alone had no effect on vaginal engorgement in one study (Wilson & Lawson, 1978), but women's self-reported sexual arousal increased with intoxication despite decreasing vaginal engorgement. Vaginal engorgement and penile tumescence are not the totality of sexual response, however. In women, interoceptive stimuli arising from alcohol may cue expectancies for other aspects of sexual functioning, such as the seeking of, and interaction with, sexual partners. In addition, decreased penile response arising from moderate alcohol doses may increase sexual pleasure by prolonging intercourse. What this line of research has established, however, is that the sexual story cannot be completed with just an understanding of the direct chemical effects of alcohol.

Aggression has been highly associated with alcohol use in common folk-lore and in sociological surveys. Alcohol has a demonstrated connection with assaultive behavior (Mayfield, 1976), homicide (Virkkunen, 1974), suicide (Buglass & McCulloch, 1979), stabbings (Shupe, 1954), and crimes of all types (Sobell & Sobell, 1975). Unfortunately, good empirical studies of al-cohol and aggression are even fewer in number than the studies on sex and alcohol, and much work remains to be done. One major problem in the literature is that aggressive behavior is itself far from unitary. Without an adequate basis, researchers have compared verbal and physical forms of aggression, and have often failed to take into account whether the subject is provoked, who is the target of the aggression, the setting for the aggression, and so forth. The interested reader is referred to Carpenter and Armenti (1972) and Nathan and Lisman (1976) for thorough reviews of this literature. In this chapter, a few recent studies that strongly suggest the involvement of expectancies on aggressive behavior will be highlighted.

In a study that brought the expectancy concept foursquare into the in-vestigation of alcohol and aggression, Lang, Goeckner, Adesso, and Marlatt (1975) used the standard 2 × 2 balanced placebo design but added a factor in which subjects were either provoked to aggress by exposing them to an insulting confederate, or not provoked. Aggression was assessed by the in-tensity and duration of "shocks" supposedly administered to a confederate of the experimenter on a Buss aggression apparatus. The results showed that subjects who believed they had consumed alcohol were more aggressive than subjects who believed they had consumed a nonalcoholic beverage, whether or not they actually received alcohol. Dose levels were in the 100 mg/100 ml range. Provocation increased aggression in all conditions, but was unrelated to the beverage administered.

However, while the Lang et al. (1975) study has unequivocally indicated that an instructional set manipulation can be responsible for increasing ag-gressive behavior, efforts to tease apart pharmacologic versus expectancy effects in relation to aggression are far from complete. For example, Lang, Goeckner, Adesso, and Marlatt (1975) have left open the possibility that higher alcohol doses directly produce aggression. These higher doses are, of course, very difficult to study in a balanced placebo design because they produce strong interoceptive cues that may contradict the instructional set. Studies have shown increased aggression after provocation at higher than 100 mg% doses (Schmutte & Taylor, 1980; Zeichner & Pihl, 1979, 1980), but expectancy effects were, unfortunately, not assessed.

As noted earlier, expectancy effects also may be operative even in the presence of clear interoceptive cues for alcohol. That is, expectancy effects may be responsible for certain behaviors rather than biological drug actions even at doses that are pharmacologically active. For example, Babor, Berglas, Mendelson, Ellingbow, and Miller (1983) showed that hostile verbal interaction and aggressive thematic content were greater during alcohol intoxication than during placebo administration, even though these measures were unrelated to changes in the blood alcohol curve (ascent and descent) as time passed. Since hostility remained constant while blood alcohol did not, it was inferred that pharmacologic effects of alcohol were not directly responsible for the hostility and aggressiveness. Instead, the cues given off by alcohol on the ascending and descending side of the BAL curve may have triggered expectancies which were in turn responsible for the behavior observed. An additional wrinkle has been added by Rohsenow and Bachorowski (1984) in a recent series of studies that tested aggression in the presence of moderate to high doses with some subjects (1.13 mg/kg). They found that for all subjects at higher doses, and men at both the high and low dose, subjects expecting alcohol were significantly *less* aggressive. In this work, Rohsenow and Bachorowski followed up on work by Brown, Goldman, Inn, and Anderson (1980), who showed that subjects actually hold multiple expectancies at the same time. Rohsenow and Bachorowski suggested that for their subjects, expectations of social and physical pleasure at higher doses were stronger than expectations of aggressivness. Hence, these competing expectancies resulted in less aggressiveness at the higher doses. Of course, the stronger expectancy in this experimental context might not be the stronger in a different (real-world) context. As pointed out by these authors, a critical finding from their study is that the pharmacologic action of alcohol does not necessarily increase aggression at a low or even at a moderately high dose; the particular behavioral effect observed may be due to an expectancy effect triggered by interoceptive alcohol cues. Furthermore, Phil, Smith, and Farrell (1984) have shown that expectancies might change not only with alcohol dose, but also may relate to the type of beverage, in that those expecting whiskey show more aggression than those expecting beer.

***Emotion—Anxiety and Euphoria.*** If any characteristic has been seen as a central, defining aspect of alcohol use, it is the presumed capacity of alcohol to alter anxiety, depression, and other moods. In this regard, alcohol may be viewed as the commonly used mood-altering psychotropic medication. This assumption has also been popular with scientists, and many theoretical and laboratory efforts to bring this feature of alcohol use into the scientific mainstream have been made. Unfortunately, these conceptions have not easily transported from the lay world to the scientific mainstream. Does alcohol induce positive affect (euphoria), does it relieve aversive emotional states (anxiety and depression), can it do both, or perhaps neither? These questions continue to be intensely investigated. The concept of alcohol as tension-reducer has been reviewed many times (see Cappell, 1975; Cappell & Greeley, Chapter 2, this volume; Cappell & Herman, 1972) and the notion of alcohol as a mood improver has also been addressed (see Freed, 1978; Marlatt, 1984).

We certainly cannot resolve these controversies. Nor will we serve as ideologues for the expectancy concept by attempting to show that all affective changes are expectancy effects. The mood altering effects of alcohol are related to dose (Kreutzer, Schneider, & Myatt, 1984), setting of alcohol consumption (Pliner & Cappell, 1974), rate of consumption (Conners & Maisto, 1979), whether the blood alcohol level is ascending or descending (Babor *et al.*, 1983), subjects' gender (Abrams & Wilson, 1979; Wilson & Abrams, 1977), and probably a variety of other independent variables not yet clearly specified. (These variables probably relate to other alcohol effects such as sex and aggression but have been less studied in those areas.) At the least, however, expectancies can be strongly tied to these effects. More importantly, careful consideration of expectancies may give us a better handle than currently exists as to the relationship of the aforementioned independent variables to the production of mood changes.

One way to place the multiplicity of potential variables that may relate to affective responses within a workable framework is to posit expectancies as an internal mediator. That is, setting, dose (interoceptive cues), person, and so forth, may all exert their influence via expectancy mediation. For example, alcohol effects may vary with different settings because people hold different expectancies in connection with different settings. Similarly, expectancies may be different for different doses, and may vary among individuals. As discussed earlier, generalized expectancies may be applied by the individual to novel stimulus situations based upon perceived similarity or prototypicality. Hence, it would be possible for a finite and perhaps rather limited group of expectancies to produce a wide variety of mood changes.

In the first of the balanced placebo studies relating to affect and mood (recall that these studies manipulate instructional set—expectancy effects are inferred), Polivy, Schueneman, and Carlson (1976) measured self-reported anxiety in the context of an electrical shock threat. Subjects in this study who received alcohol reported themselves to be less anxious than subjects who did not receive alcohol. However, those subjects who were led to believe they had consumed alcohol gave higher ratings of anxiety than those who thought they were getting orange juice and vitamin C only. The possibility that in certain contexts the belief that one has consumed alcohol may actually increase anxiety was later confirmed in a study by Abrams and Wilson (1979). Social anxiety was measured in a situation in which females were asked to make a favorable impression on a male confederate who was neither verbally nor nonverbally responsive. In this context, female subjects who were led to believe they had consumed alcohol showed significant elevations in physiologic arousal as measured by heart rate and skin conductance, and were rated as more anxious on observational measures of social behavior, than those subjects who were not led to believe they had consumed alcohol (whether or not they were). It is important to recognie that a social anxiety manipulation may have better defined alcohol expectancies associated with it than the threat of shock which is rarely, if ever, experienced in a real-world drinking environment. Also note that this is far from the first time that alcohol use has been reported to result in tension increase (Goldman, Taylor, Carruth, & Nathan, 1973), but this is the first time that tension increase was clearly demonstrated to result from manipulation of subjects' beliefs. It is interesting, however, that in an almost identical experiment with males, Wilson and Abrams (1977) found that anxiety decreased if subjects believed they had consumed alcohol. It is likely that women felt more threatened than men in this laboratory social situation because the women believed that alcohol might cause them to lose self-control, an eventuality that women stereotypically defend against. In fact, several women in the first study reported that they found it necessary to monitor their behavior closely after drinking. Thus, these studies provided evidence not only for the relevance of expectancies to the production of alcohol-related affective behavior, but also demonstrated that expectancies may vary widely depending upon the sex of the subject and the context for alcohol use. Even the nature of the anxiety-inducing situation may affect the emotional response that occurs in the context of the belief that one has consumed alcohol.

Two investigations performed by Sobell and his colleagues at Vanderbilt University studied how self-reports of mood were affected by the balanced placebo manipulation and by parameters of alcohol consumption including fast versus slow drinking, and ascent versus descent of blood alcohol concentrations (Connors & Maisto, 1979; McCollam, Burish, Maisto, & Sobell, 1980). McCollam et al. (1980) also investigated subjects' pulse rate and skin conductance. In what was apparently a rather sterile, laboratory environment, these studies found a more profound effect for actual alcohol dosage than for the instructional manipulation. Self-reports of affects and sensations were higher on the ascending than the descending phase of the BAL curve; rate of drinking had much less effect. The two physiologic measures were influenced by both instructions and actual alcohol ·consumption. Only nonchalance, a measure the authors felt related to relaxation, was unambiguously higher in subjects who believed they had consumed alcohol. Also in a laboratory environment that included extensive psychophysiologic recording, Levinson, Sher, Grossman, Newman, and Newlin (1980), found that only alcohol influenced psychophysiologic and questionnaire measures of prestress and stress (self-disclosing speech or threat of shock) levels of "tension." One possible interpretation of all these results is that subjects do not hold expectations of affective and sensation changes from alcohol unless some clearly defined and familiar stimulus context is provided (unlike a sterile laboratory). Since it is unlikely that subjects have developed specific expectancies about the effects of alcohol in a laboratory, expectancy effects may be difficult to find in the absence of effective efforts to make the laboratory situation analogous to real life. Also likely is that rigorous monitoring of subjects' physiologic and subjective changes induces close self-attention to interoceptive sensations during alcohol consumption, thereby defusing the expectancy manipulation.

Support for these contentions comes from recent work by Sher (1985), who measured alcohol expectancies using an expectancy questionnaire (AEQ) (Brown, Goldman, Inn, & Anderson, 1980) and found that expectancies prior to the experimental manipulation operated to affect mood and physical sensations more in a group setting than when subjects drank alone. This finding is consistent with the earlier work of Pliner and Cappell (1974) who also found the typical euphoriant effects of alcohol in a group, but not in an individual setting. Furthermore, when Sobell and his colleagues (Vuchinich, Tucker, & Sobell, 1979) exposed subjects to humorous stimuli while recording laughter and self-reported mood, the instructional manipulation was prepotent in influencing subjects' laughter despite a laboratory setting. In each of these cases the experimental stimuli were sufficiently familiar so that prior expectancies could be operative and also served to distract subjects from their interoceptive cues.

*Cognitive and Motor Performance.* The study of the relationship of alcohol expectancy effects to cognitive and motor performance highlights the importance of knowing in advance whether subjects maintain expectancies about a particular behavior, before conclusions can be drawn about the relevance of alcohol expectancies to behavioral outcomes. For example, when Vuchinich and Sobell (1978) selected male subjects because of their prestated belief that alcohol disrupts motor performance, they found that both actual alcohol consumption and instructional set for alcohol increased errors on a divided attention task. Alcohol alone impaired performance on a pursuit motor task. In contrast, Miller and her colleagues, who did not preselect subjects, found no instructional set effects on free-recall memory tasks (Miller, Adesso, Fleming, Gino, & Lauerman, 1978). Similarly, Rimm, Sininger, Faherty, Whitey, and Perl (1982) found no instructional set effects on driving simulator performance. Hence, we cannot decide whether these subjects were unusual, or whether no expectancies exist in connection with memory and simulated driving. Another possible explanation for varying results in connection with cognitive and motor performance measures was suggested in a study by Williams, Goldman, and Williams (1981). In this study, performance on a number of tasks remained intact after alcohol administration but only if dose and instructional set were congruent. Hence, subjects may, in fact, expect alcohol to produce impairment on cognitive–perceptual–motor tasks, and so work harder when they believe they have been given alcohol in order to compensate.

*Other Behaviors.* A few studies that have evaluated expectancy effects do not fall readily into the above categories but are worth noting. Korytnyk and Perkins (1983), noting a reported association between vandalism and alcohol consumption, studied the possibility that alcohol expectancy effects might be responsible for graffiti production. They concluded that the belief that one had consumed alcohol was not as powerful as alcohol itself in inducing graffiti writing, and therefore, that alcohol and not expectancies was responsible for behavioral disinhibition. We have already seen the flaws in disinhibition theory and, in fact, in evaluating another behavior supposedly related to disinhibition, Abrams and Wilson (1983) showed that the belief that subjects had consumed alcohol lessened their ability to delay gratification, but alcohol itself did not.

The use of alcohol for pain reduction is a practice that goes back a long way into the history of medicine. For this reason two studies by Cutter and his colleagues on the relationship of alcohol and pain are of considerable importance. Using a cold pressor test for pain induction, Cutter, Maloof, Kurtz, and Jones (1976) reported that alcoholics' subjective pain decreased as dosage increased, whereas nonalcoholics reported no pain decrease. Since no differential physiologic response was found between the two groups, subjective pain reduction in alcoholics was attributed to expectancy factors interacting with the interoceptive cues induced by increasing dosage. In a second investigation, Brown and Cutter (1977) found that prior drinking habits greatly influenced the effects of alcohol on pain reduction. A higher dose reduced pain in alcoholics, but actually increased pain in subjects that usually drank at home with friends. As noted above, it is quite possible that prior history operates via centrally recorded expectancies.

*Expectancy Content.* Recall that placebo studies only provide indirect evidence for the operation of expectancies. The experimental manipulation is limited to an instructional set about the beverage being administered, and the provision of a variety of tangible stimulus cues such as mixing drinks from labeled bottles, alcohol odors, the use of glasses typically associated with alcohol consumption, bar settings, and so on. Because it is necessary to infer the expectancy from the behavioral outcomes observed, other interpretations are possible (e.g., classical conditioning).

Further validation of the utility of the expectancy concept requires that researchers obtain a more direct means of assessing and manipulating expectancy content itself. How might we identify expectancies and gain some knowledge of the variations in expectancies across individuals and across various dosages and settings? As indicated by Mischel (1984), the most straightforward approach may be the best: ask. In some recent work in our laboratories we have done just that, and this work along with the work of other investigators who have taken the same tack has offered promise not only for specifying variations in expectancies, but for actually using this newly acquired knowledge to predict other parameters of drinking.

The direct examination of expectancy content using mathematical procedures such as factor analysis also provides a methodology for taking the next steps in the development of expectancy theory in relation to alcohol and drug use. First, the full domain of alcohol expectancies can be explored in concert using these methods, instead of on an expectancy-by-expectancy basis. Most importantly, mathematical rules can be derived that relate expectancies to observable parameters of drinking such as frequency and amount, and those behaviors that occur under the influence of alcohol. Without quantification, the expectancy approach remains more heuristic than scientifically precise. If expectancies, once quantified, successfully predict various aspects of drinking behavior, expectancy formulations are supported as part of the causal matrix. Once such validation is obtained, the next step would be to attempt intervention into the development and operation of expectancies. The ultimate goal, of course, would be modification of problematic drinking practices.

*What are the alcohol expectancies?* For years, developers of assessment tools for measurement of alcohol use and abuse have incorporated items tapping alcohol-related expectancies. These items have usually been included as "reasons for drinking," "attitudes about alcohol," and so forth. Some of these studies shall be noted subsequently. However, because the target was not direct examination of the full range of alcohol expectancies, many contaminants appear in these studies that preclude straightforward appreciation of the operation of expectancies. For example, items included value judgments about the goodness or badness of drinking, or cognitive associations to drinking situation, such as, Drinking alcohol allows you to be with people who are drinking.

To begin the process of specifying the domain of alcohol expectancies, we undertook a study to examine directly alcohol-related expectancies across a broad range of individuals and then used multivariate procedures to process this large group of expectancies into a more limited, and hopefully useful, set of alcohol expectancy factors (Brown, Goldman, Inn, & Anderson, 1980). From interviews with 125 adults with drinking histories ranging from non-drinking to chronic alcoholism, we obtained an exhaustive list of 216 possible expectancies of behavioral and subjective outcomes from alcohol use. These 216 possible drinking consequences were converted into an agree or disagree format, and then subjected to item analysis procedures to reduce the total item pool to 90 items. These 90 items were then administered to 450 college students, and a principle components factor analysis was performed on their responses to ascertain the general expectancies underlying these items. The six independent expectancies extracted were that alcohol transforms experiences in a positive way (Drinking makes the future seem brighter; Alcohol seems like magic), enhances social and physical pleasure (Having a few drinks is a nice way to celebrate special occasions; Drinking is pleasurable because it's enjoyable to join in with people who are enjoying themselves), enhances sexual performance and experience (After a few drinks, I am more sexually responsive; I often feel sexier after I've had a few drinks), increases power and aggression (If I'm feeling restricted in any way, a few drinks make me feel better; After a few drinks it is easier to pick a fight), increases social assertiveness (If I have a couple of drinks it is easier to express my feelings; A few drinks make it easier to talk to people); and reduces tension (Alcohol enables me to fall asleep more easily; Alcohol helps me sleep better). This study thus established an initial domain of human expectancies about the reinforcing effects of moderate alcohol consumption. The fact that four of these factors—sexual enhancement, increased power and aggression, increased social assertiveness, and tension reduction—overlapped with those expectancies inferred from the findings of the placebo studies cited earlier, added convergent validation for the utility of specific alcohol expectancies. Equally important, the study demonstrated that expectancies can be verbalized. Therefore, they can be more directly assessed and, perhaps more directly manipulated, rather than merely being inferred from situations having a variety of possible interpretations.

Most striking about these results was that the first two factors, which were highly general and accounted for most of the variance, indicated the belief that alcohol is a "magical" agent that actually can *transform* experiences (particularly social and physical experiences) into much more positive ones. Perhaps the pervasiveness of alcohol use throughout human history is in part explained by the perceived capacity of alcohol to perform these magical transformations.

Remarkably, other studies that have examined expectancylike concepts have shown a great deal of overlap with the expectancies reported in Brown, Goldman, Inn, and Anderson (1980) despite methodological variations (Deardoff, Melges, Hout, & Savage, 1975; Faber, Khavari, & Douglass, 1980; Isaacs, 1979; Southwick, Steele, Marlatt, & Lindell, 1981). These expectancies have even repeated in an adolescent sample aged 12–19 (Christiansen, Goldman, & Inn, 1982). The one class of expectancies that were not picked up in the study by Brown, Goldman, Inn, and Anderson (1980) because of the emphasis of positively reinforcing effects, are expectancies relating to behavioral impairment. Studies that included such expectancies have noted both the expectation for performance impairment as well as expectations for performance improvement (Christiansen, Goldman, & Inn, 1982), particularly in relation to higher dosage levels (Southwick *et al.*, 1981) or problem drinking (Faber *et al.*, 1980; Isaacs, 1979).

As noted above, support for the utility of expectancy theory will come through the development of quantitative rules for predicting observable behavioral outcomes using expectancies. Although considerable work remains to be done, there now exist a number of studies that have demonstrated the capacity of quantified expectancies to predict observable behavior. Much of this validation is concurrent (data collected on expectancies and other aspects of drinking behavior at the same time), but nevertheless the power of expectancies to predict various aspects of drinking-related behavior has been remarkable. Furthermore, a few recent studies have shown that questionnaire assessments of expectancies can predict behavioral outcomes in the laboratory (Rohsenow & Bachorowski, 1984; Sher, 1985) and following treatment for alcohol abuse (Brown, in press).

*Individual differences in expectancies and their relation to other aspects of drinking.* Not only does multivariate methodology help reduce the number of operative expectancies to a workable range, but it also provides us with each expectancy factor in the form of a scale. Hence, we can use these scales not only to establish that an individual holds a particular expectancy, but also to measure the strength with which he or she holds that expectancy. It is perhaps not surprising to find that there is individual variation in the degree to which individuals hold these expectancies. What does provide a major step in the validation process of expectancy theory, however, is the finding that these individual variations also relate to a wide variety of self-reported drinking patterns. In a series of studies in our laboratories, we have gathered evidence that expectancy patterns can successfully predict drinking behavior at all levels of the drinking continuum, from beginning drinking in adolescents through alcoholism. Brown, Goldman, Inn, and Anderson (1980) provided preliminary evidence in this regard with the observation that global expectancy factors were related to abstinence or light consumption while heavier drinking subjects tended to expect increased levels of sexual and aggressive behavior. Additional studies since that time have increasingly clarified and expanded our understanding of the relationship between expectancies and drinking patterns. In order to explore these relationships in adolescents, Christiansen *et al.* (1982) first established the domain of alcohol expectancies of adolescents at three age groups (12- to 14-year-olds, 15- to 16-year-olds, 17- to 19-year-olds). The expectancies discerned in these groups were remarkably consistent despite varying levels of drinking experience in the different age categories. They were ultimately refined in a second study (Christiansen & Goldman, 1983) to seven expectancy factors for the entire adolescent group. In these studies negative expectancies were included. The adolescent alcohol expectancies were:

(1) Alcohol is a powerful positive transforming agent.
(2) Alcohol can enhance or impede social behavior.
(3) Alcohol improves cognitive and motor functioning.
(4) Alcohol enhances sexuality.
(5) Alcohol leads to deteriorated cognitive and behavioral functioning.
(6) Alcohol increases arousal.
(7) Alcohol promotes relaxation or tension reduction.

Remarkably, predictions of adolescent drinking patterns using these expectancies surpassed in accuracy those obtained using a variety of background/demographic variables that had been previously established in the literature as powerful predictors (age, sex, socioeconomic status, ethnic background, religious affiliation, religiosity, parental attitude and drinking behavior, the presence of an alcoholic in the family, and the respondent's alcohol attitude). In the Christiansen and Goldman (1983) study, expectations for enhanced social behavior predicted frequent social drinking, whereas expectations for improved cognitive and motor functioning predicted adolescent problem drinking. In a recent doctoral dissertation at Wayne State University, Canter (1984) followed up this work by showing that, among a set of fifty possible predictor variables the expectation for enhanced social behavior best discriminated between nondrinking and light-drinking high school drinkers. The variables included the ones noted above as well as psychiatric history and family interaction variables. Canter (1984) also found that just below variables such as the number of arrests, peer drinking behavior, and divorce or death of a parent, expectations of enhanced social behavior and enhanced sexuality best discriminated heavy-drinking high school students.

The predictive advantage afforded by quantified expectancies over background variables has been carried over into a college population as well (Brown, 1985). In this somewhat older group, expectations of enhanced social and physical pleasures were the primary effects attributed to alcohol by frequent social drinkers. In contrast, the tension reduction expectancy was the strongest predictor of problematic drinking. These predictive relationships have been cross-validated.

At the upper end of the drinking continuum in adults, Brown, Goldman, and Christiansen (1985) compared the alcohol expectancies of 171 alcoholics in treatment with those of 65 hospitalized nonalcoholic medical patients. The two groups were matched relative to age, sex, marital status, race, income, occupation, education, ethnic background, religious affiliation, and religious attendance. The medical patients were then divided into those that reported heavy drinking and those that reported nonheavy drinking. The results again demonstrated the utility of expectancies. As expected, alcoholics scored the highest on the expectancy scales, and the heavy-drinking medical patients were quite similar in response pattern. In contrast, the non-heavy-drinking medical patients scored substantially lower than these other two groups. Within the same study, this observation was replicated in relation to heavy, moderate, and occasional-drinking college students. Once again, strength of alcohol expectancy was greater in the heavier-drinking groups relative to the non-heavy–drinking groups. The repeated observation of a relationship between the strength of positive alcohol expectancies and the degree of drinking among diverse types of adult drinkers indicates the robustness of the alcohol expectancy approach. Using the AEQ developed in our laboratory (Brown, Goldman, Inn, & Anderson, 1980), other researchers also have found that alcoholics score higher on the six alcohol expectancies than medical patients (Zarantonello, unpublished manuscript, 1984) and a nonmedical adult comparison group (Connors, O'Farrell, & Cutter, 1984). This response also has been recently found in adolescent alcohol abusers in treatment as compared to demographically comparable nonabusing peers (Brown & Creamer, 1985).

Even when expectancies were assessed using a different questionnaire format, the predictive power (concurrent validity) of expectancies held up. Southwick *et al.* (1981) constructed an expectancy scale based upon adjective dimensions and derived three factors (stimulation and perceived dominance, e.g., active–passive; pleasurable disinhibition—e.g., happy–sad; behavioral improvement—e.g., clumsy–coordinated). They then asked their subjects to respond to these items twice. The first time they were to indicate how moderate amounts of alcohol would affect them and the second time they indicated how too much alcohol would affect them. Heavier drinkers reported expectancies of greater stimulation/perceived dominance and pleasurable disinhibition during moderate intoxication than did lighter drinkers. Expectancylike items were also included in a comprehensive alcohol assessment tool developed by Wanberg, Horn, and Foster (1977). In this and in other studies that included expectancylike items (Faber et al., 1980; Glynn, LoCastro, Herman, & Busse, 1983; McCarty, Morrison, & Mills, 1983; Rohsenow, 1983), predictive power for drinking patterns was also demonstrated.

RELATIONSHIP OF EXPECTANCIES TO OTHER CRITERION VARIABLES. Expectancy studies have begun to examine how well expectancies might relate to alcohol consumption variables other than simple drinking pattern. For example, Southwick, Steele, Marlatt, and Lindell (1981) found that individuals hold differing expectancies for different dosage levels of drinking. All types of drinkers except abstainers expected stimulating alcohol effects at lower doses of alcohol and more neutral or even impaired effects at higher doses. Rohsenow (1983), using a variant of our AEQ, found that individuals' expectancies for their own drinking differed from those held for others' drinking. Specifically, subjects expected others to be more strongly affected by alcohol than they themselves would be. Consistent with earlier work, heavier drinkers held stronger expectancies on most scales than did light drinkers. In a recent study by Brown (in press), alcoholics' expectations for positive global effects and increased social assertiveness successfully predicted whether they would continue in treatment or drop out early. In the same study, expectations for tension reduction, increased social assertiveness, and sexual enhancement were correlated with prognosis ratings made by the treatment staff. One-year follow-up of treatment outcome showed that the strength of the alcoholic's expectation for relaxation and tension reduction better predicted treatment outcome than traditional variables such as participation in aftercare programs, marital status, employment status, physical living environment, social living environment, social support, stress level, and activities.

Placebo studies had already indicated that expecting alcohol had differential impact on behavior as a function of gender. To summarize: expecting alcohol increased aggression in males at low and moderate doses, but at lower doses women appeared more verbally aggressive. Expecting alcohol increased subjective sexual arousal in both males and females but the physiological decrement associate with alcohol in females at all doses was counteracted in males at low doses, so that increased physiological sexual arousal was evident. In heterosexual social situations, women expecting alcohol displayed more anxiety, whereas physiologic and behavioral measures of anxiety decreased among males.

In terms of specific expectancies, females tended to expect more social pleasure with moderate alcohol consumption than men, who were more likely to expect arousal and aggressive behavior (Brown, Goldman, Inn, & Anderson, 1980; Rohsenow, 1983). After variance for drinking pattern was removed, females reported overall lower positive expectancies than male counterparts. Male alcoholics reported higher specific positive expectancies than female alcoholics but alcoholic women held comparable expectancies of sexual enhancement and higher expectancies of alcohol's negative effects. Gender differences were less apparent among adolescents showing similar drinking patterns.

In sum, we now have ample evidence that alcohol-related expectancies can predict a wide variety of drinking patterns and drinking-related behaviors. The predictive power of these expectancies is at least as good, and perhaps better than, the best demographic and drinking history variables used in earlier work. Furthermore, as we increase our data base, there is every reason to believe we will become capable of even more accurate quantitative prediction. These accomplishments of quantified expectancy instruments give considerable support to alcohol-related expectancies as a theoretical explanatory device. What remains to be accomplished, however, are experimental studies that manipulate expectancies and show consequent changes in behavioral outcomes. The next step requires considerable ingenuity, however; in our society alcohol expectancies cannot be created for the first time when a subject enters a laboratory setting, so whatever manipulations are undertaken will always occur in the face of preexisting expectancies. Unambiguous inferences, therefore, may be difficult to achieve.

We have now completed our review of expectancy theorizing and its associated data base which addresses the question "Why do people drink?" Contained in this review are partial answers to the other three questions noted earlier. At this point, however, it is useful to turn our attention specifically to each of these questions separately. Recall that we began with Question 2, and so now we must back up a step to Question 1, How is drinking initiated?

### How Is Drinking Initiated?

The research history of the alcohol field is filled with unsuccessful attempts to get animals to drink more than minor amounts of alcohol without force-feeding or extensive genetic manipulation (Goldstein, 1983; Peterson, 1983). Obviously, alcohol has little inherent appeal for animals. As noted earlier, it is also highly unlikely that a child sampling alcohol for the first time will demonstrate any degree of affinity for the taste. Hence, it would appear that some form of external incentive is necessary to induce drinking, particularly past the initial contact with alcohol. To gain some appreciation of the variables that may influence drinking styles, researchers have extensively examined the adolescent years. A review of this literature may provide insights into the initiation process.

The large number of research studies devoted to adolescent drinking have consistently shown that drinking in this age range can be predicted from parental drinking behavior and/or drinking attitudes (Barnes, 1977; Lassey & Carlson, 1980; Maddox, 1964; Smart & Fejer, 1972; Strauss & Bacon, 1953). Equally predictive of adolescent drinking are peer group attitudes and drinking patterns (Barnes, 1981; Donovan & Jessor, 1978; Harfond & Spiegler, 1983; Huba & Bentler, 1980; Jessor & Jessor, 1975; Stacey & Davies, 1970). It is still somewhat of an open question as to which influence, parents or peers, is more potent regarding which drinking phenomena (drinking onset, drinking pattern, problematic drinking). The weight of the evidence seems to favor peer influence over parental influences, especially in older adolescents (Biddle, Bank, & Marlin, 1980; Harfond & Spiegler, 1983; Margulies, Kessler, & Kandel, 1975). Other relevant variables include ethnic and religious variables (Burkett, 1980; Cahalan & Cisin, 1968; Globetti, 1967; Knupfer & Room, 1967; Landman, 1952; Maddox, 1964; Ullman, 1960; Wilsnack &

Wilsnack, 1980), socioeconomic status (Cahalan & Cisin, 1968), race (Donovan, Jessor, & Jessor, 1983; Harfond & Mills, 1978; Harfond & Spiegler, 1983; Wilsnack & Wilsnack, 1980), sex (Globetti, 1972; Harfond & Mills, 1978; Margulies, Kessler, & Kandel, 1977; Smart & Gray, 1979), age (Harfond & Mills, 1978), and delinquency (Stacey & Davies, 1979). Taken as a whole, this literature indicates groups of adolescents/children "at risk" for either problematic adolescent drinking or problematic adult drinking: (1) offspring of alcoholics, (2) children who are exposed to contradictory parental models concerning drinking attitudes and behavior, (3) children of abstaining parents who made nondrinking a very emotionally laden topic, (4) adolescents whose friends hold maladaptive alcohol attitudes or who display problematic drinking practices, (5) individuals of certain ethnic-religious groups, (6) adolescents low in religiosity, (7) delinquent adolescents, and (8) adolescents who hold maladaptive alcohol attitudes. Multivariate models that have combined these and other personality, social environment, and behavioral variables have successfully predicted onset of adolescent drinking (Jessor & Jessor, 1975), adolescent problem drinking (Donovan & Jessor, 1978), and continuation or discontinuation of problem drinking when adolescents become adults (Donovan, Jessor, & Jessor, 1983).

It is important to recognize, however, that most of the variables that correlate with adolescent drinking are not immediately present at the time that alcohol is actually consumed. Even among those variables that might be present, such as adolescent peer group interaction, the mere observation of a correlation does not by itself offer a mechanism responsible for the behavioral effects of drinking. Hence, a theoretical understanding of adolescent and adult drinking calls for postulation of intervening variables that can tie together prior experience (such as from parents and religious teachings, and so on) and actual alcohol behavior. The postulation of alcohol-related expectancies offers one such theoretical model. Thus, it may be hypothesized that a major effect of a child's accumulated experience with family, religious training, mass media, advertising, and so forth, is to provide the individual with a set of alcohol expectancies. Then, in a potential drinking situation, it is these expectancies that provide a "blueprint" for the way in which an individual will drink and the behavior they will evidence upon drinking. Empirical support for this hypothesis comes from our 1983 factor-analytic investigation of alcohol expectancies in three separate age groupings (12–14, 15–16, 17–19 years) of adolescents (Christiansen, Goldman, & Brown, 1985). Remarkably, the expectancies held by 12- to 14-year-olds were highly similar to those held by the older adolescents, and with those held by college students (Brown, Goldman, Inn, & Anderson, 1980), even though the 12- to 14-year-olds as a group had little or no direct personal experience with alcohol consumption. Evidently, such direct experience is not essential for the development of expectancies, leaving the above sources as an obvious major determinant.

That expectancies may have a potent role in mediating adolescents' decisions to drink and the behavioral effects of alcohol is already indicated by a number of empirical studies. Schlegel, Crawford, and Sanborn (1977) used an expectancy-value model originated by Fishbein (1967) to predict adolescents' intentions to drink and enjoyed moderate success (correlations of .33 with actual drinking for an entire adolescent sample and .47 for adolescents above the legal age of 18). Biddle, Bank, and Marlin (1980), using a path analysis technique, found that most parental and peer influences on drinking were indirect and were instead channeled through the adolescents' own expectations, and especially their drinking preference (enjoyment or dislike of drinking). Thus, these existing predictive models seem to favor internal and/ or proximal variables (attitudes, values, expectations, normative beliefs, preferences) as predictors of adolescent drinking over distal and/or external variables (parents, peers, religious affiliation, and so on).

The most direct evidence for the power of expectancies in the prediction of adolescent drinking comes form a recent study in our laboratories (Christiansen & Goldman, 1983). In this study, we first factor-analyzed the drinking styles of 1580 adolescents ranging in age from 12 to 19 years. The three drinking styles found among adolescents were frequent social drinking, problem drinking, and family drinking. We then set up a competition between alcohol expectancies as determined by the AEQ for Adolescents (AEQ-A) and the most powerful demographic/background variables shown in prior studies to predict adolescent drinking. These include respondent's age, respondents' degree of religiosity, maternal drinking behavior, paternal drinking behavior, socioeconomic status, and the adolescent's overall attitude about the acceptability of drinking. As expected, the demographic/background variables produced significant multiple correlations with drinking style. These correlations ranged as high as .57 for the frequent drinking style. However, for all three drinking styles, the alcohol expectancy scales added unique predictive power. That is, the alcohol expectancy scales significantly increased predictive power. For example, when the expectancy scales were added to the background variables, a multiple correlation of .67 with the frequent drinking style was achieved (compared to the .57 noted above for the demographic/background variables taken alone). These results clearly show that adolescent alcohol expectancies meet the criterion for use as an intervening variable; they provide levels of prediction beyond those that could be achieved by measuring other preexisting variables alone. Of course, the nature of this study was such that only concurrent validity could be assessed, and not true predictive validity measured after a time lag. Such data are currently being collected.

## How Does Drinking Accelerate?

Although indirectly dealt with throughout our discussion of expectancies, it is important at this point to specifically explicate how expectancy theory might explain individual differences in alcohol use; that is, why do some individuals drink more than others? Research has already indicated a limit to the number of general expectancies (Brown, Goldman, Inn, & Anderson, 1980; Christiansen, Goldman, & Inn, 1982; Christiansen & Goldman, 1983), as well as individual differences in the strength with which each of the alcohol expectancies is held. These differential strengths are related to alcohol usage and the behavioral consequences of alcohol usage (at least as self-reported). Obviously, from an expectancy viewpoint the key to individual differences in alcohol use is the development of individualized strengths and patterns of alcohol-related expectancies; once particular patterns of expectancies are in place, differential alcohol consumption patterns would ensue. Of course, a perfect linkage betwen expectancy patterns and alcohol consumption should not be anticipated. Individuals may hold similar outcome expectancies but find the value of the outcome differentially important. Two individuals may expect that alcohol will help them relax in a particular situation; only one may find relaxation a desirable outcome.

Three sources of differential strength or pattern of expectancies may be hypothesized. First, each individual's own particular life experiences prior to alcohol use (usually in childhood) may provide differential expectancies. For example, usage of alcohol by family members, or even in the absence of alcohol usage, parents' expectations about alcohol use may teach children their individualized set of expectancies (via modeling). Peer group modeling and mass media may also play a role in this training process. It is evident that from this view, the groundwork for differential alcohol usage patterns is already laid down prior to any actual alcohol use.

Second, once alcohol consumption begins, different experiences with alcohol may serve to differentially strengthen alcohol expectancies. For example, if a teenage drinks frequently in a party situation, expectations of alcohol as a modifier of social and physical pleasure may be strengthened. Recall from our earlier discussion that these behaviors might occur even if alcohol itself is not chemically responsible for these behavioral outcomes. Thus, expectancies can be differentially strengthened in the absence of any direct pharmacologic effect. Imbedded in this second process is the possibility that alcohol consumption might come to be seen as an essential component of a complex response leading to a desired stimulus outcome. For example, if an individual believed that his or her social skills were inadequate for achieving desired social outcomes at a party, but that their skills augmented by alcohol consumption would enable the achievement of these outcomes, it would always be necessary to drink at parties. In this way, individual differences in behavioral skills might interact with expectations to determine the level of alcohol use.

Finally, individual physiologic differences may interact with pharmacologic effects to determine differential expectations. This process may be direct or indirect. Hence, alcohol may actually pharmacologically produce an effect that, with repetition, becomes an expectancy. For example, some individuals may achieve greater tension reduction than others from alcohol use and thereby develop different expectancies. An indirect effect on expectancies might derive from a nonspecific psychopharmacologic action. An individual with greater physiological tolerance for alcohol may drink larger amounts on more occasions and thereby have the opportunity for generation of stronger expectancies. Conversely, with the development of increasing tolerance, a consistent drinker may need ever higher doses to produce the interoceptive cues necessary to trigger expectancies.

Considerable empirical evidence already exists to support the existence of differential expectancies, some of which has been cited earlier. Any of the studies that correlated expectancies with levels of alcohol consumption offer support. The aforementioned recent report from our laboratory (Brown, Goldman, & Christiansen, 1985) has shown that heavier drinkers hold stronger alcohol expectancies, whether they are alcoholics, medical patients who are not diagnosed as alcoholic, or college students. Furthermore, heavy-drinking college students held expectancies less strong than the heavy-drinking medical patients, and the heavy-drinking medical patients held expectancies less strong than the alcoholics. Heavy-drinking subjects in each of these groups held stronger expectations than lighter-drinking members of the same group.

## Relationship of Expectancies to Alcoholism

Expectancy theorizing demands a continuity position on the development of alcohlism; that is, alcoholism is regarded as stemming from a greater number, or greater potency of the elements already discussed. In this view, expectations of positive effects of alcohol consumption become associated with more and more life contexts. Hence, individuals come to consume alcohol in more situations (and at higher doses due to tolerance) and therefore are increasingly at risk for the development of physiologic addiction. Thus, "alcoholism" is simply a term we apply when drinking has accelerated to the point of severe and multiple negative physical, psychological, and social consequences, rather than requiring some special physical disease process.

Of course, many argue for the presence of a specialized biological condition in alcoholism. Evidence for this special biological state usually comes from genetic studies supposedly showing familial transmission independent of environment (Murray, Clifford, & Gurling, 1983) or in the form of physiologic markers in those individuals at high risk for alcoholism (Swinson, 1983). It is beyond our present scope to thoroughly review this evidence but let us note that the evidence may support a biological exclusionary principle rather than indicating a necessary and sufficient biological determinant. Genetic and physiologic differences in the ability to tolerate (be comfortable with) the use of alcohol do seem to occur. Hence, some individuals may be excluded from the pool of potential alcoholics due to their initial discomfort with alcohol. From the remaining group of individuals who are comfortable with alcohol use, some subset might eventually develop the condition we call alcoholism. Understood this way, the biological evidence is quite compatible with expectancy theorizing. That is, biological factors may place an individual within a population at risk for developing alcoholism; within this population, psychological factors such as expectancy may determine the specific individuals that then go on to become alcoholics. Alcoholism researchers increasingly recognize the possibility of different subsets of alcoholics, with different etiologies. Differential combinations of biological factors and expectancies may play a role in determining these subsets. Note that even if biology was a direct and immediate cause of alcoholism, the operation of psychological factors would not be excluded. Alcoholics at times begin to drink following upon a period of abstinence. Sometimes this abstinence period may be lengthy. At such times, it is necessary to postulate some mechanism such as expectancies to explain why drinking is initiated. The need for postulating such a mechanism would be evident even if there were some strong biological urge to drink. The individual would still have to choose to drink based upon an expectation of relief from this urge.

Consistent with this logic, Brown, Goldman, and Christiansen (1985) found that alcoholics had the strongest alcohol expectancies when compared with heavy and non-heavy-drinking medical patients and college students, and these findings have since been essentially replicated (Zarantonello, unpublished manuscript). Furthermore, we have traced a possible expectancy "marker" for development of problem drinking in alcoholism (Christiansen, Goldman, & Brown, in press). In this study, it was found that, unlike their low and moderate drinking peers, adolescent problem drinkers expect improved cognitive and motor functioning under the influence of alcohol. Adolescent alcohol abusers in treatment also hold this expectancy (Creamer & Brown, 1985). A reanalysis of adult alcohol expectancies then revealed this same strong expectancy for improved cognitive and motor functioning in adult alcoholics, which was not present in nonalcoholics. Also recall that placebo studies have also suggested that alcoholics maintain expectations of craving and loss of control in the presence of alcohol (Merry, 1966) and that such expectations may even determine excessive drinking (Engle & Williams, 1972; Marlatt, Demming, & Reid, 1973).

## Expectancies and the Pharmacology of Alcohol

To this point we have minimized our discussion of alcohol pharmacology. Our initial adolescent study (Christiansen, Goldman, & Inn, 1982) begs, however, for a role for pharmacology. While demonstrating that expectancies are largely acculturated prior to alcohol consumption, these results also threaten an infinite regress paradox. That is, if children learn expectancies from parents, peers, and mass media, and expectancies alone determine the behavioral effects of alcohol, then how did alcohol expectancies ever develop in the first place? One possibility is an actual pharmacologic substrate for expectancies, but a substrate that is weak or intermittent. Hence, in the laboratory, identifying specific alcohol effects may be difficult. But we have also seen that expectancies are not uniform across individuals and that the behavioral effects of alcohol vary widely across cultures (MacAndrew & Edgerton, 1969).

At present, therefore, most compelling is the possibility that alcohol produces a generalized pharmacological effect and not the specific effects indicated by expectancies. This generalized effect has been loosely described as "behavioral plasticity" (Wilson, 1983, p. 512), but attempts to specify this effect are few in number. In a recent review, Marlatt (1984) has suggested generalized arousal from low doses and depressant effects from higher doses. Goldman has postulated alcohol-induced eccentricity of response selection by the nervous system resulting in relatively more frequent emissions of low-probability responses (Weintraub & Goldman, 1983). In contrast, Brown, Mansfield, and Skurdal (1980) have argued that alcohol eliminates low-probability responses. In any case, these generalized pharmacologic effects may then interact with the sociocultural environment to produce specific expectancies.

## Other Psychological Theories of Alcohol Use and Abuse

Given that expectancy theory has been applied to all of learned behavior (Bolles, 1972), it should come as no surprise that expectancy theory can replace most psychological theories of alcoholism. Such comprehensiveness should recommend expectancy theory to alcohol researchers, especially given its fundamental parsimony. However, the lack of a formal statement of the theory impedes clear empirical comparisons. Some brief conceptual comparisons may be made, however, using a few examples from the theories offered in this volume.

### Personality Approaches

Expectancy theorizing is readily compatible with personality theories and has even been employed as a central concept in personality theory (Mischel, 1984).

In this view, expectancies are merely one of the operative mechanisms responsible for the observed consistency in behavior that is called personality. Two examples: In power theory (McClelland, Davis, Kalin, & Wanner, 1972), alcohol as a power increaser may be viewed as a major alcohol expectancy. Rotter's (1966) locus of control theory *is* an expectancy theory; internal versus external locus of control refers to expectations of the most probable sources of controlling contingencies.

### Tension Reduction Theory

We have seen that humans expect that alcohol reduces tension and we know that such effects can occur independent of alcohol pharmacology (Wilson & Abrams, 1977); hence, expectancies may be one source of tension-reducing effects when they occur. It is also possible that inconsistent findings in the animal research occurs because animals hold no prior expectancies of alcohol effects.

### Deviance Theory

Deviance theory (Jessor & Jessor, 1975) already employs expectancy concepts, albeit in a less central role. However, prior research (Christiansen & Goldman, 1983) has shown that expectancies alone may be as good a predictor as many of the other variables employed in deviance theory.

### Self-Handicapping

Self-handicapping (Jones & Berglas, 1978) is easily conceived as an expectancy or combination of expectancies of one's own nonability plus expectancies of alcohol as a producer of performance impairment.

### Summary and Evaluation

Despite insufficient formalization, expectancy theorizing has led to the uncovering of phenomena (nonpharmacologic effects in balanced placebo designs) that might not have been uncovered otherwise, has been consistent with a wide variety of other data not specifically designed to assess expectancy concepts, and has led to prediction strategies that would not be possible otherwise (expectancy assessment instruments). As we shall see next, new intervention strategies also issue from expectancy theorizing. Expectancy theorizing is quite compatible with biological mechanisms and therefore could integrate easily with a diverse body of literature.

It is also evident, however, that increased formalization is needed to permit unique predictions that would permit comparative tests with other theories. If possible, studies that deliberately manipulate expectancies should also be designed so that causal inferences can be made. One decade of attention to expectancy mechanisms in relation to alcohol and other substance use has been highly productive; it remains to be seen how far the model can go.

## Prevention and Treatment Implications

Expectancy theorizing offers a number of unique directions for prevention and treatment. First, successful intervention depends on accurate targeting of intervention resources. We have already noted that expectancy response patterns on such instruments as the AEQ and the AEQ-A (Brown, Goldman, Inn, & Anderson, 1980; Christiansen & Goldman, 1983) had predictive power equal to or greater than that of major demographic/background variables. Hence, assessment of expectancies in both adolescents and young adults may identify high-risk individuals without the need for obtaining sensitive personal information. Since there may be a relationship between alcohol expectancies and subsequent drinking patterns, it might be possible to intervene and head off later problems before they develop.

Expectancy assessments can suggest intervention strategies. Attempts might be made to modify those expectancies that are strongest in a particular individual, or which research has shown to be most predictive of later problem drinking. The expectancy for improved cognitive and motor functioning falls in this latter category. The task now is for clinical researchers to develop treatment strategies designed to modify these expectancies. Since many of these expectancies are at least in part nonpharmacologic, it should be possible to devise means to undermine their potency. In any case, this is a direction for intervention researh that has not yet been pursued. For expectancies such as those for increased relaxation, it may be possible to train individuals to achieve desired ends without recourse to alcohol or other substances (Goldman & Klisz, 1982).

Beyond the clinical level, expectancy theorizing also offers new vistas for society-wide prevention work. The current prevailing strategy for prevention efforts through the mass media and in schools is to use "scare tactics" that attempt to discourage drinking and other drug use by sensitizing individuals to the negative effects of abusing such substances. Scare tactics have rarely discouraged any sort of problematic behavior, particularly in adolescents and young adults who readily feel that such messages do not apply to them. An empirical demonstration of this failure came from Christiansen and Goldman (1983) who found a virtual absence of relationship between awareness of the deleterious effects of alcohol and amount of alcohol consumption. The debunking of positive expectancies may be superior to "scare" messages in undermining the motivational matrix for alcohol use.

Of course, there is already some suggestion in the literature that existing expectancies may be difficult to modify (Rotter, 1954). Therefore, celebrations in advance of positive developments are surely premature. Nevertheless, this line of thinking opens a new door that has yet to be entered in relation to this enormous social problem.

## Acknowledgments

Portions of this work were supported by Grant No.06132 to Mark S. Goldman and Bruce A. Christiansen, Grant No. AA05946 to Mark S. Goldman, and Grant No.AA06143 to Sandra A. Brown, from the National Institute on Alcohol Abuse and Alcoholism.

Appreciation is also expressed to the Veterans Administration Hospital in Allen Park, Michigan; the Henry Ford Hospital Detroit, MI—Maplegrove Treatment Center; the Salvation Army Harbor Light Center in Detroit; Scripps Memorial Hospital of La Jolla, California; and Veterans Administration Medical Center, Cabrillo Doctors Hospital, Crossroads, and Pathfinders of San Diego, California from which subjects were selected who participated in various studies included in this chapter. We would like to thank Greg Smith, who reviewed the manuscript, and Anne Knox, who did the typing.

Portions of this work were completed at Wayne State University in Detroit.

## References

Abrams, D. B., & Wilson, G. T. (1979). Effects of alcohol on social anxiety in women: Cognitive versus physiological processes. *Journal of Abnormal Psychology, 88,* 161–173.

Abrams, D. B., & Wilson, G. T. (1983). Alcohol, sexual arousal, and self-control. *Journal of Personality and Social Psychology, 45,* 188–198.

Adler, L. L., & Adler, H. E. (1977). Ontogeny of observational learning in the dog (*Canis familiaris*). *Developmental Psychobiology, 10*(3), 267–271.

Ajzen, I., & Fishbein, M. (1973). Attitudinal and normative variables as predictors of specific behaviors. *Journal of Personality and Social Psychology, 27,* 41–57.

Babor, T. F., Berglas, S., Mendelson, J. H., Ellingbow, J., & Miller, K. (1983). Alcohol, affect, and the disinhibition of verbal behavior. *Psychopharmacology, 80,* 53–60.

Bandura, A. (1977). *Social learning theory.* Englewood Cliffs, NJ: Prentice Hall.

Bandura, A. (1984). Representing personal determinants in causal structures, *Psychological Review, 91,* 508–511.

Bandura, A., Ross, D., & Ross, S. A. (1963). Vicarious reinforcement and imitative learning. *Journal of Abnormal and Social Psychology, 67,* 601–627.

Barnes, G. M. (1977). The development of adolescent drinking behavior: An evaluative review of the impact of the socialization process within the family. *Adolescence, 12,* 572–589.

Barnes, G. M. (1981). Drinking among adolescents: A subcultural phenomenon or a model of adult behavior. *Adolescence, 16,* 211–299.

Biddle, B. J., Bank, B. J., & Marlin, M. M. (1980). Social determinants of adolescent drinking. *Journal of Studies on Alcohol, 41*, 215–241.

Bolles, R. C. (1972). Reinforcement, expectancy, and learning. *Psychological Review, 79*, 394–409.

Briddell, D. W., Rimm, D. C., Caddy, G. K., Krawitz, G., Sholis, D., & Wunderlin, J. (1978). Effects of alcohol and cognitive set on sexual arousal to deviant stimuli. *Journal of Abnormal Psychology, 87*, 418–430.

Briddell, D. W., & Wilson, G. T. (1976). Effects and expectancy set on male sexual arousal. *Journal of Abnormal Psychology, 85*, 225–234.

Brown, S. A. (1985). Expectancies versus background in the prediction of college drinking patterns. *Journal of Consulting and Clinical Psychology, 53*, 123–130.

Brown, S. A. (in press). Reinforcement expectancies and alcohol treatment outcome after one year. *Journal of Studies on Alcohol.*

Brown, S. A., & Creamer, V. (1985). *Alcohol expectancies in adolescents: Familial and drinking experience influences.* Unpublished manuscript, University of California at San Diego.

Brown, R. A., & Cutter, H. S. (1977). Alcohol, customary drinking behavior, and pain. *Journal of Abnormal Psychology, 86*, 179–188.

Brown, S. A., Goldman, M. S., & Christiansen, B. A. (1985). Do alcohol expectancies mediate drinking patterns of adults? *Journal of Consulting and Clinical psychology, 53*, 512–519.

Brown, S. A., Goldman, M. S., Inn, A., & Anderson, L. (1980). Expectations of reinforcement from alcohol: Their domain and relation to drinking patterns. *Journal of Consulting and Clinical Psychology, 48*, 419–426.

Brown, J. S., Mansfield, J. G., & Skurdal, A. J. (1980). An inference-reduction interpretation of the effects of ethanol on conflict behavior. *Physiological Psychology, 8*, 423–432.

Buglass, D., & McCulloch, J. W. (1979). Further suicidal behavior: The development and validation of predictive scales. *British Journal of Psychiatry, 116*, 483–491.

Burkett, S. R. (1980). Religiosity, beliefs, normative standards and adolescent drinking. *Journal of Studies on Alcohol, 41*, 662–671.

Cahalan, D., & Cisin, I. H. (1968). American drinking practice: A summary of findings from a national probability sample. I. Extent of drinking by population subgroups. *Quarterly Journal of Studies on Alcohol, 29*, 130–151.

Canter, W. H. (1984). *Adolescent problem drinkers: An analysis of a social learning model.* Doctoral dissertation, Wayne State University, Detroit.

Cappell, H. (1975). An evaluation of tension models of alcohol consumption. In R. J.Gibbons, Y. Israel, H. Kalant, R. E. Popham, W. Schmidt, & R. G. Smart (Eds.), *Research Advances in Alcohol and Drug Problems* (Vol. 2, pp. 177–210). New York: John Wiley & Sons.

Cappell, H. L., & Herman, C. P. (1972). Alcohol and tension reduction: A review. *Quaterly Journal of Studies on Alcohol, 33*, 33–64.

Carpenter, J. A. (1968). Contributions from psychology to the study of drinking and driving. *Quaterly Journal of Studies on Alcohol* (Suppl. 4), 234–251.

Carpenter, J. A., & Armenti, N. P. (1972). Some effects of ethanol on human sexual and aggressive behavior. In B. Kissen & H. Begleiter (Eds.), *The biology of alcoholism: Physiology and behavior* (Vol. 2, pp. 509–543). New York: Plenum Press.

Christiansen, B. A., & Goldman, M. S. (1983). Alcohol related expectancies vs. demographic/background variables in the prediction of adolescent drinking. *Journal of Consulting and Clinical Psychology, 51*, 249–257.

Christiansen, B. A., Goldman, M. S., & Brown, S. A. 1985. The differential development of adolescent alcohol expectancies may predict adult alcoholism. *Addictive Behaviors, 10*, 299–306.

Christiansen, B. A., Goldman, M. S., & Inn, A. (1982). The development of alcohol-related expectancies in adolescents: Separating pharmacological from social learning influences. *Journal of Consulting and Clinical Psychology, 50*, 336–344.

Conger, J. J. (1956). Reinforcement theory and the dynamics of alcoholism. *Quarterly Journal of Studies on Alcohol, 17*, 296–305.

Connors, G. J., & Maisto, S. A. (1979). Effects of alcohol, instructions, and consumption rate on affect and physiological sensations. *Psychopharmacology, 62,* 261–266.

Connors, G. J., O'Farrell, T. J., & Cutter, H. S. G. (1984, August). *Alcohol expectancies among alcoholics, problem drinkers, and nonproblem drinkers.* Paper presented at the 92nd Annual Convention of the American Psychological Association, Toronto, Ontario, Canada.

Creamer, V., & Brown, S. A. (1985, April). Presentation at Western Psychological Conference, San Jose, Cal.

Cutter, H. S., Maloof, B., Kurtz, H. R., & Jones, W.C. (1976). "Feeling no pain." Differential responses to pain by alcoholics and non-alcoholics before and after drinking. *Journal of Studies on Alcohol, 37,* 273–277.

Deardoff, C. M., Melges, F. T., Hout, C. N., & Savage, D. J. (1979). Situations related to drinking alcohol: A factor analysis of questionnaire responses. *Journal of Studies on Alcohol, 39,* 1499–1505.

Donovan, J. E., & Jessor, R. (1978). Adolescent problem drinking; psychosocial correlates in a national sample study. *Journal of Studies on Alcohol, 39,* 1506–1524.

Donovan, J. E., Jessor, R., & Jessor, L. (1983). Problem drinking in adolescence and young adulthood. A follow-up study. *Journal of Studies on Alcohol, 44,* 109–137.

Engle, K. B., & Williams, T. K. (1972). Effect of an ounce of vodka on alcoholics' desire for alcohol. *Quarterly Journal of Studies on Alcohol, 33,* 1099–1115.

Faber, P. D., Khavari, K. A., & Douglass, F. M. (1980). A factor analytic study of the reasons for drinking: Empirical validation of positive and negative reinforcement dimensions. *Journal of Consulting and Clinical Psychology, 48,* 780–781.

Farkas, G. M., & Rosen, R. C. (1976). Effect of alcohol on elicited male sexual response. *Journal of Studies on Alcohol, 37,* 265–272.

Fishbein, M. (1967). Attitude and the prediction of behavior. In M. Fishbein (Ed.), *Readings in attitude theory and measurement* (pp. 477–492). New York: John Wiley & Sons.

Freed, E. X. (1978).Alcohol and mood: An updated review. *International Journal of the Addictions, 13,* 173–200.

George, W. H., & Marlatt, G. A. (1983). Alcoholism: The evaluation of a behavioral perspective. In M. C. Galanter (Ed.), *Recent developments in alcoholism* (Vol. 1, pp. 105–138). New York: Plenum Press.

Globetti, G. (1967). *Journal of Alcohol Education, 13,* 21.

Globetti, G. (1972). Problem and no problem drinking among high school students in abstinence communities. *International Journal of the Addictions, 7,* 511–523.

Glynn, R. J., LoCastro, J., Hermos, J., & Busse, R. (1983). Social contexts and motives for drinking in men. *Journal of Studies on Alcohol, 44,* 1011–1025.

Goldman, M. S., & Klisz, D. K. (1982). Behavioral treatment of an alcoholic: The unvarnished story. In W. M. Hay, & P. E. Nathan, (Eds.), *Clinical case studies in the behavioral treatment of alcoholism* (pp. 23–48). New York: Plenum Press.

Goldman, M. S., Taylor, H. A., Carruth, M. L., & Nathan, P. E. (1973). Effects of group decision making on group drinking by alcoholics. *Quarterly Journal of Studies on Alcohol, 34,* 807–822.

Goldstein, D. B. (1983). *Pharmacology of alcoholism.* New York: Oxford University Press.

Harfond, T. C., & Mills, G. S. (1978). Age-related trends in alcohol consumption. *Journal of Studies on Alcohol, 39,* 207–210.

Harfond, T. C., & Spiegler, D. L. (1983). Developmental trends of adolescent drinking. *Journal of Studies on Alcohol, 44,* 181–188.

Harvey, J. H., & Weary, G. (1984). Current issues in attribution theory and research. In M. R. Rosenzweig & L. W. Porter (Eds.), *Annual review of psychology* (Vol. 35), Palo Alto, CA: Annual Reviews.

Heider, F. (1958). *The psychology of interpersonal relations.* New York: John Wiley & Sons.

Huba, G. J., & Bentler, P. M. (1980). The role of peer and adult models for drug taking at different stages in adolescence. *Journal of Youth and Adolescence, 9,* 449–465.

Irwin, F. W. (1971). *Intentional behavior and motivation.* New York: Lippincott.

Isaacs, M. (1979). College students' expectations of the results of drinking. *Journal of Studies on Alcohol, 40*, 476–479.

Jessor, R., & Jessor, S. L. (1975). Adolescent development and the onset of drinking: A longitudinal study. *Journal of Studies on Alcohol, 36*, 21–51.

Jones, E. E., & Berglas, S. (1978). Control of attributions about the self through self-handicapping strategies: The appeal of alcohol and the role of unachievement. *Personality and Social Psychology Bulletin, 4*, 200–206.

Jones, E. E., & Nisbett, R. E. (1971). *The actor and the observer: Divergent perceptions of the causes of behavior.* Morristown, NJ: General Learning Press.

Kelley, H. H. (1967). Attribution theory in social psychology. *Nebraska Symposium on Motivation, 15*, 192–238.

Knupfer, G., & Room, R. (1967). Drinking patterns and attitudes of Irish, Jewish and White Protestant American men. *Quarterly Journal of Studies on Alcohol, 28*, 676–699.

Korytnyk, N. X., & Perkins, D. V. (1983). Effects of alcohol versus expectancy for alcohol on the incidence of graffiti following an experimental task. *Journal of Abnormal Psychology, 92*, 382–385.

Kreutzer, J. S., Schneider, H. G., & Myatt, C. R. (1984). Alcohol, aggression and assertiveness in men: Dosage and expectancy effects. *Journal of Studies on Alcohol, 45*, 275–278.

Kruglinski, A. W. (1979). Causal explanation, teleological explanation: On radical particularism in attribution theory. *Journal of Personality and Social Psychology, 37*, 1447–1457.

Landman, R. H. (1952).Studies of drinking in Jewish culture. III. Drinking patterns of children and adolescents attending religious schools. *Quarterly Journal of Studies on Alcohol, 13*, 87–94.

Lang, A. R., Goeckner, D. J., Adesso, V. T., & Marlatt, G. A. (1975). The effects of alcohol on aggression in male social drinkers. *Journal of Abnormal Psychology, 84*, 508–518.

Lang, A. R., Searles, J., Lauerman, R., & Adesso, V. (1980). Expectancy, alcohol, and sex guilt as determinants of interest in and reaction to sexual stimuli. *Journal of Abnormal Psychology, 89*, 644–653.

Lansky, D., & Wilson, G. T. (1981). Alcohol, expectations, and sexual arousal in males: An information processing analysis. *Journal of Abnormal Psychology, 90*, 35–45.

Lassey, M. L., & Carlson, J. E. (1980). Drinking among rural youth: The dynamics of parental and peer influences. *International Journal of the Addictions, 15*, 61–75.

Levinson, R. W., Sher, K. J., Grossman, L. M., Newman, J., & Newling, D. B. (1980). Alcohol and stress response dampening: Pharmacological effects, expectancy, and tension reduction. *Journal of Abnormal Psychology, 89*, 528–538.

Lewin, K. (1951). The nature of field theory. In M. H. Marx (Ed.), *Psychological Theory* (pp. 299–314). New York: Macmillan.

Ludwig, A. M., Wikler, A., & Stark, L. H. (1974). The first drink; psychobiological aspects of craving. *Archives of General Psychiatry, 30*, 539–547.

MacAndrews, C., & Edgerton, R. B. (1969). *Drunken comportment: A social explanation.* Chicago: Aldine Publishing Company.

MacCorquodale, K. M., & Meehl, P. E. (1954). Preliminary suggestions as to a formalization of expectancy theory. *Psychological Review, 60*, 53–60, 125–129.

Maddox, G. L. (1964). Adolescence and alcohol. In R. G. McCarthy (Ed.), *Alcohol education for classroom and community. A sourcebook for education* (pp. 32–47). New York: McGraw-Hill.

Margulies, R. Z., Kessler, R. C., & Kandell, D. B. (1977). A longitudinal study of onset of drinking among high school students. *Quarterly Journal of Studies on Alcohol, 38*, 879–912.

Marlatt, G. A. (1984, March). *Alcohol, the magic elixir: Stress, expectancy, and the transformation of emotional states.* Paper presented at the 7th Annual Coatesville Jefferson Conference, *Stress: Alcohol and Drug Interaction,* Coatesville, PA.

Marlatt, G. A., Demming, B., & Reid, J. B. (1973). Loss of control drinking in alcoholics: An experimental analogue. *Journal of Abnormal Psychology, 81*, 233–241.

Marlatt, G. A., & Rohsenow, D. J. (1980). Cognitive processes in alcohol use: Expectancy and the balanced-placebo design. In N. K. Mello (Ed.), *Advances in substance abuse: Behavioral and biological research* (Vol. 1, pp. 159–199). Greenwich, CT: JAI Press.

Mayfield, D. (1976). Alcoholism, alcohol intoxication, and assaultive behavior. *Diseases of the Nervous System, 37,* 288–291.

McCarty, D., Morrison, S., & Mills, K. C. (1983). Attitudes, beliefs and alcohol use. *Journal of Studies on Alcohol, 44,* 328–341.

McClelland, D. C., Davis, W. N., Kalin, R., & Wanner, E. (1972). *The drinking man.* New York: Free Press.

McCollam, D. C., Burish, T. G., Maisto, S. A., & Sobell, M.B. (1980). Alcohol's effect on physiological arousal and self-reported affect and sensations. *Journal of Abnormal Psychology, 89,* 244–233.

Merry, J. (1966). The "loss of control" myth. *Lancet, 1,* 1257–1258.

Miller, M. E., Adesso,V. J., Fleming, J. P., Gino, A., & Lauerman, R. (1978). The effects of alcohol on the storage and retrieval processes of heavy social drinkers. *Journal of Experimental Psychology: Human Learning and Memory, 4,* 246–255.

Mischel, W. (1973). Toward a cognitive social learning reconceptualization of personality. *Psychological Review, 80,* 252–283.

Mischel, W. (1984). Convergences and challenges in the search for consistency. *American Psychologist, 39,* 351–364.

Mischel, W., & Peake, P. K. (1982). Beyond deja vu in search of cross-situational consistency. *Psychological Review, 89,* 730–755.

Murray, R. M., Clifford, C. A., & Gurling, H. M. D. (1983). Twin adoption studies: How good is the evidence for genetic role? In M. Galanter (Ed.), *Recent developments in alcoholism* (Vol. 1, pp. 25–48). New York: Plenum Press.

Nash, F. H., Frank, J.D., Imber, S. D., & Stone, A. R. (1964). Selected effects of merit medication on psychiatric outpatients. *American Journal of Psychotherapy, 18,* 33–48.

Nathaṇ, P. E., & Lisman, S. A. (1976). Behavioral and motivational patterns of chronic alcoholics. In R. E. Tarter & A. A. Sugerman (Eds.), *Alcoholism—Interdisciplinary approaches to an enduring problem* (pp. 479–522). Reading, MA: Addison-Wesley.

Nisbett, R. E., & Wilson, T. D. (1977). Telling more than we know: Verbal responses on mental processes. *Psychological Review, 84,* 231–259.

Peterson, D. R. (1983). Pharmocogenetic approaches to the neuropharmacology of ethanol. In M. Galanter (Ed.), *Recent developments in alcoholism* (Vol. 1, pp. 49–68). New York: Plenum Press.

Pihl, R. O., Smith, M., & Farrell, B. (1984). Alcohol and aggression in men: A comparison of brewed and distilled beverages. *Journal of Studies on Alcohol, 45,* 278–282.

Pliner, P., & Cappell, H. (1974). Modification of affective consequences of alcohol: A comparison of social and solitary drinking. *Journal of Abnormal Psychology, 85,* 607–610.

Polivy, J., Schueneman, A. L., & Carlson, K. (1976). Alcohol and tension reduction: Cognitive and physiological effects. *Journal of Abnormal Psychology, 85,* 595–606.

Quattrone, G.A. (1982). Over attribution and unit formation: When behavior engulfs the person. *Journal of Personality and Social Psychology, 42,* 593–607.

Rimm, D.C., Sininger, R. A., Faherty, J. D., Whitey, M. D., & Perl, M. B. (1982). A balanced placebo investigation of the effects of alcohol vs. alcohol expectancy on simulated driving behavor. *Addictive Behaviors, 7,* 27–32.

Rohsenow, D. J. (1983). Drinking habits and expectancies about alcohol's effects for self versus others. *Journal of Consulting and Clinical Psychology, 51,* 752–756.

Rohsenow, D. J., & Bachorowski, J. A. (1984). Effects of alcohol and expectancies on verbal aggression in men and women. *Journal of Abnormal Psychology, 93,* 418–432.

Ross, L. (1977). The intuitive psychologist and his shortcomings: Distortions in the attribution process. *Advances in Experimental and Social Psychology, 10,* 174–220.

Ross, S., Krugman, A. D., Lyerly, S. B., & Clyde, D. J. (1962). Drugs and placebos: A model design. *Psychological Report, 10,* 383–392.

Ross, M., & Olson, J. M. (1981). An expectancy attribution model of the effects of placebos. *Psychological Reviews, 88*, 408–437.

Rotter, J. B., (1954). *Social learning and clinical psychology.* New York: Prentice-Hall.

Rotter, J. B. (1966). Generalized expectancies for internal versus external control of reinforcement. *Psychological Monographs, 80* (Whole No. 608).

Rotter, J. B. (1981). The psychological situation in learning theory. In D. Magnusson (Ed.), *Toward a psychology of situations: An interactional perspective.* Hillsdale, NJ: Lawrence Erlbaum.

Schacter, S. (1964). The interaction of cognitive and physiological determinants of emotional state. In L. Berkowitz (Ed.), *Advances in experimental social psychology* (Vol. 1, pp. 49–80). New York Academic Press. p. 49–80.

Schacter, S., & Singer, J. E. (1962). Cognitive, social, and physiological determinants of emotional state. *Psychological Review, 69*, 379–399.

Schlegel, R. P., Crawford, C. A., & Sanborn, M. A. (1977). Correspondence and mediational properties of the Fishbein Model: An application to adolescent alcohol use. *Journal of Experimental and Social Psychology, 13*, 421–430.

Schmutte, G. T., & Taylor, S. P. (1980). Physical aggression as a function of alcohol and pain feedback. *Journal of Social Psychology, 110*, 235–244.

Shapiro, A. K. (1978). The placebo effect. In W. G. Clark & J. del Giudice (Eds.), *Principles of Psychopharmacology* (2nd ed., pp. 441–459). New York: Academic Press.

Shapiro, A. K., & Morris, L.A. (1978). Placebo effects in medical and psychological therapies. In S. L. Garfield & A. K. Bergin (Eds.), *Handbook of psychotherapy and behavior change* (2nd ed., pp. 369–410). New York: John Wiley & Sons.

Sher, K. J. (1985). Subjective effects of alcohol: The influence of setting and individual differences in alcohol expectancies. *Journal of Studies on Alcohol, 46*, 137–146.

Shomer, R. W. (1966). *Effects of chance and skill outcomes on expectancy recall and distributive allocations.* Unpublished doctoral dissertation, University of California, Los Angeles.

Shupe, L. M. (1954). Alcohol and crime: A study of the urine concentration found in 882 persons arrested during or immediately after commission of a felony. *Journal of Criminal Law, Criminology, and Police Science, 44*, 661–664.

Smart, R. G., & Fejer, D. (1972).Drug use among adolescents and their parents: Closing the generation gap in mood modification. *Journal of Abnormal Psychology, 79*, 153–160.

Smart, R. G., & Gray, G. (1979). Parental and peer influences as correlates of problem drinking among high school students. *International Journal of the Addictions, 14*, 905–918.

Sobell, M. B., & Sobell, L. C. (1975). Drunkenness, a "special circumstance" in crime and violence, sometimes. *International Journal of the Addictions, 10*, 869–882.

Southwick, L. L., Steele, C. M., Marlatt, G.A., & Lindell, M. (1981). Alcohol-related expectancies: Defined by phase of intoxication and drinking experience. *Journal of Consulting and Clinical Psychology, 49*,713–721.

Stacey, B., & Davies, J. (1970). Drinking behaviour in childhood and adolescence: An evaluative review. *British Journal of the Addictions, 65*, 203–212.

Staddon, J. E. R. (1984). Social learning theory and the dynamics of interaction. *Psychological Review, 91*, 502–507.

Storms, M., & Nisbett, R. (1970). Insomnia and the attribution process. *Journal of Personality and Social Psychology, 16*, 319–328.

Strauss, R., & Bacon, S. D. (1953). *Drinking in college.* Westport, CT: Greenwood.

Swinson, R. P. (1983). Genetic markers and alcoholism. In M. Galanter (Ed.), *Recent developments in alcoholism* (Vol. 1, pp. 9–24). New York: Plenum Press.

Tolman, E. G. (1932). *Purposive behavior in animals and man.* New York: Appleton-Century-Crofts.

Ullman, A. D. (1960). Ethnic differences in the first drinking experience. *Social Problems, 8*, 45–56.

Valins, S. (1966). Cognitive effects of false heart-rate feedback. *Journal of Personality and Social Psychology, 4*, 400–408.

Valins, S., & Nisbett, R. E. (1972). Attribution processes in the development and treatment of emotional disorders. In E. E. Jones, D. E. Kanouse, H. H. Kelley, R. E. Nisbett, S. Valins, & B. Weiner (Eds.), *Attribution: Perceiving the causes of behavior* (pp. 137–150). Morristown, NJ: General Learning Press.

Virkkunen, M. (1974). Alcohol as a factor precipitating aggression and conflict behavior leading to homicide. *British Journal of the Addictions, 69,* 149–154.

Vuchinich, R. E., & Sobell, M. B. (1978).Empirical separation of physiologic and expected effects of alcohol on complex perceptual-motor performance. *Psychopharmacology, 60,* 81–85.

Vuchinich, R. E., Tucker, J. A., & Sobell, M.B. (1979). Alcohol, expectancy, cognitive labeling, and mirth. *Journal of Abnormal Psychology, 88,* 641–651.

Wanberg, K. W., Horn, J. L., & Foster, F. M. (1977). A differential assessment model for alcoholism: The scales of the Alcohol Use Inventory. *Journal of Studies on Alcohol, 38,* 512–543.

Weintraub, A., & Goldman, M. S. (1983). Alcohol and proactive interference: A test of response eccentricity theory of alcohol's psychological effects. *Addictive Behaviors, 8,* 151–166.

Wicker, A. W. (1969). Attitudes vs. actions; the relationship of verbal and overt behavioral responses to attitude objects. *Journal of Social Issues, 25,* 41–47.

Williams, R. M.,Goldman, M. S., & Williams, D. L. (1981). Expectancy and pharmacological effects of alcohol on human cognitive and motor performance: The compensation for alcohol effect. *Journal of Abnormal Psychology, 90,* 267–270.

Wilsnack, R. W., & Wilsnack, S. C. (1980). Drinking and denial of social obligations among adolescent boys. *Journal of Studies on Alcohol, 41,* 1118–1133.

Wilson, G. T. (1983). Self-awareness, self-regulation, and alcohol consumption: An analysis of J. Hull's Model. *Journal of Abnormal Psychology, 92,* 505–513.

Wilson, G. T., & Abrams, D. (1977). Effects of alcohol on social anxiety and physiological arousal: Cognitive versus pharmacological processes. *Cognitive Therapy and Research, 1,* 195–210.

Wilson, G. T., & Lawon, D. M. (1976). Expectancies, alcohol, and sexual arousal in male social drinkers. *Journal of Abnormal Psychology, 85,* 587–594.

Wilson, G. T., & Lawson, D. M. (1978). Expectancies, alcohol and sexual arousal in women. *Journal of Abnormal Psychology, 87,* 358–367.

Wilson, G. T., Lawson, D. M., & Abrams, D. B. (1978). Effects of alcohol on sexual arousal in male alcoholics. *Journal of Abnormal Psychology, 87,* 609–616.

Zajonc, R. B. (1980). Feeling and thinking: Preferences need no inferences. *American Psychologist, 35,* 151–175.

Zarantonello, M. (1984). *Expectations for reinforcement from alcohol use, anxiety, depression, and drinking habits in a clinical sample.* Unpublished manuscript, Loyola University, Chicago.

Zeichner, A., & Pihl, R. O. (1979). Effects of alcohol and behavior contingencies on human aggression. *Journal of Abnormal Psychology, 88,* 153–160.

Zeichner, A., & Pihl, R. O. (1980). Effects of alcohol and instigator intent on human aggression. *Journal of Studies on Alcohol, 41,* 265–276.

Zucker, R. A. (1976). Parental influences on the drinking patterns of their children. In M. Greenblatt & M.S. Schuckit (Eds.), *Alcoholism problems in women and children* (pp. 211–238). New York: Grune & Stratton.

# 7 Stress Response Dampening

KENNETH J. SHER

## Background

### *The Tension Reduction Hypothesis*

It is undoubtedly true that most people believe alcohol consumption reduces stress, and that stress reduction is a common motive for drinking. These everyday notions of alcohol's psychological effects and of why humans (and some animals) drink were first addressed in an explicit scientific theory by Conger (1956). Based on his own work on alcohol's behavioral effect on learned conflict in rats (Conger, 1951) and Masserman and Yum's (1946) finding that cats drink more when exposed to an approach–avoidance conflict situation, Conger (1956) hypothesized that alcohol consumption is reinforced because of its drive-reducing properties. Later theorists and investigators replaced the term "drive" with "tension" and Conger's formulation has come to be known as the tension reduction hypothesis (TRH). Experiments exploring the TRH can be classified into two types: (1) those that attempt to demonstrate that changes in the level of "tension" result in changes in the level of alcohol consumption, and (2) those that attempt to show that alcohol consumption or administration results in reduced tension.

### Definitional and Theoretical Problems

A major difficulty of the TRH has nothing to do with the hypothesis as it was originally proposed but rather with the way it has been interpreted by later researchers. The original work on the TRH was carried out with animals using an approach–avoidance paradigm; alcohol was thought to act by reducing the fear associated with the avoidance component. However, most

KENNETH J. SHER. Department of Psychology, University of Missouri, Columbia, Missouri human studies purporting to "test" the TRH have not used a conflict situation. Instead, "tension" has been equated with a wide range of self-report, behavioral, physiologic, and biochemical indices and it would seem that the original specificity of the TRH in terms of drive reduction has been lost. An unfortunate consequence of this diversity of definition is a lack of consensus concerning what constitutes an adequate test of the TRH. For example, a number of investigators (Logue, Gentry, Linnoila, & Erwin, 1978; Steffen, Nathan, & Taylor, 1974) have used self-reported anxiety and/or alcohol-related changes in tonic levels of muscular tension to evaluate the tension reducing properties of alcohol and have concluded either that the TRH is true or that it is false on the basis of these studies. However, change in anxiety or a physiological concomitant could not by itself be construed to offer support for or against the theory that Conger (1956) originally proposed since he explicitly stated that *alcohol can produce conflict and increase anxiety:*

> alcohol might be expected to have different effects if the relative strengths of the two incompatible response tendencies are different. [Earlier] we have assumed a relatively balanced conflict. But . . . in some situations the restraining tendencies are initially so great that a person never comes close enough to a potentially tempting goal for effective tendencies to be aroused. Thus there is no conflict and no heightened drives. Alcohol, however, may reduce these restraining tendencies enough for the person to be aroused but not enough to permit achieving the goal. The net effect of alcohol then would be to produce conflict and an increase in anxiety as the individual is tempted to approach nearer the dangerous goal. Such reasoning may help to account for the fact that some individuals find alcohol not tension-reducing but tension-increasing. (pp. 304–305)

It is clear that Conger did not view alcohol as a simple tension-reducer robust across individuals and situations (although this view is often attributed to him). The original TRH proposed by Conger does not yield simple predictions that are independent of a Hullian understanding of the underlying dynamics of a specific situation. Further complexities in analyzing alcohol effects in approach–avoidance and similar conflict situations are discussed by Brown and Crowell (1974).

Thus, it does not seem that the TRH makes many straightforward predictions about the relations between alcohol and stress. For the purposes of the present chapter I will take the position that at our current level of understanding it is more useful to simply examine the relationships between stress (as defined by an explicit experimental manipulation known to produce a reliable response) and alcohol, and not rely heavily upon vague and difficult to define constructs such as tension.

The present review attempts to assess the current state of knowledge and build on the observations and conclusions of earlier writers. In recent years there has been a wealth of psychological and biomedical research relevant to an understanding of alcohol and stress. In undertaking an integration of such a massive literature, the present review focuses on areas of consistency in the stress and alcohol literature and proposes a model of alcohol–stress relations that is congruent with available data.

## General Overview of Research on Acute Effects of Alcohol

The stress response dampening model is based upon an analysis of alcohol's effect on stress response. Thus before describing the model, we will selectively review the literature on the subjective and autonomic effects of alcohol on the stressed organism. However, in order to provide a context for understanding the effect of alcohol on response to stress, a brief review of the effect of alcohol on the nonstressed organism is helpful.

### The Effect of Alcohol on the Nonstressed Organism

Studies falling into this first category cover a wide range of psychological, behavioral, and physiologic phenomena. Phenomena most relevant to the study of alcohol and stress include the effects of alcohol on affect and on autonomic nervous system (ANS) activity.

The *affective consequences* of alcohol consumption appear inconsistent, with some studies finding increased positive affect (e.g., Kastl, 1969), other studies negative affective consequences (e.g., Berg, 1971), and still other studies concomitant negative and positive mood changes (Warren & Raynes, 1972). A number of factors have been shown to be important in determining alcohol's effect on subjective state, including dose (e.g., Williams, 1966), the time elapsed since drinking (presumably because of changes in blood alcohol concentration; Sher, 1985), mood of the individual prior to drinking (Mayfield, 1968), and the individual's expectancies concerning alcohol effects (Sher, 1985). Published studies of the effect of prolonged drinking on alcoholics consistently demonstrate increased levels of anxiety and dysphoric states (e.g., McNamee, Mello, & Mendelson, 1968; Mendelson, LaDou, & Solomon, 1964; Steffen *et al.*, 1974). However, in these experiments alcoholics are required to drink in a medical/research setting and the question must be raised if similar results would be obtained in a more natural and less conflictual environment. In any event, these studies convincingly demonstrate that alcoholics do not necessarily show positive mood effects and that, in fact, the opposite may be more likely. Perhaps one of the strongest statements that can be made concerning the effect of alcohol on mood is that it is closely dependent upon the context in which drinking occurs (Kalin, McClelland, & Kahn, 1965; Pliner & Cappell, 1974; Sher, 1985; Warren & Raynes, 1972).

Both Russell and Mehrabian (1975) and Sher (1985) have concluded that the effect of alcohol on mood is a complex function of social setting, state and trait aspects of the individual, and pharmacologic factors such as dose and limb of the blood alcohol curve. For this reason, simple generalizations concerning the affective consequences of alcohol consumption on nonstressed individuals are problematic and likely to be inaccurate or of limited use.

The *physiologic* consequences of alcohol consumption on the nonstressed organism have been shown to be wide-ranging. Perhaps most relevant to notions of stress are studies of alcohol's effects on the ANS. These effects are specific to the ascending limb [i.e., when the blood alcohol concentration (BAC) is rising] and cannot necessarily be generalized to more delayed effects of alcohol.

One of the most consistent ANS effects of alcohol is an increase in resting heart rate (HR). In an earlier review, Naitoh (1972) concluded "without any exception, HR has increased with ingestion of alcohol" (p. 414) and most subsequent research has tended to support this claim although failures to replicate have been reported (e.g., Sher, 1984; Wilson & Abrams, 1977). Other cardiovascular effects of alcohol include reduced cardiac contractility (Child, Levisman, & Pearce, 1979; Knott & Beard, 1972) and increased cutaneous vasodilation (cf. Wallgren & Barry, 1970). In addition to these cardiovascular effects, alcohol consumption increases skin conductance level (SCL; e.g., Jones, Parsons, & Rundell, 1976), another important index of autonomic activity.

A number of investigators (cf. Van Thiel, 1983a, 1983b) have shown that alcohol consumption results in an increase in plasma cortisol, probably due to a hypothalamic stress reaction and pituitary release of adrenocorticotropic hormone (ACTH). That is, alcohol consumption by itself results in a pattern of endocrine and physiologic (HR and SCL) response that in several key respects resembles the response to various physical and psychological stressors.

However, the characterization of the physiologic repsonse to ethanol as a stress response is not wholly satisfactory. While certain psychobiological functions change in an arousal direction, cardiac contractility and muscle tension (e.g., Schuckit, Engstrom, Alpert, & Duby, 1981; Steffen *et al.*, 1974) are decreased, that is change in a relaxation direction. As Levenson, Sher, Grossman, Newman, and Newlin (1980) have noted, this is a complex pattern in that it includes responses that often reflect psychophysiologic arousal as well as relaxation. This pattern might explain the seeming paradox that social drinkers expect alcohol to be both relaxing and stimulating (Southwick, Steele, Marlatt, & Lindell, 1981).

The effects of alcohol on resting state have usually been viewed as a simple function of dose and occasionally of limb of the blood alcohol curve. However, there is a relatively large literature in animals (Reed, 1977) and humans (e.g., Schaeffer, 1981; Schuckit, 1980b) indicating that there are large individual differences in physiologic effects of alcohol even among organisms with similar drinking histories. The picture is further complicated because tolerance clearly develops to many alcohol effects with repeated alcohol exposure.

To summarize, the effects of alcohol on the nonstressed state defy a simple psychophysiologic description. Alcohol consumption results in a complex physiologic state that interacts with a number of individual difference variables and the social context to create a relatively unique, situationally specific phenomenological experience. The relevance of alcohol's effects on the nonstressed state to the understanding of the relation between alcohol and stress is not clear. To focus on the finding of increased HR following alcohol consumption and conclude that alcohol consumption leads to increased stress (as some writers have done) is to distort the multidimensional characteristics of alcohol intoxication. Changes in autonomic indices, by themselves, without reference to situational variables do not necessarily indicate psychological stress.

While the effects of alcohol on the nonstressed organism are of interest in their own right, they are also of great methodological interest. Since alcohol appears to have direct effects on indices used to assess stress response (e.g., HR and SCL), assessment of the effect of alcohol on response to stress must take these direct stimulus effects into account.

## The Effect of Alcohol on Stress Response

Two basic paradigms can be described that investigate the effect of alcohol on stress response. In the first, an organism is stressed, and then the extent to which stress response is reduced by subsequent alcohol consumption is assessed. Noel, Lisman, Schare, and Lederer (1981) have termed this effect *stress response recovery* (SRR). Stress response recovery effects are difficult to document experimentally since in order for such an effect to be achieved, subjects must first be exposed to a stressor that produces long-acting stress responses. Consequently, there have been few recent human studies of this effect (Noel & Lisman, 1981; Sutker, Allain, Brantley, & Randall, 1982) and only one of these (Noel & Lisman, 1981) would appear to meet the requirement of demonstrating that stress responses were still present at the time of beverage consumption.

The second paradigm involves assessing the extent to which stress response is dampened by alcohol. A number of studies have assessed stress-response-dampening (SRD) effects. Although there are several contradictory findings, the following conclusions seem justified based on recent research.

1. A fairly consistent finding is that of reduced HR responding following a relatively large (around 1 g/kg) dose of alcohol (Cummings & Marlatt, 1983; Levenson *et al.*, 1980; Sher & Levenson, 1982; Wilson, Abrams, & Lipscomb, 1980; Zeichner, Feurstein, Swartzman, & Reznick, 1983[1]). Findings surrounding electrodermal responding are less consistent, with many published studies reporting nonsignificant effects (Bradlyn, Strickler, & Maxwell, 1981; Levenson *et al.*, 1980; Sher & Levenson, 1982; Wilson *et al.*, 1980) although significant electrodermal dampening has been reported (Cummings & Marlatt, 1983; Lindman, Alexanderson, & Kvarnstrom, 1980; Lienert & Traxel, 1959; Greenberg & Carpenter, 1957).

2. As Bandura (1969) noted more than 15 years ago, the effectiveness of lower doses of ethanol is inconsistent, with some studies finding reduced stress responsiveness (Bradlyn *et al.*, 1981; Rimm, Briddell, Zimmerman, & Caddy, 1981; Noel & Lisman, 1981), some finding increased stress responsiveness (e.g., Keane & Lisman, 1980), and some finding no alteration (Abrams & Wilson, 1979; Keane & Lisman, 1980; Wilson & Abrams, 1977). Studies by Sher and Walitzer (1986) and Wilson *et al.* (1980) are of particular interest in that they clearly demonstrate that the cardiovascular SRD effects of alcohol are dose dependent with significantly greater effects at higher dose levels.

3. Although expectancy for alcohol has been shown to be an important variable in understanding many alcohol-related behaviors, particularly those related to disinhibition of a variety of appetitive/approach behaviors, its importance in understanding SRD effects of alcohol appears limited. Although Wilson and Abrams (1977) reported that the expectancy for alcohol reduces stress response, other studies have demonstrated nonsignificant (Alexanderson & Lindman, 1980; Bradlyn *et al.*, 1981; Keane & Lisman, 1980; Levenson *et al.*, 1980; Rimm *et al.*, 1981; Sutker *et al.*, 1982; Wilson, Perold, & Abrams, 1981) or contradictory effects (Abrams & Wilson, 1979; Polivy, Schueneman, & Carlson, 1976; Sutker *et al.*, 1982). The finding that the expectancy of alcohol can increase stress response is an important one and will be discussed

---

[1] Zeichner *et al.* (1983) do not report a significant effect of alcohol on dampening of the HR response to a stressor. However, examination of their data reveals pronounced SRD effects (the HR response to the stressor is reduced more than 60%). The data analyses are not reported in enough detail to determine why a significant finding was not reported.

further in the section Nonpharmacologic Effects: The Role of Expectancy, below.

4. Individual differences in drinkers appear to be important predictors of the magnitude of alcohol's SRD effects (Eddy, 1979; Lipscomb, Nathan, Wilson, & Abrams, 1980; Sher & Levenson, 1982; Sher & Walitzer, 1986). Eddy's (1979) findings suggest that stress-reducing effects are more pronounced in problem drinkers and Sher and Levenson's (1982) findings suggest that social drinkers with characteristics of prealcoholics (i.e., traits related to impulsiveness, aggressiveness, and extroversion) show more pronounced SRD effects than those who do not have these characteristics. It is important to point out that individual differences in SRD effects of alcohol do not appear to be attributable to individual differences in stress or anxiety proneness. In the two experiments in our laboratory documenting personality correlates of SRD effects, no evidence was found to support the theory that individual differences in trait anxiety were related to alcohol-related stress response dampening.

### Overview of the Model

Before proposing a model of alcohol effects and drinking based on SRD effects, it is first necessary to define how the term stress is to be used. For our purposes, we can begin by adopting Folkman and Lazarus's (1985) definition of a stressor as a situation or stimulus appraised as a "threat, challenge or harm-loss. Threat refers to the potential for harm or loss; challenge refers to the potential for growth, mastery, or gain; and harm-loss refers to injury, already done" (p. 152).

However, Folkman and Lazarus's (1985) definition of stress seems overly broad for the purpose of building a model based around the effects of alcohol on stress. Earlier research summarized by Gray (1977, 1979) suggests that the effect of alcohol and other central nervous system (CNS) depressants on stress response is specific to a neuropharmacologic system related to punishment (within the Lazarus framework, threat and possibly harm-loss stressors) and so the relevance of "challenge" stressors is questionable. It is our assumption that both threat and harm-loss stressors are experienced as aversive, that is involving Gray's punishment system, while challenge stressors are not unless they are also appraised as threatening. Thus, social situations involving potential rejection or physically dangerous situations would be considered stressors, while erotic stimuli or impending athletic competition would not be considered stressors except under threatening conditions, for example, in situations that might lead to performance anxiety. Stress cannot be inferred merely on the basis of physiologic arousal unless such arousal can be linked to emotions of threat ("worry," "fear," "anxiety") and possibly emotions of harm ("anger," "sadness," "disappointment," "disgust").

## Stress Response Dampening Model of Drinking and Alcoholism

### *Statement of the Model*

The SRD model is fundamentally a modest, pared-down TRH. *Alcohol is posited to dampen stress response and thus is seen as being particularly reinforcing when it is consumed in a stressful context. Because of this, individuals who experience SRD effects are likely to drink with increased frequency and possibly in greater quantity when stressed.* However, in some situations alcohol consumption and/or intoxication is likely to be punished or proscribed, and the SRD model does not predict that alcohol consumption will reduce stress (although it should dampen the stress responsivity of the individual[2]) when consumed in these situations, nor does it predict that all stressful situations will tend to elicit drinking behavior. These important qualifications are discussed below.

Some of the individual differences we have observed in our laboratory suggest that persons who show prealcoholic personality characteristics (i.e., traits such as antisociality and impulsiveness) are particularly susceptible to SRD effects and consequently might be particularly prone to developing a pattern of drinking under stressful situations. With sufficient alcohol intake, dependence processes (such as tolerance to SRD and other alcohol effects, withdrawal symptoms, and craving) may become more important determinants of drinking behavior than stress-related motives. Even in the nondependent drinker, stress-related drinking may only represent a very minor category of drinking behavior. Nevertheless, for a variety of reasons, we believe that stress-related drinking may be etiologically linked to drinking problems in a substantial proportion of individuals. This is based on the observation that persons believed to be at risk for alcoholism have demonstrated pronounced stress reduction when drinking, and the finding that persons suffering from anxiety and stress-related disorders and who report pro-

---

[2] The notion that alcohol consumption can simultaneously increase stress and reduce stress derives from the hypothesis that alcohol can have several stress-related effects. Alcohol consumption can lead to increased stress indirectly via real or anticipated behavioral or cognitive impairment or punishment of signs of intoxication. However, if the individual has consumed a sufficient dose of alcohol, his or her responses to these alcohol-related stressors should be dampened.

nounced SRD effects from drinking seem to be especially susceptible to developing drinking problems. These findings are discussed later in the chapter.

### Parameters and Boundary Conditions

Dose-Related Parameters

We have previously argued (Levenson *et al.*, 1980; Sher & Levenson, 1982) that existing literature suggested that a relatively large dose (around 1.0 g/kg) was necessary for demonstrating cardiovascular SRD effects in an unselected population of social drinkers. A study by Wilson *et al.* (1980) documented clear evidence for dose-dependency with significant SRD effects being found at a 1.0 g/kg dose but not a 0.5 g/kg dose. More recent data (Sher & Walitzer, 1986) suggest that significant SRD effects can be seen at lower doses (e.g., 0.85 g/kg) and some individuals demonstrate SRD effects at doses as low as 0.425 g/kg. Although the findings of dose-dependency of SRD effects are consistent, the minimum dosage necessary to demonstrate a dampening of stress responsiveness is most probably a function of a number of variables including the time since drinking (i.e., the BAC and rate of change in BAC) and the nature and severity of the stressor. Existing literature suggests a monotonic relation between dose and SRD effects within a dose range likely to be consumed by social drinkers. Whether this relation holds across the entire range of possible dose effects concluding with a hypnotic dose, or whether there is a nonmonotonic relation with decreasing SRD effects at very high doses, has not been determined.

The Negative Consequences of Intoxication

In our society, alcohol consumption often brings with it a variety of negative social consequences. Situations may arise in which the intoxicated indvidual recognizes these consequences and experiences stress. To illustrate this point, consider the drunk driver who has just been pulled over to the side of the road by a police cruiser; the driver realizes that he or she is obviously drunk, will probably lose his or her license, and may go to jail. This situation is likely to elicit a large stress response (which is still somewhat diminished by the SRD effects of alcohol already in the driver's system). In this scenario, alcohol intoxication can be viewed as both stress producing and stress dampening. While it is probably more accurate to say that it is expectancies regarding alcohol and not intoxication per se that are stressful, in this and many other real-life situations (particularly those involving relatively high doses of alcohol) it may be difficult to distinguish between pharmacologic and expectancy effects. This pattern, of alcohol expectancy increasing stress and the pharmacological effect of alcohol dampening stress, has been experimentally demonstrated in a different context by Polivy *et al.* (1976).

The drunk driving incident is only an extreme example of how the consequences of alcohol consumption can be stress inducing. The social drinker at a party may realize that he or she is slurring words and alienating the date he or she is trying to impress. The executive may realize, or even be told, that he or she is drinking excessively and is making a bad impression. Were we to take physiologic and self-report measures of stress response on the party-goer or executive we might find that alcohol consumption appeared to result in increased stress. There are undoubtedly numerous other kinds of situations where consequences of intoxication (e.g., behavioral impairment, nausea) are stress inducing. These situations do not discredit the SRD model but they do illustrate that SRD effects are not the only stress-related effects of alcohol. This perspective perhaps explains why some studies (Abrams & Wilson, 1979; Polivy *et al.*, 1976; Sutker *et al.*, 1982) have found that the expectancy of alcohol can be stress increasing.

Most individuals, including drinkers, are reasoning social beings. Because of this, they modulate their drinking behavior across situations in accordance * with social custom and in ways that presumably minimize negative consequences of intoxication. Recognizing these constraints, the SRD model does not predict that the individual will drink in every stressful situation. Some of the most stressful situations that we encounter (job interviews, public speaking engagements, school or licensing examinations, and so forth) are also those that are likely to explicitly or implicitly punish drinking or intoxicated behavior. The degree to which individuals are likely to drink for stress relief in a given situation is probably a function of the perceived consequences of drinking and intoxicated behavior in that situation as well as of their experience with SRD effects. Also, because most individuals are aware that intoxication can last for relatively long periods of time (i.e., hours), events that are relatively remote temporally might still be expected to exert an influence on drinking behavior.

### Domains of Stress Response Affected

The SRD model was based on the empirical findings that physiologic stress response, especially cardiovascular responding, is dampened by alcohol. As noted above, much of the research has failed to demonstrate significantly dampened electrodermal responsivity. However, in light of some positive findings (e.g., Cummings & Marlatt, 1983; Greenberg & Carpenter, 1957), it might be premature to conclude that electrodermal responsivity is not dampened. Furthermore, because alcohol has direct effects on basal levels of skin conductance and skin temperature that are known to affect measurement of electrodermal responsivity, interpretation of findings in intoxicated subjects can be problematic.

The issue of the breadth of alcohol's effects on electrodermal versus cardiovascular responding is very important. If alcohol's SRD effects are specific to the cardiovascular system (as some data suggest) the potential psychologic importance of cardiovascular SRD effects is probably quite limited. Specific dampening of HR (and other cardiovascular responses) and no other autonomic response systems would suggest that cardiovascular SRD effects are mediated peripherally, perhaps by blocking of beta-adrenergic receptors on the heart. An abundant literature on the effect of beta-blocking drugs such as propranolol on anxiety and panic (Reisenzein, 1983) indicates that in general these drugs are poor at reducing subjective distress despite being effective at reducing cardiovascular responsivity. Alternatively, some theorists might interpret decreased HR responding in the absence of decreased skin conductance (SC) responding as indicating a reduction in active-avoidance activities (Fowles, 1980). This alternative explanation is discussed at somewhat greater length below.

However, it does not seem likely that the SRD effects observed with HR are limited to this measure and are the result of local influences of alcohol on the heart. Animal studies have shown alcohol-mediated SRD effects in plasma and brain catecholamines, and plasma nonsterified fatty acids and corticosterone (Vogel & DeTurck, 1983; Pohorecky, Rassi, Weiss, & Michalak, 1980). These findings suggest that the SRD properties of ethanol are very general and are probably mediated centrally. Although it is almost certainly true that many alcohol effects are mediated peripherally, and that SRD effects on different measures might be mediated by different pharmacologic and physiologic mechanisms, the conclusion that alcohol brings about a generalized dampening of stress response (rather than one specific to cardiovascular measures) seems plausible given the animal data. Concurrent measurement of plasma catecholamines and cortisol in human SRD studies would do much to clarify this issue, and would help locate the mechanism of the cardiovascular dampening that we and others have observed.

Whether or not subjective stress response dampening occurs concomitantly with, or is secondary to physiologic changes, is uncertain. The finding that beta-blocking drugs failed to reduce anxiety in hyperaroused individuals suggests that theories of stress-reducing effects based on reduction of peripheral arousal rest on shaky empirical foundations (Reisenzein, 1983). Whatever the mechanism, the reliability of findings of self-reported SRD effects is less than that of physiologic findings. While alcohol consumption often leads to decreased report of anxiety (Alexanderson & Lindman, 1980; Eddy, 1979; Levenson *et al.*, 1980; Lindman & Alexanderson, 1980; Lindman *et al.*, 1980; Polivy *et al.*, 1976; Rimm *et al.*, 1981), a number of negative findings at several dosage levels demonstrates that the effect is not robust across a variety of experimental situations (Abrams & Wilson, 1979; Keane & Lisman, 1980; Sher & Levenson, 1982; Wilson & Abrams, 1977; Wilson *et al.*, 1980). The reason for the greater variability of findings for affective self-report measures than for physiologic measures might be a function of the different assessment strategies used and variation in the demand characteristics associated with different experiments. Furthermore, there are many reasons to suspect that the validity of self-reports of intoxicated subjects differ from the validity of sober subjects. Alcohol intoxication might interact with processes such as self-report biases, sensitivity to demand characteristics, the ability to introspect, and possibly even the ability to scale experience in the way required by many of the Likert-type scales used in contemporary research. Given this perspective, the frequent (albeit not universal) findings of reduced self-report of distress become more impressive. It is surprising that the issue of differential validity of drunken and sober self-reports has not been addressed in the literature.

There is also significant variability across studies employing behavioral indices of stress and anxiety. In discussing behavioral indices, it is helpful to distinguish two general categories of behavioral response. The first is what we might call *emotional behavior*. Examples of emotional behavior include observable consequences of emotional arousal such as tremor, sweating, hyperactivity, hesitation and blocking in speech, and so on. The second can be called *avoidance behavior*. Examples of the latter include latency to engage in punished behaviors or the extent to which approach toward aversive stimuli is carried out (e.g., performance on a behavioral avoidance test; see Lang, 1968). The effect of alcohol on passive-avoidance has served as a primary test of the TRH in a variety of studies using an approach–avoidance conflict paradigm. These two general categories of stress behavior are not congruent; for instance, complete approach to an aversive stimulus (i.e., apparently little stress) can be accompanied by high levels of emotional behavior.

There have been relatively few published reports examining the effect of alcohol on emotional behavior under stress. Two such studies were carried out by Wilson and his colleagues. Abrams and Wilson (1979) reported expectancy-related effects on emotional behavior, but the effect was not clear-cut and was part of a higher-order interaction involving the sex of the raters. Similarly, Wilson *et al.* (1980) reported dose-related effects on emotional behavior that again were part of a higher-order interaction involving rater sex. The results of the latter investigation offer limited support for the hypothesis that SRD effects are discernible in emotional behavior. More direct support that alcohol reduces emotional behavior under stress comes from the study by Bradlyn *et al.* (1981) who found that subjects who received an alcoholic beverage were rated as less anxious while giving a speech than subjects given a nonalcoholic beverage.

In seeming contradiction to these generally positive findings, Keane and Lisman (1980) reported that alcohol significantly decreased the amount of verbal production and increased the amount of pausing among subjects making a stressful self-presentation. Both of these have been found to be useful nonverbal indices of anxiety. However, interpretation of these data is not unambiguous. Although reduced output and hesitation in spontaneous speech might indicate anxiety in sober individuals, similar behavior by intoxicated subjects cannot be interpreted in this way. Alcohol disrupts speech production in nonstressed individuals (e.g., Sher, 1985) and Keane and Lisman's design does not allow for an assessment of the independent contributions of stress and alcohol consumption on disrupted speech production. Thus, although it is clear that the intoxicated men in this study were less socially and verbally competent than their sober counterparts, it is not clear that they displayed more emotional behavior. An overall evaluation of the effect of alcohol on emotional behavior under stress suggests that alcohol might have a stress dampening effect but that further replication and clarification is needed.

The data on the effect of alcohol behavior on approach (i.e., reduction of passive-avoidance) in an approach–avoidance conflict paradigm is one of the few areas where earlier reviewers (e.g., Cappell & Herman, 1972; Hodgson, Stockwell, & Rankin, 1979; Steele & Southwick, 1983) agreed that there was consistent support for the TRH (although see Brown & Crowell, 1974). Recent investigations by Lindman (1980) and his colleagues have yielded a great deal of new human data consistent with this (although one recent investigation, that of Rimm *et al.*, 1981, failed to demonstrate significant approach to an avoided stimulus following alcohol consumption) and there seems little reason to question this conclusion.[3]

It is important to note that the SRD model does not necessarily predict how alcohol consumption will affect *adaptive* behavioral responses to any of a variety of stressors (e.g., efforts to terminate or minimize the impact of a stressor). These behaviors are undoubtedly under the control of more than just the subjective response to the painful stimulus and thus cannot be predicted by the SRD model alone. Furthermore, the adaptive capacity of the organism may affect the degree to which a stress response is elicited by a

[3] An additional recent study by Thyer and Curtis (1984) investigating the effect of alcohol on avoidance behavior in phobic patients concluded that alcohol has no effect on approach towards a phobic object on a behavioral avoidance test. However, the statistical tests they use to support this conclusion appear faulty (e.g., incorrect degrees of freedom are reported, the error term apparently shifts from one related test to another). In fact, the cell means reported by these authors (p. 606) *are* consistent with reduced avoidance behavior after alcohol consumption. Consequently, the results of this investigation should not be viewed as inconsistent with earlier studies showing reduced avoidance behavior following alcohol consumption.

stressor. For example, in active-avoidance situations it is likely that relatively little stress response is aroused by a discriminative stimulus for punishment and it is doubtful that alcohol would result in stress reduction. In fact, it is possible that the cognitive and motor impairing effects of alcohol might disrupt effective active avoidance and result in increased exposure to a stressor and increased stress response. Consequently, in situations where clear adaptive coping responses are readily available, alcohol may not be stress reducing. However, we hypothesize that if all effective coping behaviors were blocked, SRD effects of alcohol could be observed. We would thus expect that alcohol would result in dampening of the stress response to a learned helplessness manipulation, a prediction largely confirmed by Noel et al. (1981).

## Types of Stressor

As noted above, the SRD model attempts to limit itself to stressors that elicit reliable patterns of physiological response and that are considered subjectively aversive. These criteria are very broad and would appear to cover a wide variety of stressors ranging from evaluative threat to physical danger. In one of the only studies to compare SRD effects across stressors, Levenson et al. (1980) found comparable alcohol-related SRD effects on the responses to making a self-disclosing speech and to receiving a painful electric shock, indicating that SRD effects were not limited to a specific type of stressor. Thus, existing evidence suggests that alcohol SRD effects are robust across a number of stressful conditions. Although usually not considered in the general alcohol and stress literature, subjective responses to physically painful stimuli also appear to be dampened by alcohol (Cutter, Maloof, Kurtz, & Jones, 1976).

However, we suspect that the SRD model as currently proposed will probably be shown to be overly broad. Recent data (Ekman, Levenson, & Friesen, 1983) indicate that emotional states appear to have distinct physiologic correlates. This suggests that different forms of stress response (e.g., a fear response or a disgust response) may have different physiologic determinants in the CNS and thus alcohol, and most other psychoactive compounds, could be expected to have very different effects on different emotional states. Further study of the effects of alcohol on a variety of stressors would help to clarify these issues. For example, it would be useful to study response to stressors such as blood stimuli, which are known to produce a parasympathetic stress response (in contrast with the vast literature using stressors producing sympathetic stress reactions).

## Individual Differences in Stress Response Dampening

Claridge (1970) was one of the first to point out that the average effect of a drug is as much a function of subject characteristics as of the drug's pharmacologic properties. This would certainly appear to be the case when considering stress reducing effects of alcohol. To date, several different types of subject characteristics have been identified that appear to relate to the magnitude of SRD effects.

The importance of *gender* in moderating SRD effects has been investigated by Wilson and Abrams (1977; Abrams & Wilson, 1979) and Sutker *et al.* (1982) who have examined differences in the stress-reducing function of alcohol in men and women, using balanced placebo designs. Although the methods and results of these investigations were different, in both studies it appeared that the expectancy for alcohol was more stress inducing for women than men while the pharmacologic effects, when present, were comparable across sexes. These intriguing findings suggest that cognitive factors may be responsible for some observed differences between the males and females in stress-related drinking or regarding stress-related effects of alcohol. For example, the perceived social consequences of intoxication might be viewed as negative by women and consequently a woman's belief that she has consumed alcohol might result in increased stress.

Although the gender variable appears to relate more to expectancy effects than pharmacologic effects, other subject characteristics appear more closely tied to pharmacologic effects. Lipscomb *et al.* (1980) examined the relation between *tolerance* to a challenge dose of alcohol and the cardiovascular SRD effect of alcohol consumption. Simply put, the degree to which a person's standing stability is disturbed by alcohol predicts the degree to which, in terms of HR response, alcohol is found to be stress reducing for the person. The effect of alcohol on standing stability might represent a useful marker for persons who are susceptible to reinforcing properties of alcohol, and additional research using this index is warranted. It is important to note that what Lipscomb *et al.* refer to as "tolerance" appears to be more a function of constitutional than experiential factors since individual differences in the effect of alcohol on standing stability is not a function of drinking pattern, and thus might be more aptly termed a measure of alcohol sensitivity.

In an experiment comparing problem-drinking and non-problem-drinking female subjects, Eddy (1979) found that problem drinkers experienced greater stress reduction from alcohol than non-problem drinkers. These experimental findings are consistent with the findings from representative national surveys indicating that self-reported stress reduction from alcohol is associated with problem-drinking status (Cahalan, 1970; Cahalan, Cisin, & Crossley, 1969). Miller, Hersen, Eisler, and Hilsman's (1974) finding that alcoholics are more likely than nonalcoholics to increase alcohol consumption when stressed is certainly consistent with the notion that alcohol consumption is especially stress reducing for this population. While there is a substantial body of literature demonstrating that chronic alcoholics report increased anxiety and other dysphoric states after drinking (McNamee *et al.*, 1968; Mendelson *et al.*, 1964; Steffen *et al.*, 1974) these findings should not be interpreted as indicating that alcohol is not stress reducing for alcoholics. These studies do not address the issue of stress response and, as already noted, the distinction between the effects on the stressed and nonstressed organism is a crucial one.

Sher and Levenson (1982) have reported that persons with traits such as aggressiveness, impulsivity, and extroversion, which longitudinal studies (Jones, 1968; McCord & McCord, 1960; Robins, Bates, & O'Neal, 1962; Vaillant & Milofsky, 1982) have shown to be characteristic of the prealcoholic, are particularly sensitive to stress reducing properties of alcohol. In two studies, personality measures such as the Socialization scale of the California Psychological Inventory (Gough, 1969) and the MacAndrew (1965) Alcoholism Scale, which appear to sample prealcoholic traits, were found to predict the magnitude of cardiovascular stress response in intoxicated but not in sober subjects. However, the association between SRD effects and prealcoholic personality characteristics does not appear to be robust across investigations. Using a similar methodology, Cummings and Marlatt (1983) failed to replicate this finding and Sher and Walitzer (1986) was only able to partially replicate the earlier findings of Sher and Levenson (1982). Further investigation is needed to determine the boundary conditions of the relation between prealcoholic personality traits and individual differences in SRD effects.

Existing research literature does not suggest that proneness to anxiety or other aversive states relate to individual differences in SRD effects. Although not extensive, there are some data concerning the relation between *anxiety proneness* and drinking behavior. Post hoc analyses of the experiments reported by Sher and Levenson (Sher, 1982) failed to indicate greater SRD effects in persons prone to experiencing anxiety, although anxiety proneness was found to relate to the degree of stress response. In a more recent study (Sher, 1984), anxiety proneness appeared negatively related to SRD effects. In an experiment with socially anxious young men, Keane and Lisman (1980) failed to find stress-reducing effects attributable to alcohol. Finally, in a stress-induced drinking study, Holroyd (1978) found that high-trait-anxiety subjects drank less alcohol than low-trait-anxiety subjects. These experimental findings are consistent with data from the national drinking studies (Cahalan, 1970; Cahalan & Room, 1974) that show that anxiety was not a potent predictor of heavy-drinking or problem-drinking status. Thus, these data suggest that anxiety proneness is not a particularly important individual difference variable in determining either SRD effects or stress-related drinking behavior. An important exception to the apparent lack of relation between drinking behavior and stress may be found in the drinking behavior of persons suffering from severe anxiety disorders. This phenomenon will be discussed in the section below entitled Possible Mechanisms of Stress Response Dampening Effects, subsection Clinical Studies.

## Stress-Response-Dampening Effects of Selected Other Drugs

A number of commonly used drugs, both licit and illicit, appear to have stress-reducing properties, and many individuals apparently use these substances to achieve stress reduction. The following brief review of some commonly used substances with possible stress-reducing properties serves to illustrate that SRD effects are not limited to alcohol and the SRD model may be applicable to a number of substances.

### Nicotine

Many smokers report that their primary motivations for smoking are to reduce negative affect and to increase relaxation (Tomkins, 1966). Experimental studies tend to demonstrate that nicotine does have stress-reducing properties (e.g., Nesbitt, 1973; Pomerleau, Turk, & Fertig, 1984). In fact, in two key respects the effect of nicotine is similar to the effects of alcohol (Gilbert, 1979): (1) nicotine appears to have reliable effects in reducing emotional distress (i.e., stress-reducing properties) and has muscle relaxant properties; and (2) nicotine appears to also have the seemingly paradoxical effect of increasing basal levels of autonomic arousal. This is not to say that the effects of nicotine and alcohol are comparable across all physiologic measures. For example, nicotine is a potent peripheral vasoconstrictor, in contrast to alcohol which acts as a vasodilator in the periphery. Pharmacologically, both nicotine and alcohol appear to have wide-ranging effects on a number of organ systems, which defy a simple summary. Although not conclusive, existing evidence supports the position that nicotine does function as a stress reducer and that people smoke to achieve stress-reducing effects.

### Anxiolytic Drugs

The most frequently used drugs with demonstrated antianxiety actions are the benzodiazepines. Benzodiazepines have well-documented effects in reducing anxiety and response to stress (Gray, 1978; Rickels, 1978). In addition to having anxiolytic action, these drugs also have hypnotic, muscle relaxant, and anticonvulsant properties (Tallman, Paul, Skolnick, & Gallager, 1980). These anxiolytic effects appear to be mediated centrally, and specific sites of action of the benzodiazepine compounds have been identified in the brain. Because of the anxiolytic effects of these drugs they appear to be high in reinforcement value and, as noted by Tyrer (1980, p. 576), "patients have the habit of coming back and asking for more." Until recently, diazepam (Valium) was the most widely used prescription drug in the United States, with 54 million prescriptions written in 1977 (National Academy of Sciences,

1979). Despite the high rate of use, the extent to which these drugs are "abused" is a matter of some controversy since the distinction between true addiction and effective therapy is not an easy one to make (Hollister, 1981). However, existing data do support the notion that these drugs have stress-reducing properties and are consumed for SRD effects. A similar case could probably be made for other classes of anxiolytic compounds such as the barbiturates and meprobamate (e.g., Gray, 1978; Lienert & Traxel, 1959).

### Opiates

While opiate drugs are used medically primarily for their analgesic effects and may be abused for these effects, it is generally believed that most regular opiate users consume these drugs for euphoriant effects, the assumption being that these substances are intrinsically positively reinforcing. This view has not gone unchallenged, however. The effect of morphine in the pain-free individual can be one of dysphoria and not euphoria (Jaffe, 1985). There is a rather substantial sociological and clinical literature suggesting that opiates are often used and abused for coping with psychological distress (Alexander & Hadaway, 1982). As Sutker and Archer (1984) have recently pointed out, however, there is little experimental data directly assessing the extent to which opiates reduce stress responsiveness and to which stress elicits opiate intake.

The pharmacologic basis of opiate effects is becoming well known and specific sites of action in the brain, known as opiate receptors, have been identified (e.g., Pert & Snyder, 1973). It is important to point out that, although not an opiate, alcohol does have certain effects similar to opiates, such as analgesia (Cutter *et al.*, 1976), and may have similar indirect effects (Davis & Walsh, 1970; Triana, Frances, & Stokes, 1980). The possibility that alcohol-related SRD effects are mediated via the effect of ethanol on endogenous opiate systems will be discussed in the section Possible Mechanisms of Stress Response Dampening Effects, subsection Central Effects.

### Summary

It appears that several drugs, including nicotine, the benzodiazepines, and possibly the opiates, have stress-reducing properties and that people may consume these drugs for their stress-reducing effects. Thus the SRD model may be applicable to a number of substances. However, the extent to which stress reduction is a primary motivation for consuming any of these drugs is an open question, and, in practice, one that is difficult to answer.

### Direct Comparisons of the Stress-Reducing Properties
### of Alcohol and Other Drugs

Relatively few direct comparisons of the effect of alcohol versus other drugs have been published. In the only relevant human study in the literature of which we are aware, Lienert and Traxel (1959) compared the effects of a small dose of alcohol, a small dose of meprobamate, and a placebo on the magnitude of electrodermal responses to a sentence association test in male .social drinkers. These findings indicated reduced electrodermal responding following both alcohol and meprobamate consumption. Drawing from a large body of animal data, Gray (1977) has argued that the effects of the benzodiazepines, the barbiturates, and alcohol on the behavioral aspects of anxiety are virtually identical, and that all of these substances "block the behavioural effects of stimuli which warn of impending punishment, of stimuli which warn of frustrative non-reward, and of novel stimuli" (Gray, 1979, p. 606). Whether or not these generalizations are equally applicable to humans is presently unclear.

### Concurrent Use of Alcohol and Other Drugs

It is of interest that many of the commonly used substances that appear to have stress-reducing properties are often consumed concurrently with alcohol (Freed, 1973; Kaufman, 1982). There is a strong correlation between alcohol consumption and tobacco use in the general population, while the overwhelming majority of alcoholics (over 90%) are smokers, many of them heavy smokers (Istvan & Matarazzo, 1984). In fact, the association between alcoholism and smoking is so strong that some writers have suggested that alcoholics who do not smoke might represent an etiologically distinct subgroup (Walton, 1972).

It is clear that benzodiazepines are often used concurrently by persons with drinking problems, especially women. For example, Curlee (1970) reported 20% of the male alcoholics and 43% of the female alcoholics in her sample used minor tranquilizers and sedatives. In a more recent report, Corrigan (1980) found that 34% of her sample reported using tranquilizers and 20% reported using sleeping pills (presumably barbiturates).

There also seems to be a strong association between alcohol use and heroin use. Alcohol abusers appear to be relatively likely to use opiates when these are readily available, and opiate addicts are frequently heavy users of alcohol, especially when the purity of the opiate drugs is decreased (Kaufman, 1982). The high mortality associated with heroin abuse is often alcohol-related (Green & Jaffe, 1977; Ruttenberg & Luke, 1984).

There are a number of reasons why individuals who drink might also be particularly likely to use or abuse other substances. Istvan and Matarazzo (1984) suggest several possibilities: (1) there may exist reciprocal activation mechanisms whereby the use of one substance might serve as a cue to use the other; (2) general activation resulting from the use of one drug could lead to an increase in the use of other drugs; (3) alcohol and other substances might be used to moderate the effects of each other via antagonistic, additive, or synergistic effects; (4) a common motivation (e.g., stress reduction, sensation seeking) might lead to the use of two or more different substances with similar effects. Because of the wide range of effects produced by drugs such as the benzodiazepines, alcohol, opiates, and nicotine, and the lack of relevant empirical tests, it is not possible to definitively explain the observed associations seen in the patterns of use of various drugs. However, the apparent association between alcohol and substances with stress-reducing properties is certainly consistent with the notion that these drugs are all used, in part, for their stress-reducing effects. It would be extremely useful for future researchers to ascertain specific "reasons for using" various compounds in individuals who use multiple drugs, and to undertake careful time-series analyses relating environmental circumstances to the use of multiple substances, in order to determine how environmental circumstances relate to use of different drugs.

## Possible Mechanisms of Stress Response Dampening

### Pharmacologic Mechanisms

Direct Effects on Physiologic Responsiveness

**Artifactual.** The most consistent finding of alcohol in reducing stress response occurs on HR. A number of studies have reported that a moderate to large dose of alcohol reduces the HR response to a stressor (Cummings & Marlatt, 1983; Levenson *et al.*, 1980; Sher & Levenson, 1982; Sher & Walitzer, 1986; Wilson *et al.*, 1980; Zeichner *et al.*, 1983). Before considering physiologic mechanisms that can explain such an effect, the possibility that these findings are artifactual must first be considered. Because alcohol is often found to increase resting levels of HR, it is possible that findings of dampened HR reactivity to a stressor following alcohol consumption might be due to an initial values effect (Wilder, 1950). However, significant SRD effects have been obtained in the absence of effects on resting HR (Sher & Walitzer, 1986), and individual differences in SRD effects do not appear to be a function of individual differences in the effect of alcohol on resting HR (Sher & Levenson, 1982). Thus it does not seem likely that the frequent findings of dampened HR reactivity are caused by initial values effects.

*Peripheral Effects.* The findings of dampened HR responsivity in the absence of comparably consistent effects of other indices of stress response suggest that alcohol might have an effect on peripheral beta-adrenergic mechanisms,[4] since these are involved in the mediation of HR but not electrodermal increases under stress. Consistent with this hypothesis are the findings of reduced cardiac contractility, a beta-adrenergic function, following a dose of ethanol (Child *et al.*, 1978) and reduced responsiveness of an indirect measure of cardiac contractility (Levenson *et al.*, 1980).

Before evaluating this hypothesis further, it might be useful to consider the effects of drugs that selectively block beta-adrenergic receptor activity, the beta-blockers. Reviews of the effects of beta-blockers (Reisenzein, 1983) have concluded that although these drugs are effective at reducing peripheral *cardiovascular* indices of arousal, they are ineffective at reducing anxiety and other symptoms of subjective distress except perhaps in those individuals for whom symptoms of physiologic arousal (e.g., heart palpitation, tremor) are themselves a major source of distress.

Thus, the extent to which the effect of alcohol in dampening cardiovascular stress responsivity is similar to that of beta-blocking drugs, is unclear at the present time. It has previously been suggested (Sher & Levenson, 1982) that SRD effects might be mediated via beta-adrenergic blocking action, possibly in the periphery. However, the relatively frequent findings of reduced self-report of stress and anxiety following alcohol consumption noted earlier and the animal literature on stress-reducing effects seem to argue against a simple isolated effect of alcohol on beta-receptors in the ANS. The experimental literature on the effects of beta-blockers does not suggest that reduced cardiovascular arousal leads to reduced self-report of anxiety. In respect to electrodermal responsiveness, peripheral beta-adrenergic mechanisms are not involved in the regulation of this sympathetic index of arousal. The effects of alcohol in dampening stress response across a number of biochemical indices in animals argues further against a simple, isolated effect on beta-receptors in the ANS. Thus, although a direct effect of alcohol on beta-adrenergic transmission is consistent with the findings of reduced HR responding and the known effects on cardiac contractility, it is not consistent with other relevant data. Given the potential problems inherent when interpreting both self-report and electrodermal measures in intoxicated subjects discussed earlier, the number of positive findings with these measures becomes more impressive.

[4] Although electrodermal activity and HR *under stress* are largely a function of the activity of the sympathetic branch of the autonomic nervous system, these two indices of sympathetic arousal are regulated by different neurotransmitters at the target organ, acetylcholine in the case of the sweat glands and norepinephrine in the case of the heart. Beta-adrenergic receptors, a class of norepinephrine receptors, are important in regulating the rate and force of contraction of the heart but are not associated with the activity of the sweat glands in the *periphery*.

The author knows of no studies directly attempting to assess whether SRD effects are mediated by beta-adrenergic receptor blockade. While there have been a number of psychopharmacologic investigations of the interactive effects of alcohol and beta-blockers (but not on their joint effects on stress response), these studies yield a confusing pattern (Alkana & Noble, 1979; Kissin, 1974) with findings of both antagonistic and additive effects across different measures.[5] Future studies could directly determine the extent to which SRD effects are mediated by beta-adrenergic mechanisms and whether or not such effects are mediated peripherally.

***Central Effects.*** Most speculation concerning the mechanisms of stress response dampening focuses on the CNS. Gray (1977, 1978, 1979) has produced a theory of the pharmacologic mechanisms of stress reduction resulting from the use of a variety of anxiolytic compounds including alcohol, the benzodiazepines, the barbiturates, and related substances such as meprobamate. According to Gray, all of these drugs exert their influence by their effects on the behavioral inhibition system (BIS). As conceived by Gray, the BIS inhibits behavior likely to lead to aversive consequences and can be thought of as an anxiety system. Antianxiety agents are posited to disrupt the BIS and consequently reduce anxiety and behavioral inhibition. Gray has postulated that the BIS is centered in the septal and hippocampal regions of the brain and is closely related to noradrenergic functioning (Gray, 1977, 1978) and possibly gamma-aminobutyric acid (GABA)-ergic functioning (Gray, 1979). A rather large body of data indicates that the benzodiazepines bind to receptors in the brain that interact with receptors for GABA (Tallman *et al.*, 1980), facilitating GABA-ergic neurotransmission. It is therefore of great interest that alcohol has been found to facilitate GABA-ergic neurotransmission in cat cortex (Nestoros, 1980). Antianxiety effects associated with the noradrenergic system have been well documented in animals by Gray (1977) but the extent to which these drugs act primarily on these systems is open to some question (Hoehn-Saric, 1982). However, tests of anxiety reduction by an alpha-2-adrenergic agonist (clonidine) in humans have been partially supportive of a noradrenergic locus of some antianxiety drug effects (Hoehn-Saric, 1982). (As noted above, propranolol, a beta-adrenergic antagonist that crosses the blood–brain barrier, has not been shown generally

---

[5] To add to this confusion, there are beta-adrenergic receptors in the central nervous system as well as the autonomic nervous system, and the drug most commonly used to block beta-adrenergic receptors, propranolol, crosses the blood–brain barrier. Future studies on the interaction of alcohol and beta-blockers should attempt to contrast the effects of beta-blockers that do and do not cross the blood–brain barrier so that the locus of Alcohol × Beta-blocker interactions can be better localized.

effective in reducing stress in nonalcoholics). However, propranolol might be more effective in reducing stress in alcoholics (Carlsson & Fasth, 1976). Thus, at present, it seems reasonable to hypothesize that antianxiety drugs, including alcohol, exert their effects on brain centers associated with the neurotransmitter GABA and possibly those associated with norepinephrine as well. Direct tests of this hypothesis are possible by studying the effectiveness of GABA and norepinephrine antagonists on alcohol-related SRD effects.

Extending Gray's model to psychophysiologic assessment, Fowles (1980) has suggested that electrodermal responding reflects BIS activity (i.e., activation of a punishment/anxiety system) while HR responding is indicative of an appetitive, instrumental motivational system—the behavioral activation system (BAS). If Fowles is correct, then the data reported by a number of investigators including Levenson *et al.* (1980) and Wilson *et al.* (1980) suggest a primary effect of alcohol *not* on the BIS (i.e., not on stress and anxiety) but rather on instrumental responding, since HR and not electrodermal activity appears to be dampened by ethanol. We believe that this interpretation is probably not correct. First, in the experimental paradigms used by these investigators, these measures are found to covary in a positive direction, suggesting that they are reflecting a similar process, not one that is orthogonal or compensatory. Second, the interpretation of SC changes might be problematic because of the initial effects of alcohol on the values of resting SCL and its effects on skin temperature, which could effect measures of electrodermal responsivity. Although Fowles's (1980) theory concerning the interpretation of HR and SC patterning might be applicable to psychopaths and might also be applied to people more generally, generalization of Fowles's findings to intoxicted subjects might be hazardous because of direct effects of alcohol on the skin which could conceivably affect the interpretation of these measures. Greater support for an interpretation along the lines suggested by Fowles (1980) would be provided by experiments specifically designed to determine if alcohol affected active coping efforts or some other process linked to the BAS, and if this was more related to HR than SC responding.

Several researchers have noted similarities between the effects of alcohol and opiate drugs (Altshuler, 1982). Naloxone, an opiate antagonist, reverses some alcohol-related effects but not others (Mendelson, 1980). If SRD effects were mediated only via effects on endogenous opiate systems, we would predict that naloxone would block these effects. In a recent investigation, Ewing and McCarty (1983) failed to find evidence of an ethanol–naloxone interaction on various measures of stress responsiveness. Unfortunately, alcohol was not found to reliably reduce response to stress in the absence of naloxone and so any conclusions regarding the ability of opiate antagonists to block alcohol-related SRD effects are not warranted on the basis of this study. Replication using a somewhat higher dose of ethanol (subjects reached a peak BAC of 63 mg/100 ml) would certainly aid in clarifying this issue.

### Direct Effect of Alcohol on Cognitive Processes and Resulting Indirect Effect on Stress Responsivity

Levenson *et al.* (1980) previously suggested that alcohol might affect the cognitive processes necessary for evaluating a situation as stressful. Although there is little in the way of data bearing directly on this hypothesis, Sher and Levenson (1982) did find that alcohol can affect the appraisal of the anticipated affective response to a stressor, and it would seem worthwhile to attempt to replicate this finding and determine its generality.

In a related vein, Hull (1981) has hypothesized that alcohol exerts its effects via the cognitive processes subserving the self-aware state. Although Hull (1981) presents an impressive array of findings supporting the contention that alcohol impairs cognitive abilities and is stress reducing, critical links between these sets of findings are lacking. Although it would appear that alcohol does reduce self-awareness (Hull, Levenson, Young, & Sher, 1983), it has yet to be shown that the magnitude of stress reduction is a function of the magnitude of reduced self-awareness. While data on the interaction between negative, self-relevant life events, and self-consciousness on alcoholic relapse (Hull & Young, 1983a) and on the interaction between failure feedback and self-consciousness on stress-induced drinking (Hull & Young, 1983b) are consistent with the self-awareness theory, these findings do not demonstrate that stress-reducing effects of alcohol are mediated by levels of self-awareness or that individual differences in stress reducing effects are mediated by differences in self-consciousness. The most relevant data bearing on the self-awareness theory of stress reduction have been collected in a recent experiment by Yankofsky, Wilson, Adler, Hay, and Vrana (1984). These authors found that alcohol reduced the perception of negative interpersonal feedback. However, as Yankofsky *et al.* (1984) note, it appeared that alcohol did not affect the amount of self-evaluative activity. Furthermore, since no attempt was made to relate self-evaluative activity to stress responsiveness, causal links between self-awareness and SRD effects have yet to be established. Nevertheless, the data just cited must be considered partially supportive.

However, there are some data that would seem inconsistent with the model. The finding that alcohol was equally effective at reducing the response to a physical threat and response to social stressors (Levenson *et al.*, 1980) seems inconsistent with the self-awareness theory. Since the social stressor should depend more upon the perception and encoding of negative information about the self, the self-awareness theory would predict greater dampening of the response to the speech than to the shock (especially since content analyses of these speeches suggested that alcohol was effective at reducing self-awareness; Hull *et al.*, 1983). In addition, Sher and Walitzer (1986) failed to find a relation between public or private self-consciousness and the magnitude of SRD effects at either of two dose levels of alcohol.

Levenson *et al.* (1980) suggested that alcohol might serve to make persons feel more competent at dealing with an upcoming stressor. The research of McClelland and his colleagues (McClelland, Davis, Kalin, & Wanner, 1972) indicating increased power fantasies following alcohol consumption and Yankofsky *et al.*'s (1984) finding that alcohol consumption protected subjects' feelings of power and control after an aversive heterosocial interaction, are certainly consistent with this viewpoint. However, alcohol consumption has not been found to lead to heightened levels of "competence" or "skillfulness" in coping with social stressors (Keane & Lisman, 1980; Sher & Levenson, 1982). Thus the extent to which alcohol consumption might directly lead to increased self-efficacy expectations is unclear. Future studies should attempt to measure possible alcohol effects on self-competency and self-efficacy to evaluate this hypothesis more carefully and determine the relation between these potential mediators and stress responsiveness.

A final hypothesis suggested by Levenson *et al.* (1980) is that alcohol might increase distractibility, leading one to attend less to a stressor. To date critical tests of this hypothesis are lacking although both the self-awareness hypothesis and the increased power/efficacy hypothesis are consistent with this more general cognitive disruption perspective.

### *Nonpharmacologic Effects: The Role of Expectancy*

Although one influential study (Wilson & Abrams, 1977) has found that the belief one has consumed alcohol was stress reducing, most published studies suggest that this expectancy is either unimportant (Bradlyn *et al.* 1981; Levenson *et al.*, 1980; Rimm *et al.*, 1981; Wilson *et al.*, 1981) or stress increasing (Abrams & Wilson, 1979; Polivy *et al.*, 1976; Sutker *et al.*, 1982). This should not be taken to mean, however, that expectancies are unimportant in determining drinking behavior since expectancies for alcohol-related stress reduction might be important in predicting individual differences in stress-related drinking behavior. However, there is not much empirical literature available on this last point. Although expectancies for reinforcement from alcohol, including expectancies for stress-reducing effects, appear to correlate with drinking behavior (e.g., Brown, Goldman, Inn, & Anderson, 1980), reliable associations with stress-related drinking have not yet been reported. On a somewhat related point, the strength of individually held expectancies for stress reduction from alcohol have not been found to correlate with actual SRD effects (Sher & Walitzer, 1986).

## Empirical Demonstration of Stress-Related Drinking

The foregoing discussion documents the fact that alcohol consumption can lead to stress reduction, and that this appears to be due to pharmacologic mechanisms and is not attributable to expectancy effects. However, if the SRD model proposed here is to have any explanatory power as a theory of drinking behavior, it must be able to make predictions concerning the relation between stress and voluntary alcohol consumption. As noted above, the SRD model does not predict that all stressful situations will generate alcohol consumption since drinking on a given occasion is likely to be a function of a number of factors, some of which might be substantially more influential than the intensity of a stressor. The following literature review indicates that stressful situations are likely to lead to increased alcohol consumption when actual consumption or intoxication is unlikely to be punished, and when more effective methods for coping with the stressor are not available.

*Studies of Stress-Inducing Drinking.* In stress-induced drinking studies, some stressor manipulation occurs and the effect this has on some aspect of drinking behavior (usually amount consumed) is then assessed. According to the SRD model, stress should lead to increased consumption of alcoholic beverages under certain stressful conditions. Although few consistent patterns emerge from a review of the stress induced drinking literature, several general principles governing the relationship between stress and drinking behavior are suggested.

To date, a number of different stressors including heterosocial evaluation (Higgins & Marlatt, 1975), criticism (Marlatt, Kosturn, & Lang, 1975; Miller *et al.*, 1974), difficult (or insoluble) intellectual tasks (Hull & Young, 1983b; Noel & Lisman, 1980; Tucker, Vuchinich, Sobell, & Maisto, 1980), and public speaking (Strickler, Tomaszewski, Maxwell, & Suib, 1979) have been shown capable of eliciting drinking behavior. However, stressors differ in the extent to which they tend to elicit drinking behavior. Although Higgins and Marlatt's (1973, 1975) findings demonstrating stress-induced drinking to an interpersonal stressor and not to an impersonal stressor have led to speculation that interpersonal and not impersonal threats can motivate drinking, this distinction does not seem tenable. Social stressors can lead to reduced beverage consumption (e.g., Holroyd, 1978) and impersonal stressors can lead to increased levels of consumption (e.g., Noel & Lisman, 1980). A study by Gabel, Noel, Keane, and Lisman (1980) further explored the issue of stressor type raised by previous investigators. These researchers found high levels of alcohol consumption following erotic stimuli but not following stimuli depicting mutilation.

Additionally, autonomic arousal (assessed by HR and electrodermal measures) was not related to alcohol consumption. These findings seem contradictory to the SRD model. However, the model does not posit that physiologic arousal will predict drinking behavior *across* individuals since the tendency to experience SRD effects and to drink under stress is not viewed as a simple function of distress. Additionally, the physiologic response to scenes of mutilation might represent a fundamentally different physiologic state than that caused by most other stressors. The literature on blood and injury fears suggests a predominantly parasympathetic rather than a sympathetic response to this class of stimuli (Marks, 1981). Thus generalization from studies employing blood- and injury-related stimuli should probably be made cautiously.

The findings of Pihl and Yankofsky (1979) and Holroyd (1978) appear to demonstrate that social-evaluative stresses lead to decreases in drinking, findings in seeming contradiction to the SRD model. However, it should be noted that both sets of findings were in comparison not to a neutral but to a success, or esteem-enhancing, control group. Conceivably, these negative findings might be more attributable to high levels of consumption following an esteem-enhancing manipulation than to low levels of consumption following a stress.[6] Future studies are needed to be able to rule out this type of alternative hypothesis.

The notion that drinking alcohol as a response will vary as a function of the individual's beliefs about how alcohol will affect him in a specific situation seems self-evident. In the extreme, one would not expect stressful situations where alcoholic behavior is proscribed (e.g., on the job) to elicit drinking to the same extent as stressful situations where alcohol behavior is condoned (e.g., at certain social gatherings). Until quite recently, these nonstressor aspects of the environment have been neglected in laboratory investigations of stress-induced drinking. A notable exception to this is Tucker *et al.*'s (1980) study examining the effect of the opportunity for drinking at a later time on stress-induced drinking. These authors found that subjects who knew of the opportunity to drink following a difficult intellectual task appeared to restrict their pretask drinking, presumably to minimize impairment on the task. This study demonstrates the importance of understanding situational demands fac-

---

[6] The use of an esteem-enhancing manipulation can even lead to interpretive difficulties when stress-induced drinking is demonstrated. For example, in the experiment by Hull and Young (1983), high self-conscious individuals who experienced failure feedback consumed more alcohol than high self-conscious individuals who experienced success feedback. However, it is not clear if this difference is due to relatively high levels of consumption in the failure group or relatively low levels of consumption in the success group.

ing the drinker and how opportunities for consuming alcohol vary across these demands. This implies that greater attention to the demand characteristics of drinking in the laboratory might reveal more potent determinants of drinking behavior.

Previous drinking history may influence the extent to which an individual will drink when stressed. Based on the limited evidence acquired to date (Miller *et al.*, 1974; Pihl & Yankofsky, 1979), drinking history appears to interact with degree of stress to affect amount of alcohol consumed (although Rohsenow, 1982a, Experiment 1, reports a negative finding). Future studies should be directed to assessing differences in stress-induced drinking as a function of problem-drinking status and drinking pattern.

Probably the most important finding to emerge from the stress-induced drinking literature is that the degree to which a stressor will elicit drinking is determined in part by the availability of effective alternative coping responses (Marlatt *et al.*, 1975; Stricker *et al.*, 1979; Tucker, Vuchinich, & Sobell, 1981). Although not a universal finding (Rohsenow, 1982a, Experiment 1), the demonstration that the opportunity for effective coping moderates drinking in the face of stress seems fundamental to an understanding of alcohol and stress relations, particularly since alcohol consumption can lead to cognitive impairment and can disrupt attempts to cope effectively. The coping opportunities that might influence the occurrence of stress-related drinking appear diverse, ranging from the opportunity to retaliate against an aggressor (Marlatt *et al.*, 1975), to reducing physiologic arousal through relaxation (Stricker *et al.*, 1979), to preparing oneself appropriately for the demands of a challenging task (Tucker *et al.*, 1981). That is, the "opportunity for coping" appears to be a general finding, replicable across experimental demands and types of coping activities.

Before concluding this section, discussion of an overlooked methodological point is in order. In order to infer that a stress manipulation results in increased alcohol consumption as opposed to beverage consumption more generally, the availability of a control beverage is desirable. Several studies have compared alcoholic beverage to nonalcoholic beverage consumption (e.g., Gabel, Noel, Keane, & Lisman, 1980; Noel & Lisman, 1980) and found effects specific for alcohol. Strictly speaking, these differential effects for alcohol must be considered suspect unless alcoholic and control beverages are first matched for desirability in a nonstressed sample. Otherwise, the experiment can be interpreted as indicating that the stressor merely increases consumption of any preferred beverage.

Our reading of the literature is that alcohol is generally stress reducing but that whether or not someone drinks on a given occasion appears to be a function of a number of contributing factors that go far beyond the stress-reducing pharmacologic effects. Stress-related drinking is a function of a number of psychological and social factors, especially the ability to cope effectively with the stressor without alcohol and the potentially negative consequences of alcohol consumption. Furthermore, people drink for a number of reasons and careful attention needs to be paid to the nature of the control groups and tasks employed in stress-induced-drinking studies so that clear interpretations of results of experimental investigations are possible.

*Field Studies.* A number of studies have surveyed drinkers and assessed variables relevant to the SRD model. Although these studies are correlational and lack the methodological control of laboratory investigations, they are valuable for a number of reasons:

1. Participants in these studies may be more typical of persons in the general population. Although no one has yet characterized the type of person who volunteers for an experiment in which he or she may have to experience a stressful situation and consume an alcoholic beverage, it seems quite likely that at the very least, these will be unusually adventuresome people. In fact, these people may be the least likely to experience stress since the very act of volunteering for this type of experiment implies a certain boldness.
2. Because laboratory alcohol research with humans is labor intensive and expensive, experiments typically employ limited numbers of subjects; this results in limited statistical power. Field studies, which are usually less expensive on a cost per subject basis, are not as restricted with regard to feasible sample sizes.
3. Drinking-related behavior or attitudes are not sampled in "atypical" or "unnatural" laboratory situations.

Although a detailed review of field and survey studies is beyond the scope of this chapter (and the interested reader can refer to Cappell & Greeley, Chapter 2, this volume), the empirical literature is generally supportive of the SRD model and the following conclusions seem warranted. First, most social drinkers expect alcohol to reduce anxiety (e.g., Brown *et al.*, 1980; Southwick *et al.*, 1981) and other negative mood states, and stress-reduction from drinking is more often reported by problem drinkers than nonproblem drinkers (Cahalan, 1970; Cahalan *et al.*, 1969). Second, cross-sectional studies of nonalcoholics have shown that various indices of stress or tension are related to alcohol consumption but the magnitude of this relationship typically is not great (e.g., Cahalan, 1970; Cahalan & Room, 1974; Margolis, Kroes, & Quinn, 1974; Neff & Husaini, 1982; Pearlin & Radabaugh,1976; Sadava, Thistle, & Forsyth, 1978; Wells-Parker, Miles, & Spencer, 1983) and negative findings have been reported (e.g., Rohsenow, 1982b). Finally, individual differences may play an important role in mediating alcohol–stress relationships (Conway, Vickers, Ward, & Rahe, 1981). Much work needs to be done investigating the relationship between alcohol and stress in the "real world," particularly longitudinal research which has been noticeably lacking. However, it should be pointed out that at least as far as "problem drinking" goes, it would appear that psychological symptoms such as anxiety are weak predictors compared with such variables as social environment. Future studies should address this complexity if they wish to elucidate the nature of alcohol–stress relationships.

*Clinical Studies.* While a detailed review of the clinical literature on alcohol and stress is beyond the scope of this chapter (and the interested reader might wish to refer to Cappell and Greeley, Chapter 2, this volume), studies with clinical populations are generally supportive of the SRD model. Clinical observations suggest that the coexistence of alcohol problems and phobias is a relatively frequent occurrence, that the phobia often precedes the alcohol problem, and that for some phobics alcohol is seen as an aid to coping with a high level of anxiety (e.g., Bowen, Cipwynyk, D'Arcy, & Keegan, 1984; Chambless, Caputo, & Cherney, 1984; Mullaney & Trippett, 1979; Smail, Stockwell, Canter, & Hodgson, 1984). These data seem to contradict those findings that suggest that psychological distress is not a useful predictor of alcohol consumption. The literature on stress-induced drinking does not indicate that trait anxious individuals are prone to drink when stressed (Holroyd, 1978) and, as a group, alcoholics do not appear to be particularly high on trait anxiety (e.g., MacAndrew, 1982). Although no clear explanation of this seeming contradiction is readily apparent, one can hypothesize that at moderate to low levels of distress, anxiety level is not a useful predictor of individual differences in stress-related drinking behavior. As anxiety becomes debilitating, however, some sufferers more readily turn to alcohol.

There appears to be a relation between life events and increases in alcohol consumption and/or relapses in alcoholics (e.g., Marlatt & Gordon, 1980; Tucker, Vuchinich, & Harris, 1985). Longitudinal studies are needed to better characterize the alcohol–stress relation in problem drinkers and alcoholics, and to determine how individual difference variables such as personality (Hershenson, 1965), perceived social support (Rosenberg, 1983), coping abilities (Marlatt & Gordon, 1980), and self-consciousness (Hull & Young, 1983a) might mediate this relation.

**Evaluation of the Model**

*Overview of the Model*

The SRD model of alcohol use/abuse posits that, in sufficient dosage, alcohol consumption leads to decreased stress responsiveness and is thus reinforced.

These effects are posited to be mediated via pharmacologic mechanisms and to affect central mechanisms in the brain sensitive to aversive stimulation. Individual differences in these effects are seen to be more a function of vulnerability to experiencing stress reduction from alcohol than the tendency to experience stress.

Because drinking behavior is conceived as being determined by a number of variables and because alcohol consumption can lead to negative consequences, stressful circumstances are viewed as neither necessary nor sufficient causes of alcohol consumption. Thus the SRD model is not viewed as a comprehensive theory of drinking behavior. Drinking is most likely to occur in response to a stressor when the probability that drinking behavior or intoxication will be punished is low and when alternative effective coping responses are not readily available. Presumably, when stress levels become intolerably high and individuals have limited coping resources, drinking behavior may occur even in the face of punishment. It would also seem likely that impulsive individuals (i.e., persons who have problems inhibiting behaviors that are immediately reinforced but later punished) might also be particularly vulnerable to drink when stressed.

It is acknowledged that alcohol might exert SRD effects via a number of different mechanisms. For example, it is possible that for certain women, alcohol might be used to cope with menstrual distress because of either analgesic or diuretic effects. The recent finding of an association between alcoholism and family history of essential tremor (Nasrallah, Schroeder, & Peetty, 1982; Schroeder & Nasrallah, 1982) coupled with demonstration of alcohol's antitremor effects (Landauer, 1981) suggest that alcohol might be stress reducing for some individuals because of an antitremor effect. Persons with post-traumatic stress disorders might abuse alcohol in order to achieve hypnotic effects (LaCoursiere, Godfrey, & Ruby, 1980). Although these and other possibilities can be considered, it is hypothesized that alcohol has direct effects on brain centers involved in the regulation of anxiety and aversive stimulation. It is these effects that have been the focus of this chapter and are probably of greatest relevance when attempting to understand the pharmacologic basis of most stress-induced drinking.

## Relation of the Stress-Response-Dampening Model to Other Models

### Conger's (1956) Tension Reduction Hypothesis

The SRD model bears a close resemblance to the TRH. This is not surprising since the SRD model was derived from the results of empirical studies probing the TRH. The major distinction between the two models/theories is that the SRD model does not adopt the concepts of drive, inhibition, and conflict and consequently a number of predictions which might be made from the TRH would not be made by the SRD model. Thus, the SRD model can be considered a narrower, more molecular model which relies on fewer hypothetical constructs than the TRH. Perhaps it would be most accurate to think of the SRD model as a psychobiological minitheory which can be embedded in the context of a broader cognitive–social learning framework.

### Self-Awareness Model of Hull (1981)

Hull (1981) hypothesizes that alcohol interferes with the cognitive processes underlying self-awareness. Consequently, the impact of certain stressors (e.g., those conveying negative information about the self) is likely to be attenuated by alcohol-related reductions in self-awareness. Although Hull (1981; Hull et al., 1983) convincingly argues that alcohol can reduce self-awareness, it has yet to be demonstrated that alcohol-related reductions in self-awareness result in stress reduction. Data supporting a self-awareness mechanism of stress-response dampening were reviewed above, and it was concluded that at present, support for the model is limited. Support for the self-awareness theory in respect to stress induced drinking was provided by Hull and Young (1983) who showed that high-self-conscious individuals receiving failure feedback on an intellectual task drank more wine on a "taste-rating task" than high-self-conscious individuals receiving success feedback. However, the interpretation of this finding is not clear-cut since high-self-conscious subjects receiving failure feedback did not drink any more than low-self-conscious subjects receiving either failure or success feedback. While Hull and Young's data (1983b) support the hypothesis that high-self-conscious persons might modulate their drinking more as a function of success and failure experiences, the hypothesis that high-self-conscious persons are more likely to drink more when stressed (by self-relevant stressors) is not supported.

The SRD model and the self-awareness model appear to differ in their predictions concerning the type of person most likely to experience pronounced SRD effects. The SRD model posits that individuals who show certain undercontrolled personality traits such as aggressiveness and impulsivity are the most likely to experience SRD effects and to drink when stressed. This individual difference model is not based on theoretical considerations but instead on observed empirical relations. The self-awareness model predicts that persons high in dispositional self-awareness are most likely to experience stress reducing effects of alcohol and drink under stress. Although there is some evidence to suggest that high-self-aware recovering alcoholics might be more likely to relapse following self-relevant, negative life events (Hull & Young, 1983a) and drink when stressed (Hull & Young, 1983, but see comments in previous paragraph), this general perspective does not seem consistent with other available data (e.g., Holroyd, 1978; Sher & Walitzer,

1986). Hull (1981) argues that the prealcoholic personality pattern noted by several investigators (e.g., Jones, 1968; Hoffman, Loper, & Kammeier, 1974) is consistent with the hypothesis of high dispositional self-awareness. However, examination of Hull's (1981) argument reveals that he has misread the important findings of Hoffman *et al.* (1974) and the characteristics he attributes to prealcoholic personality are actually attributable to the clinical alcoholic personality (see Barnes, 1979). In fact, the portrait of the prealcoholic personality painted by Hoffman *et al.* (1974) appears inconsistent with the hypothesis of high self-awareness.

The foregoing was meant only as a critique of the relevance of the self-awareness theory to stress response dampening effects and not to other potentially important alcohol effects on aggression and social behavior. Until direct tests of the self-awareness model and stress reduction from alcohol are undertaken, the relevance of the model for explaining alcohol-related SRD effects is uncertain.

## Models of Stress-Induced Drinking

A number of models of stress-induced drinking have been proposed including a simple learning model (e.g., Conger, 1956), an expectancy model (Marlatt, 1976), and the self-handicapped model (Jones & Berglas, 1978). The SRD model is compatible with all of these models, but clearly differs in emphasis. Alcohol is posited to be reinforcing because of SRD effects, and consequently drinking under stress is likely to be reinforced. Thus the SRD model proposes a basis of reinforcement for certain types of drinking behavior, and drinking under stress can be thought of, in part, as a learned phenomenon. However, as noted above, drinking under stress appears to be a multidetermined phenomenon. Although providing a foundation for understanding stress-induced drinking, a simple learning formulation based on pharmacologically based reinforcement is likely to be inadequate since it fails to readily account for the numerous situational variables that influence the occurrence and extent of stress-induced drinking.

The expectancy model of stress-induced drinking emphasizes the importance of an individual's beliefs about how drinking will help that individual cope with a difficult stressor. The model posits that an individual is likely to drink when stressed if he or she expects alcohol to help him or her cope more effectively with a stressor and when more effective coping strategies are not readily available. As is obvious from the above, the expectancy model has been incorporated in the SRD model of stress-induced drinking proposed here. It is important to point out, however, that existing evidence suggests that SRD effects are mediated via pharmacologic mechanisms and so the expectancy model is seen as relevant to understanding why someone is likely to drink on a given occasion, but not why such drinking is likely to be maintained.

The self-handicapping model predicts that individuals will drink when anticipating an upcoming task if they expect to perform poorly on the task and if alcohol intoxication would provide a reasonable excuse for poor performance. It would certainly seem like this model is consistent with many views of stress-induced drinking in that if the behavioral act of drinking is likely to be reinforcing for any reason (including a purely psychological one such as esteem-protecting attributions), then the individual would be more likely to drink when stressed. That is, the opportunity for self-handicapping might reasonably be expected to increase the likelihood of stress-induced drinking. However, there would appear to be a variety of situations that might elicit stress-induced drinking and not be easily subjected to a self-handicapping analysis. Furthermore, when self-handicapping alcohol consumption does occur it would seem likely that it could be reinforced not only by the positive effects of esteem-protecting attributions (as hypothesized by the model) but also by SRD effects. Thus, the self-handicapping model is compatible with explanations of stress-induced drinking derived from the SRD model but, in isolation, applies to only a limited subset of stress-induced drinking situations and/or is an incomplete explanation. Hopefully, the empirical foundations of this model will be expanded so that the extent to which alcohol actually serves self-handicapping functions can be determined.

**Critical Tests of the Model**

There are three types of research investigations that together would provide critical tests of the SRD model. These include studies comparing the effectiveness of alcohol (in commonly used doses) with the effectiveness of "established" drugs with stress-reducing/anxiolytic effects (such as the benzodiazepines), studies examining the relation of SRD effects to actual voluntary drinking behavior, and studies using ethanol antagonists to selectively block stress-reducing effects of alcohol and then examining the effect that this pharmacologic antagonism has on voluntary drinking behavior. If the SRD model is correct, we would expect alcohol to show effects similar to other drugs with known stress-reducing effects, we would expect a correlation between the magnitude of SRD effects and various indices of drinking behavior, and we would expect that blockade of SRD effects would result in reduced frequency and/or quantity of alcohol. Unfortunately, to date these tests have not been carried out. Nevertheless, outlining these tests is useful in illustrating the kinds of additional evidence needed to validate the SRD model as a compelling explanation of some types of drinking behavior.

*Comparisons of the Effects of Alcohol with Established "Stress Reducers"*

Although it has been shown in animals that alcohol has a number of stress-reducing effects comparable to those of established stress reducers such as the benzodiazepines (Gray, 1978), the author is not aware of comparable data from studies with humans. In the only relevant study of which the author is aware, Lienert and Traxel (1959) found that alcohol and meprobamate were both effective at reducing the electrodermal responses to certain words (although in the doses employed the meprobamate produced slightly larger effects than ethanol). Similar studies comparing alcohol with benzodiazepines and perhaps beta-adrenergic blocking agents and employing more relevant stressors would be extremely helpful in evaluating the effectiveness of alcohol in producing SRD effects.

*Relating Stress-Response-Dampening Effects to Drinking Behavior*

Although the results of the national surveys of Cahalan (1970) and Cahalan *et al.* (1969) indicate that heavy alcohol consumers and problem drinkers report that alcohol is an effective stress reducer more than light consumers and nonproblem drinkers, the correlational and self-report nature of these data limits confidence in these findings. Unfortunately, there is little experimental evidence assessing this important relation. One recent investigation (Cummings & Marlatt, 1983) examined the relation between SRD effects and *ad lib.* drinking behavior in the laboratory. The results of this study were not supportive of the hypothesis that persons prone to SRD effects are particularly likely to drink when stressed. It should be pointed out that the *ad lib.* consumption in this study could not strictly be considered "stress-induced" since the physiological and self-report data collected by Cummings and Marlatt (1983) indicated recovery from the stressor prior to the *ad lib.* drinking opportunity *and* because stressed subjects drank no more than nonstressed subjects. Given this context, it is not too surprising that the best predictor of amount consumed was the amount of stress (state and trait anxiety) the subject brought to the experiment since this might be a more accurate reflection of stress at the time of drinking. Grossman (1983) found evidence of a negative relation between the magnitude of SRD effects and stress-induced drinking. That is, persons who were vulnerable to SRD effects drank *less* under stress. Should this result prove replicable, it would suggest an alternative individual difference model of SRD effects. This alternative model would predict that individuals who are relatively insensitive to SRD effects are those most likely to drink in quantity under stress since they need to consume more to achieve adequate stress reduction. A similar model of risk for alcoholism based on sensitivity to intoxicating effects has been proposed by Schuckit (1980a). Future studies should not only examine the relation between sensitivity to SRD effects and careful laboratory evaluations of stress-induced drinking, but also "real world" stress-induced drinking since the drinking behavior of subjects on a single drinking occasion is likely to be of low reliability. Even if these data were reliable (i.e., highly generalizable to drinking behavior in similar situations), they would provide little information on the frequency of occurrence of stress-related drinking episodes.

### Examining the Effect of Blocking Stress-Response-Dampening Effects on Drinking Behavior

Convincing support of a model of stress-induced drinking based on SRD effects would be provided by studies demonstrating that selective blockade of the mechanism responsible for stress reduction and observing a decrease in stress-related drinking behavior. Although blockade is usually brought about by pharmacologic antagonism of a drug effect, psychological blockade could also be attempted if SRD effects were shown to be mediated primarily via cognitive processes. At present, we do not have the knowledge base for attempting such studies since the mechanisms responsible for SRD effects have yet to be elucidated. Additional studies that attempt to examine specific mechanisms of SRD effects (e.g., Ewing & McCarty, 1983; Yankofsky et al., 1984) are needed to advance our understanding of the effect of alcohol on stress.

## Implications for Treatment and Prevention

### Treatment

Several implications can be drawn from the research on alcohol and stress. First, since many problem drinkers claim that alcohol is very helpful in coping with stress, it is important to determine if stress reduction is a motive for drinking for a given client. For those clients who report significant stress-related drinking, psychotherapeutic approaches that attempt to foster coping skills, such as relaxation training and assertion training, are seen as having particular promise (Chaney, O'Leary, & Marlatt, 1978; Marlatt, 1980; Parker, Gilbert, & Thoreson, 1978).

The pharmacotherapeutic approaches are less clear. Biologically oriented physicians have argued that the benzodiazepine compounds should be prescribed more frequently in clients who are using alcohol for stress reduction

[Stress, distress, and drug treatment (editorial), 1978] since the "problems of alcohol abuse are far greater than the mild degree of dependence that may result from abusing the alternatives" (p. 1347). Others have advocated that specific antipanic agents should be used in cases of alcoholism secondary to panic disorder/agoraphobia (Hudson & Perkins, 1984). However, some alcohol treatment approaches [e.g., Alcoholics Anonymous (A.A.)] view the use of most psychoactive compounds as a "crutch" and incompatible with productive recovery. Certainly, given the frequent abuse of tranquilizers by alcoholics, use of these substances as a substitute must be recommended cautiously. Should a pharmacologic basis of SRD effects be established, drugs that selectively antagonize SRD effects might be shown to be useful therapeutic agents.

*Prevention*

Although there is some evidence suggesting that stress-reduction from alcohol is an important etiological factor in the development of alcoholism (Sher & Levenson, 1982), the critical prospective investigations have yet to be conducted. Nevertheless, two implications can be derived from the literature on the stress reducing properties of alcohol. The first concerns identification of high-risk individuals. If individuals who are at high risk for alcoholism are either particularly sensitive (Sher & Levenson, 1982) or insensitive (Grossman, 1983) to SRD effects, then the evaluation of SRD effects for an individual might prove to be a useful assessment of vulnerability to alcoholism and preventive interventions might be targeted at this population. The second implication concerns the potential preventive utility of training high-risk individuals in stress reduction techniques and coping skills.

**Summary**

Alcohol appears to dampen response to stress. This assertion cannot be made unequivocally since alcohol consumption may only reduce certain aspects of stress response, may only have stress reducing properties in sufficient dosage, and may not be equally effective in dampening the response to all stressors. Furthermore, since alcohol consumption can lead to a variety of negative consequences ranging from physical discomfort to behavioral and cognitive impairment, alcohol consumption can at times be stress inducing. Perhaps for these reasons, many reviewers have found the alcohol and stress literature confusing and inconclusive.

Although most people expect alcohol to reduce stress, and alcohol does appear to have SRD properties, drinking in response to stress is a complex phenomenon. Whether or not someone drinks on a given occasion appears to be a function of a number of contributing factors that go far beyond the stress-reducing pharmacologic effects. Stress-related drinking is determined by a variety of psychological and social factors, especially the perceived ability to cope effectively with the stressor without alcohol. Rather than invalidating the notion of stress-induced drinking, these other important determinants of stress-induced drinking provide a context for understanding the nature of the alcohol–stress relation.

## Acknowledgment

Preparation of this chapter was supported in part by Grant No. AA6182 from the National Institute of Alcohol Abuse and Alcoholism.

## References

Abrams, D., & Wilson, G. T. (1979). Effects of alcohol on social anxiety in women: Cognitive versus physiological arousal. *Journal of Abnormal Psychology, 88,* 161–173.

Alexander, B. K., & Hadaway, P. F. (1982). Opiate addiction: The case for an adaptive orientation. *Psychological Bulletin, 92,* 367–382.

Alexanderson, G., & Lindman, R. (1980). Of mice and women. 2. Differential effects of dose information and administration of alcohol on fear. In R. Lindman (Ed.), *Anxiety and alcohol: Limitations of tension reduction theory in alcoholics* (Monograph Suppl. 1, pp. 75–82). Abo, Finland: Abo Akademi, Department of Psychology.

Alkana, R. L., & Noble, E. P. (1979). Amethystic agents: Reversal of acute ethanol intoxication in humans. In E. Majchrowicz & E. P. Noble (Eds.), *Biochemistry and pharmacology of ethanol* (Vol. 2, pp. 349–374). New York: Plenum Press.

Altshuler, H. L. (1982). Ethanol reinforcement: Self-administration and discriminative stimulus parameters. In S. Saito & T. Yanagita, Eds. *Learning and Memory: Drugs as Reinforcers* (pp. 240–256). Amsterdam: Excerpta Medica.

Bandura, A. (1969). *Principles of behavior modification.* New York: Holt, Rinehart and Winston.

Barnes, G. A. (1979). The alcoholic personality: A reanalysis of the literature. *Journal of Studies on Alcohol, 40,* 571–634.

Berg, N. (1971). Effects of alcohol intoxication on self-concept. *Quarterly Journal of Studies on Alcohol, 32,* 442–453.

Bowen, R. C., Cipywnyk, D., D'Arcy, C., & Keegan, D. (1984). Alcoholism, anxiety disorders, and agoraphobia. *Alcoholism: Clinical and Experimental Research, 8,* 48–50.

Bradlyn, A. S., Strickler, D. P., & Maxwell, W. A. (1981). Alcohol, expectancy and stress: Methodological concerns with the expectancy design. *Addictive Behaviors, 6,* 1–8.

Brown, J. S., & Crowell, C. R. (1974). Alcohol and conflict resolution: A theoretical analysis. *Quarterly Journal of Studies on Alcohol, 35,* 66–85.

Brown, S. A., Goldman, M. S., Inn, A., & Anderson, L. (1980). Expectations of reinforcement from alcohol: Their domain and relation to drinking patterns. *Journal of Consulting and Clinical Psychology, 48,* 419–426.

Cahalan, D. (1970). *Problem drinkers.* San Francisco: Jossey-Bass.

Cahalan, D., Cisin, I., & Crossley, H. M. (1969). *American drinking practices: A national study of drinking behavior and attitudes* (Monograph No. 6). New Brunswick, NJ: Rutgers Center of Alcohol Studies.

Cahalan, D., & Room, R. (1974). *Problem Drinking among American Men.* New Brunswick, N.J.: Rutgers Center on Alcohol Studies.

Cappell, H., & Herman, C. P. (1972). Alcohol and tension reduction: A review. *Quarterly Journal of Studies on Alcohol, 33,* 33–64.

Carlsson, C., & Fasth, B.-G. (1976). A comparison of the effects of propranolol and diazepam in alcoholics. *British Journal of Psychiatry, 119,* 605–606.

Chambless, D. L., Caputo, G. C., & Cherney, J. (1984, November). *Anxiety disorders in alcoholic inpatients.* Paper presented at the meeting of the Association for Advancement of Behavior Therapy, Philadelphia.

Chaney, E. F., O'Leary, M., & Marlatt, G. A. (1978). Skill training with alcoholics. *Journal of Consulting and Clinical Psychology, 46,* 1092–1104.

Child, J. S., Levisman, J. A., & Pearce, M. L. (1979). Cardiac effects of acute ethanol ingestion unmasked by autonomic blockade. *Circulation, 59,* 120–125.

Claridge, G. (1970). *Drugs and human behavior.* New York: Praeger.

Conger, J. J. (1951). The effects of alcohol on conflict behavior in the albino rat. *Quarterly Journal of Studies on Alcohol, 12,* 1–29.

Conger, J. J. (1956). Reinforcement theory and the dynamics of alcoholism. *Quarterly Journal of Studies on Alcohol, 17,* 296–305.

Conway, T. L., Vickers, R. R., Ward, H. W., & Rahe, R. H. (1981). Occupational stress and variation in cigarette, coffee, and alcohol consumption. *Journal of Health and Social Behavior, 22,* 155–165.

Corrigan, E. M. (1980). *Alcoholic women in treatment.* New York: Oxford University Press.

Cummings, C. C., & Marlatt, G. A. (1983). *Stress-induced alcohol consumption.* Paper presented at the 91st Annual Convention of the American Psychological Association, Anaheim, CA.

Curlee, J. (1970). A comparison of male and female patients at an alcoholism treatment center. *Journal of Psychology, 74,* 239–247.

Cutter, H., Maloof, B., Kurtz, N., & Jones, W. (1976). "Feeling no pain": Differential responses to pain by alcoholics and nonalcoholics before and after drinking. *Journal of Studies on Alcohol, 37,* 273–277.

Davis, V., & Walsh, M. (1970). Alcohol, amines, and alkaloids: A possible biochemical basis for alcohol addiction. *Science, 167,* 1005–1007.

Eddy, C. C. (1979). The effects of alcohol on anxiety in problem- and nonproblem-drinking women. *Alcoholism: Clinical and Experimental Research, 3,* 107–114.

Ekman, P., Levenson, R. W., & Friesen, W. (1983). Autonomic nervous system activity distinguishes among emotions. *Science, 221,* 1208–1210.

Ewing, J. A., & McCarty, D. (1983). Are the endorphins involved in mediating the mood effects of ethanol? *Alcoholism: Clinical and Experimental Research, 7,* 271–275.

Folkman, S., & Lazarus, R. S. (1985). If it changes it must be a process: Study of emotion and coping during three stages of a college examination. *Journal of Personality and Social Psychology, 48,* 150–170.

Fowles, D. (1980). The three-arousal model: Implications of Gray's two-factor learning theory for heart rate, electrodermal activity, and psychopathy. *Psychophysiology, 17,* 87–104.

Freed, E. X. (1973). Drug abuse by alcoholics: A review. *International Journal of the Addictions, 8,* 451–473.

Freed, E. X. (1978). Alcohol and mood: An updated review. *International Journal of the Addictions, 8,* 451–473.

Gabel, P., Noel, N., Keane, T., & Lisman, S. (1980). Effects of sexual versus fear arousal on alcohol consumption in college males. *Behaviour Research and Therapy, 18,* 519–526.

Gilbert, D. G. (1979). Paradoxical tranquilizing and emotion-reducing effects of nicotine. *Psychological Bulletin, 86,* 643–661.

Gough, H. (1969). *Manual for the California Psychological Inventory.* Palo Alto, CA: Consulting Psychologists Press.

Gray, J. (1977). Drug effects on fear and frustration: Possible limbic site of action of minor tranquilizers. In L. L. Iverson, S. D. Iverson, & S. H. Snyder (Eds.), *Handbook of Psychopharmacology* (pp. 433–529). New York: Plenum Press.

Gray, J. (1978). The neuropsychology of anxiety. *British Journal of Psychology, 69*, 417–434.

Gray, J. (1979). Anxiety and the brain: Not by neurochemistry alone. *Psychological Medicine, 9*, 605–609.

Green, J., & Jaffe, J. H. (1977). Alcohol and opiate dependence: A review. *Journal of Studies on Alcohol, 38*, 1274–1293.

Greenberg, L., & Carpenter, J. (1957). The effect of alcoholic beverages on skin conductance and emotional tension. I: Wine, whiskey and alcohol. *Quarterly Journal of Studies on Alcohol, 18*, 190–204.

Grossman, L. M. (1983). Individual differences in the tension reduction effect of alcohol: Physiological correlates of stress-induced drinking (Doctoral dissertation, Indiana University, 1983). *Dissertation Abstracts International, 44*, 910B.

Hershenson, D. B. (1965). Stress-induced use of alcohol by problem drinkers as a function of their sense of identity. *Quarterly Journal of Studies on Alcohol, 26*, 213–222.

Higgins, R., & Marlatt, G. (1973). Effects of anxiety arousal on the consumption of alcohol by alcoholics and social drinkers. *Journal of Consulting and Clinical Psychology, 41*, 426–433.

Higgins, R., & Marlatt, G. (1975). Fear of interpersonal evaluation as a determinant of alcohol consumption in male social drinkers. *Journal of Abnormal Psychology, 84*, 644–651.

Hodgson, R. J., Stockwell, T. R., & Rankin, H. J. (1979). Can alcohol reduce tension? *Behaviour Research and Therapy, 17*, 459–479.

Hoehn-Saric, R. (1982). Neurotransmitters in anxiety. *Archives of General Psychiatry, 39*, 735–742.

Hoffman, H., Loper, R., & Kammeier, M. (1974). Identifying future alcoholics with the MMPI alcoholism scales. *Quarterly Journal of Studies on Alcohol, 35*, 490–498.

Hollister, L. E. (1981). Management of the anxious patient prone to drug abuse. *Journal of Clinical Psychiatry, 42*, 35–38.

Holroyd, K. (1978). Effects of social anxiety and social evaluation on beer consumption and social interaction. *Journal of Studies on Alcohol, 39*, 737–744.

Hudson, C. J., & Perkins, S. H. (1984). Panic disorder and alcohol misuse. *Journal of Studies on Alcohol, 45*, 462–464.

Hull, J. G. (1981). A self-awareness model of the causes and effects of alcohol consumption. *Journal of Abnormal Psychology, 90*, 586–600.

Hull, J. G., Levenson, R. W., Young, R. D., & Sher, K. J. (1983). Self-awareness-reducing effects of alcohol consumption. *Journal of Personality and Social Psychology, 44*, 461–473.

Hull, J. G., & Young, R. D. (1983a). The self-awareness reducing effects of alcohol consumption: Evidence and implications. In J. Suls & A. G. Greenwald (Eds.), *Social psychological perspectives on the self* (Vol. 2, pp. 159–190). Hillsdale, NJ: Lawrence Erlbaum.

Hull, J. G., & Young, R. D. (1983b). Self-consciousness, self-esteem, and success-failure as determinants of alcohol consumption in male social drinkers. *Journal of Personality and Social Psychology, 44*, 1097–1109.

Istvan, J., & Matarazzo, J. D. (1984). Tobacco, alcohol, and caffeine use: A review of their interrelationships. *Psychological Bulletin, 95*, 301–326.

Jaffe, J. H. (1985). Drug addiction and drug abuse. In L. S. Goodman & A. Gilman (Eds.), *The pharmacological basis of therapeutics* (pp. 532–581). New York: Macmillan Publishing Company.

Jones, B., Parsons, O., & Rundell, O. (1976). Psychophysiological correlates of alcoholism. In R. E. Tarter & A. Sugarman (Eds.), *Alcoholism: Interdisciplinary approaches to an enduring problem* (pp. 435–477). Reading, MA: Addison-Wesley.

Jones, E. E., & Berglas, S. (1978). Control of attributions about the self through self-handicapping strategies: The appeal of alcohol and the role of unachievement. *Personality and Social Psychology Bulletin, 4*, 200–206.

Jones, M. C. (1968). Personality correlates and antecedents of drinking patterns in adult males. *Journal of Consulting and Clinical Psychology, 32*, 2–12.

Kalin, R., McClelland, D. C., & Kahn, M. (1965). The effect of male social drinking on fantasy. *Journal of Personality and Social Psychology, 1*, 441–452.

Kastl, A. (1969). Changes in ego functioning under alcohol. *Quarterly Journal of Studies on Alcohol, 30*, 371–383.

Kaufman, E. (1982). The relationship of alcoholism and alcohol abuse to the abuse of other drugs. *American Journal of Drug and Alcohol Abuse, 9*, 1–17.

Keane, T., & Lisman, S. (1980). Alcohol and social anxiety in males: Behavioral, cognitive, and physiological effects. *Journal of Abnormal Psychology, 89*, 213–223.

Kissin, B. (1974). The pharmacodynamics and natural history of alcoholism. In B. Kissin & H. Begleiter (Eds.), *The biology of alcoholism: Vol. 3. Clinical pathology* (pp. 1–36). New York: Plenum Press.

Knott, D., & Beard, J. (1972). Changes in cardiovascular activity as a function of alcohol intake. In B. Kissin & H. Begleiter (Eds.), *The biology of alcoholism: Vol 2. Physiology and behavior* (pp. 345–366). New York: Plenum Press.

LaCoursiere, R., Godfrey, K., & Ruby, L. (1980). Traumatic neurosis in the etiology of alcoholism: Viet Nam combat and other trauma. *American Journal of Psychiatry, 137*, 966–968.

Landauer, A. A. (1981). Alcohol drinking reduces hand tremor. *British Journal of Addiction, 76*, 429–430.

Lang, P. J. (1968). Fear reduction and fear behavior: Problems in treating a construct. In J. M. Schlien (Ed.), *Research in psychotherapy* (Vol. 3, pp. 90–102). Washington, DC: American Psychological Association.

Levenson, R. W., Sher, K., Grossman, L., Newman, J., & Newlin, D. (1980). Alcohol and stress response dampening: Pharmacological effects, expectancy, and tension reduction. *Journal of Abnormal Psychology, 89*, 528–538.

Lienert, G., & Traxel, W. (1959). The effects of meprobamate and alcohol on galvanic skin response. *Journal of Psychology, 48*, 329–344.

Lindman, R. (Ed.). (1980). *Anxiety and alcohol: Limitations of tension reduction theory in nonalcoholics* (Monograph Suppl. 1). Abo, Finland: Abo Akademi, Department of Psychology.

Lindman, R., & Alexanderson, G. (1980). The effect of alcohol on motor hesitation in man. In R. Lindman (Ed.), *Anxiety and alcohol: Limitations of tension reduction theory in nonalcoholics* (Monograph Suppl. 1, pp. 45–55). Abo, Finland: Abo Akademi, Department of Psychology.

Lindman, R., Alexanderson, G., & Kvarnstrom, B. (1980). Skin conductance as a function of alcohol during motor approach towards a noxious goal. In R. Lindman (Ed.), *Anxiety and alcohol: Limitations of tension reduction theory in nonalcoholics* (Monograph Suppl. 1, pp. 56–66). Abo, Finland: Abo Akademi, Department of Psychology.

Lipscomb, T., Nathan, P., Wilson, G. T., & Abrams, D. (1980). Effects of tolerance on the anxiety-reducing function of alcohol. *Archives of General Psychiatry, 37*, 577–582.

Logue, P., Gentry, W., Linnoila, M., & Erwin, C. (1978). Effect of alcohol consumption on state anxiety changes in male and female nonalcoholics. *American Journal of Psychiatry, 135*, 1079–1081.

MacAndrew, C. (1965). The differentiation of male alcoholic outpatients from nonalcoholic psychiatric outpatients by means of the MMPI. *Quarterly Journal of Studies on Alcohol, 26*, 238–246.

MacAndrew, C. (1982). An examination of the relevance of the individual differences (A-Trait) formulation of the tension-reduction theory to the etiology of alcohol abuse in young males. *Addictive Behaviors, 7*, 39–46.

Margolis, B. L., Kroes, W. H., & Quinn, R. P. (1974). Job stress: An unlisted occupational hazard. *Journal of Occupational Medicine, 16*, 659–661.

Marks, I. (1981). *Cure and care for neurosis*. New York: John Wiley & Sons.

Marlatt, G. A. (1976). Alcohol, stress and cognitive control. In I. G. Sarason & C. D. Spielberger (Eds.), *Stress and anxiety* (Vol. 3, pp. 271–296). Washington, DC: Hemisphere.

Marlatt, G. A. (1980). *Relapse prevention: A self-control program for the treatment of addictive behaviors*. Unpublished manuscript, University of Washington, Seattle.

Marlatt, G. A., & Gordon, J. R. (1980). Determinants of relapse: Implications for the maintenance of behavior change. In P. O. Davidson & S. M. Davidson (Eds.), *Behavioral Medicine: Changing Health Lifestyles* (pp. 410–452). New York: Brunner/Mazel.

Marlatt, G. A., Kosturn, C. F., & Lang, A. (1975). Provocation to anger and opportunity for retaliation as determinants of alcohol consumption in social drinkers. *Journal of Abnormal Psychology*, 8, 652–659.

Masserman, J., & Yum, K. (1946). An analysis of the influence of alcohol on experimental neuroses in cats. *Psychosomatic Medicine*, 8, 36–52.

Mayfield, D. (1968). Psychopharmacology of alcohol. I. Affective change with intoxication, drinking behavior and affective state. *Journal of Nervous and Mental Disease*, 146, 314–321.

McClelland, D. C., Davis, W. M., Kalin, R., & Wanner, E. (1972). *The drinking man.* New York: Free Press.

McCord, W., & McCord, J. (1960). *Origins of alcoholism.* Stanford, CA: Stanford University Press.

McNamee, H., Mello, N., & Mendelson, J. (1968). Experimental analysis of drinking patterns of alcoholics: Concurrent psychiatric observations. *American Journal of Psychiatry*, 124, 1079–1081.

Mendelson, J. H. (1980). The search for alcohol antagonists: New research possibilities. *Advances in Alcoholism*, 1(23).

Mendelson, J., La Dou, J., & Solomon, P. (1964). Experimentally induced chronic intoxication and withdrawal in alcoholics: Part 3, Psychiatric findings. *Quarterly Journal of Studies on Alcohol* (Suppl. No. 2), 40–52.

Miller, P., Hersen, M., Eisler, R., & Hilsman, G. (1974). Effects of social stress on operant drinking of alcoholics and social drinkers. *Behaviour Research and Therapy*, 12, 67–72.

Mullaney, J. A., & Trippett, C. (1979). Alcohol dependence and phobias: Clinical description and relevance. *British Journal of Psychiatry*, 135, 565–573.

Naitoh, P. (1972). The effect of alcohol on the autonomic system of humans: Psychophysiological approach. In B. Kissin & H. Begleiter (Eds.), *The biology of alcoholism: Vol. 2. Physiology and behavior* (pp. 367–433). New York: Plenum Press.

Nasrallah, H. A., Schroeder, D. J., & Peetty, F. (1982). Alcoholism secondary to essential tremor. *Journal of Clinical Psychiatry*, 4, 163–164.

National Academy of Sciences (1979). *Sleeping pills, insomnia and medical practice: Report of a study of the Institute of Medicine.* Washington, D.C.: National Academy of Sciences.

Neff, J. A., & Husaini, B. A. (1982). Life events, drinking patterns, and depressive symptomatology: The stress-buffering role of alcohol consumption. *Journal of Studies on Alcohol*, 43, 301–318.

Nesbitt, P. (1973). Smoking, physiological arousal, and emotional response. *Journal of Personality and Social Psychology*, 25, 137–144.

Nestoros, J. (1980). Ethanol specifically potentiates GABA mediated neurotransmission in feline cerebral cortex. *Science*, 209, 708–710.

Noel, N., & Lisman, S. A. (1980). Alcohol consumption by college women following exposure to unsolvable problems: Learned helplessness or stress-induced drinking? *Behaviour Research and Therapy*, 18, 429–440.

Noel, N., Lisman, S. A., Schare, M., & Lederer, J. (1981, April). *Effects of alcohol before or after unsolvable puzzles: Prevention or alleviation of stress reactions.* Presented at meeting of the Eastern Psychological Association, New York.

Parker, J., Gilbert, G., & Thoreson, R. (1978). Reduction of autonomic activity in alcoholics: A comparison of relaxation and meditation techniques. *Journal of Consulting and Clinical Psychology*, 46, 879–886.

Pearlin, L. I., & Radabaugh, C. W. (1976). Economic strains and the coping functions of alcohol. *American Journal of Sociology*, 82, 652–663.

Pert, C. B., & Snyder, S. H. (1973). Opiate receptor: Demonstration in nervous tissue. *Science*, 179, 1011–1014.

Pihl, R., & Yankofsky, L. (1979). Alcohol consumption in male social drinkers as a function of situationally induced depressive affect and anxiety. *Psychopharmacology*, *65*, 251–257.

Pliner, P., & Cappell, H. (1974). Modification of affective consequences of alcohol: A comparison of social and solitary drinking. *Journal of Abnormal Psychology*, *83*, 418–425.

Pohorecky, L. A., Rassi, E., Weiss, J. M., & Michalak, V. (1980). Biochemical evidence for an interaction of ethanol and stress: Preliminary studies. *Alcoholism: Clinical and Experimental Research*, *4*, 423–426.

Polivy, J., Schueneman, A. L., & Carlson, K. (1976). Alcohol and tension reduction: Cognitive and physiological effects. *Journal of Abnormal Psychology*, *85*, 595–600.

Pomerleau, O. F., Turk, D. C., & Fertig, J. (1984). The effects of cigarette smoking on pain and anxiety. *Addictive Behaviors*, *9*, 265–271.

Reed, T. E. (1977). Three heritable responses to alcohol in a heterogeneous randomly mated mouse strain. *Journal of Studies on Alcohol*, *38*, 618–632.

Reisenzein, R. (1983). The Schachter theory of emotion: Two decades later. *Psychological Bulletin*, *94*, 239–264.

Rickels, K. (1978). Use of antianxiety agents in anxious outpatients. *Psychopharmacology*, *58*, 1–17.

Rimm, D., Briddell, D., Zimmerman, M., & Caddy, G. (1981). The effects of alcohol and the expectancy of alcohol on snake fear. *Addictive Behaviors*, *6*, 47–51.

Robins, L., Bates, W., & O'Neal, P. (1962). Adult drinking patterns of former problem children. In D. Pittman & C. R. Snyder (Eds.), *Society, culture and drinking patterns* (pp. 395–412). New York: John Wiley & Sons.

Rohsenow, D. (1982a). Control over interpersonal evaluation and alcohol consumption in male social drinkers. *Addictive Behaviors*, *7*, 113–121.

Rohsenow, D. (1982b). Social anxiety, daily moods, and alcohol use over time among heavy social drinking men. *Addictive Behaviors*, *7*, 311–315.

Rosenberg, H. (1983). Relapsed versus non-relapsed alcohol abusers: Coping skills, life events, and social support. *Addictive Behaviors*, *8*, 183–186.

Russell, J., & Mehrabian, A. (1975). The mediating role of emotions in alcohol use. *Journal of Studies on Alcohol*, *36*, 1508–1536.

Ruttenberg, A. J., & Luke, J. L. (1984). Heroin-related deaths: New epidemiological insights. *Science*, *226*, 14–20.

Sadava, S. W., Thistle, R., & Forsyth, R. (1978). Stress, escapism and patterns of alcohol and drug use. *Journal of Studies on Alcohol*, *39*, 725–736.

Schaeffer, J. M. (1981). Firewater myths revisited: Review of findings and some new directions. *Journal of Studies on Alcohol* (Suppl. 9), 99–117.

Schroeder, D., & Nasrallah, H. A. (1982). High alcoholism rate in patients with essential tremor. *American Journal of Psychiatry*, *139*, 1471–1473.

Schuckit, M. A. (1980a). Alcoholism and genetics: Possible biochemical mediators. *Biological Psychiatry*, *15*, 437–447.

Schuckit, M. A. (1980b). Self-rating of alcohol intoxication by young men with and without family histories of alcoholism. *Journal of Studies on Alcohol*, *41*, 242–249.

Schuckit, M. A., Engstrom, D., Alpert, R., & Duby, J. (1981). Differences in the muscle-tension response to ethanol in young men with and without family histories of alcoholism. *Journal of Studies on Alcohol*, *42*, 918–923.

Sher, K. J. (1982, December). *Individual differences in the tension reducing effects of alcohol*. Presented at the Annual Meeting of the Association for Advancement of Behavior Therapy, Los Angeles, CA.

Sher, K. J. (1985). Subjective effects of alcohol: The influence of setting and individual differences in alcohol expectancies. *Journal of Studies on Alcohol*, *46*, 137–146.

Sher, K. J., & Levenson, R. W. (1982). Risk for alcoholism and individual differences in the stress-response-dampening effect of alcohol. *Journal of Abnormal Psychology*, *91*, 350–368.

Sher, K. J., & Walitzer, K. S. (1986). Individual differences in the stress-response-dampening effect of alcohol: A dose response study. *Journal of Abnormal Psychology*, *95*, 159–167.

Smail, P., Stockwell, T., Canter, S., & Hodgson, R. (1984). Alcohol dependence and phobic anxiety states. I. A prevalence study. *British Journal of Psychiatry*, *144*, 53–57.

Southwick, L., Steele, C. M., Marlatt, G. A., & Lindell, M. (1981). Alcohol-related expectancies: Defined by phase of intoxication and drinking experience. *Journal of Consulting and Clinical Psychology*, *49*, 713–721.

Steele, C. M., & Southwick, L. (1983). *The psychology of social drunkenness: The hidden role of response conflict*. Unpublished manuscript, University of Washington, Seattle.

Steffen, J., Nathan, P., & Taylor, H. (1974). Tension reducing effects of alcohol: Further evidence and some methodological considerations. *Journal of Abnormal Psychology*, *83*, 542–547.

Stress, distress, and drug treatment (editorial). (1978, December 23 and 30). *The Lancet*, pp. 1347–1348.

Strickler, D., Tomaszewski, R., Maxwell, W., & Suib, M. (1979). The effects of relaxation instructions on drinking behavior in the presence of stress. *Behaviour Research and Therapy*, *17*, 45–51.

Sutker, P. B., Allain, A. N., Brantley, P., & Randall, C. (1982). Acute alcohol intoxication, negative affect, and autonomic arousal in women and men. *Addictive Behaviors*, *7*, 17–25.

Sutker, P. B., & Archer, R. P. (1984). Opiate abuse and dependence disorders. In H. E. Adams & P. B. Sutker (Eds.), *Comprehensive handbook of psychopathology* (pp. 585–622). New York: Plenum Press.

Tallman, J. F., Paul, S. M., Skolnick, P., & Gallager, D. (1980). Receptors for the age of anxiety: Pharmacology of the benzodiazepines. *Science*, *207*, 274–281.

Thyer, B., & Curtis, G. C. (1984). The effects of ethanol intoxication on phobic anxiety. *Behaviour Research and Therapy*, *22*, 599–610.

Tomkins, S. (1966). Psychological model for smoking behavior. *American Journal of Public Health*, *56*, 17–20.

Triana, E., Frances, R., & Stokes, P. (1980). The relationship between endorphins and alcohol-induced subcortical activity. *American Journal of Psychiatry*, *137*, 491–493.

Tucker, J. A., Vuchinich, R. E., & Harris, C. V. (1985). Determinants of substance abuse relapse. In M. Galizio & S. A. Maisto (Eds.), *Determinants of substance abuse: Biological, psychological, and environmental factors* (pp. 383–421). New York: Plenum Press.

Tucker, J. A., Vuchinich, R. E., & Sobell, M. B. (1981). Alcohol consumption as a self-handicapping strategy. *Journal of Abnormal Psychology*, *90*, 220–230.

Tucker, J. A., Vuchinich, R. E., Sobell, M. B., & Maisto, S. A. (1980). Normal drinkers' alcohol consumption as a functon of conflicting motives induced by intellectual performance stress. *Addictive Behaviors*, *5*, 171–178.

Tyrer, P. (1980). Comments: Dependence on benzodiazepines. *British Journal of Psychiatry*, *137*, 576–577.

Vaillant, G. E., & Milofsky, E. (1982). The etiology of alcoholism: A prospective viewpoint. *American Psychologist*, *37*, 494–503.

Van Thiel, D. (1983a). Adrenal response to ethanol: A stress response? In L. A. Pohorecky & J. Brick (Eds.), *Stress and alcohol use* (pp. 23–27). New York: Elsevier.

Van Thiel, D. (1983b). Effects of ethanol upon organ systems other than the central nervous system. In B. Tabakoff, P. B. Sutker, & C. L. Randall (Eds.), *Medical and social aspects of alcohol abuse* (pp. 79–132). New York: Plenum Press.

Vogel, W., & DeTurck, K. (1983). Effects of ethanol on plasma and brain catecholamine levels in stressed and nonstressed rats. In L. A. Pohorecky & J. Brick (Eds.), *Stress and alcohol use* (pp. 429–438). New York: Elsevier.

Wallgren, H., & Barry, H. (1970). *Actions of alcohol* (Vols. 1 and 2). New York: Elsevier.

Walton, R. G. (1972). Smoking and alcoholism: A brief report. *American Journal of Psychiatry*, *128*, 139–140.

Warren, G., & Raynes, A. (1972). Mood changes during three conditions of alcohol intake. *Quarterly Journal of Studies on Alcohol*, *33*, 979–988.

Wells-Parker, E., Miles, S., & Spencer, B. (1983). Stress experiences and drinking histories of elderly drunken-driving offenders. *Journal of Studies on Alcohol, 44*, 429–437.

Wilder, J. (1950). The law of initial values. *Psychosomatic Medicine*, 392–401.

Williams, A. (1966). Social drinking, anxiety, and depression. *Journal of Personality and Social Psychology, 3*, 448–457.

Wilson, G. T., & Abrams, D. (1977). Effects of alcohol on social anxiety and physiological arousal: Cognitive versus pharmacological processes. *Cognitive Therapy and Research, 1*, 195–210.

Wilson, G. T., Abrams, D., & Lipscomb, T. (1980). Effects of increasing levels of intoxication and drinking pattern on social anxiety. *Journal of Studies on Alcohol, 41*, 250–264.

Wilson, G. T., Perold, E. A., & Abrams, D. B. (1981). The effects of expectations of self-intoxication and partner's drinking on anxiety in dyadic social interaction. *Cognitive Therapy and Research, 5*, 251–264.

Yankofsky, L., Wilson, G. T., Adler, J., Hay, W., & Vrana, S. (1984). *The effect of alcohol on self-evaluation and perception of negative interpersonal feedback*. Unpublished manuscript, Rutgers University.

Zeichner, A., Feuerstein, M., Swartzman, L., & Reznick, E. (1983). Acute effects of alcohol on cardiovascular reactivity to stress in Type A (coronary prone) businessmen. In L. A. Pohorecky & J. Brick (Eds.), *Stress and alcohol use* (pp. 353–368). New York: Plenum Press.

# 8 Self-Awareness Model

JAY G. HULL

The self-awareness model of alcohol use (Hull, 1981) is one of a general class of theories that assume that some of the causes and effects of alcohol consumption can be understood in terms of the pharmacologic effects of the drug. While some of these theories propose that alcohol has effects on behavior by virtue of its direct pharmacologic effects on affective and motivational states (e.g., the tension reduction model; see Conger, 1956), the self-awareness model proposes that alcohol affects behavior indirectly by virtue of its effects on cognition. Specifically, this model proposes that alcohol reduces self-awareness by inhibiting the use of information-processing strategies essential to the self-aware state. Given that self-awareness is associated with specific affective and behavioral consequences (e.g., self-regulation with respect to internal and external standards of behavior), alcohol is proposed to have the opposite effects (i.e., behavioral disinhibition). Furthermore, given that self-awareness is sometimes painful (e.g., following personal failures), self-awareness avoidance through intoxication is proposed to constitute one motive to consume alcohol.

While the self-awareness model assumes that alcohol has effects on behavior by virtue of its pharmocologic effects on cognition, it is not presented as a complete explanation of alcohol use. As stated by Hull (1981): "The complexity of the variables already associated with alcohol use and abuse suggests that no single theory will be developed that will encompass the entire field. . . . As a consequence, the most fruitful approach to theory building in the area of alcohol use appears to be to restrict the range of phenomena to be explained and at the same time formulate a model with empirical referents that contains hypotheses and assumptions that are subject to disproof (p. 586)." The present chapter will review evidence on whether the self-awareness model has met these modest, yet specific goals. I begin by consid-

JAY G. HULL. Department of Psychology, Dartmouth College, Hanover, New Hampshire.

ering some of the general research on the effects of alcohol on cognition. The specific assumptions of the self-awareness model are then detailed followed by a review of the evidence on each proposition. Finally, I consider the relation of the self-awareness model to other theories of alcohol use.

## The Effects of Alcohol on Cognition

The self-awareness model takes as a general assumption that alcohol has effects on behavior by virtue of disrupting cognitive processes. It is therefore necessary to briefly consider evidence on the effects of alcohol on cognition. In general, research suggests that memory for information processed in the intoxicated state is impaired relative to memory for information processed in the sober state. The locus of these effects appears to be in the effects of alcohol on the processes involved in the storage of information. In particular, research suggests that alcohol-induced cognitive impairment involves central information processes as opposed to more peripheral sensory or motor mechanisms (Moskowitz, 1973).

Among the central processes impaired by intoxication, the acquisition of new information would appear to be particularly vulnerable to alcohol effects (Ryback, 1971). Thus, researchers have contrasted the effects of being intoxicated while learning new information and while trying to recall old information. Differences in the effects of alcohol in these two cases are attributed to the impact of intoxication on either information storage or retrieval processes. With some exceptions, this literature has demonstrated that information storage processes are more impaired by intoxication than retrieval processes (Birnbaum & Parker, 1977; Bernbaum, Parker, Hartley, & Noble, 1978; Jones, 1973; Miller, Adesso, Fleming, Gino, & Lauerman, 1978). Furthermore, alcohol has some of its strongest effects in memory studies in which information organizational cues are neither obvious nor strong (Parker, Birnbaum, & Noble, 1976). When such cues are strengthened, alcohol has less of an effect (Birnbaum & Parker, 1977). It would seem, then, that alcohol may have its effects on memory by decreasing the use of organizational strategies during the acquisition and storage of information.

The hypothesis that alcohol impairs information processing by inhibiting the use of organizational strategies was tested in an experiment by Birnbaum et al. (1978). In keeping with the general literature, intoxicated subjects performed significantly worse than sober subjects on three trials of free recall. More importantly, cueing by the experimenter produced more improvement in recall for intoxicated than sober subjects. Such results suggest that alcohol has its greatest effects by disrupting the subject's spontaneous tendency to use associative cues. A second study by these authors demonstrated that at a level of intoxication similar to that in the first experiment, information retrieval processes were unimpaired.

Building on these studies, Birnbaum, Johnson, Hartley, and Taylor (1980) proposed that alcohol debilitates information storage by inhibiting the use of elaboration strategies or schemata. Thus, it has been shown that elaboration (i.e., the classification and integration of new information with previously acquired information) facilitates storage and retention of information. It is possible that alcohol debilitates storage by reducing the likelihood that elaborative information will be either generated or efficiently used by intoxicated subjects in processing new information. On the basis of this research, Birnbaum *et al.* (1980) concluded that in fact the alcohol-induced memory deficit involves the production of elaborative schemata.

The research and conclusions drawn by Birnbaum and her colleagues remain somewhat controversial (Hashtroudi, Parker, DeLisi, & Wyatt, 1983; Williams & Rundell, 1984). Nevertheless, there is little disagreement that alcohol impairs memory by virtue of its effects on information storage as opposed to retrieval processes. Somewhat more tentatively, it is suggested that alcohol may have its effects on information storage by disrupting organizational processes involved in the encoding of information. It is interesting to note in this regard that chronic use and abuse of alcohol also appears to result in deficits in the acquisition and storage of information, and furthermore, that these deficits appear to involve impairment of rehearsal and organizational strategies (Cermak, Butters, & Gerrein, 1973; Cermak & Reale, 1978). Such a similarity between the chronic and acute effects of alcohol is suggestive of a general effect of alcohol on cognitive impairment.

### The Self-Awareness Model of the Causes and Effects of Alcohol Consumption

Social psychological research has shown that self-awarness corresponds to a type of organizational process that one would expect to be debilitated by alcohol consumption. Thus, one efficient organizational strategy is to process information according to its self-relevance. A piece of information that is tagged as self-relevant is more easily recalled than information that is tagged using any of a variety of non-self-relevant schemes (Rogers, Kuiper, & Kirker, 1977). If alcohol functions to debilitate information storage by inhibiting the use of elaboration strategies or schema, it should function to decrease the tendency of individuals to encode information according to its self-relevance. Furthermore, it should have the opposite effects of manipulations that increase the use of self-relevant encoding schemes. Given that self-awareness depends on the use of self-relevant encoding schemes (Hull & Levy, 1979), alcohol should have the effect of decreasing self-awareness. The logical implications of such an analysis can be summarized with four basic propositions:

1. Alcohol decreases self-awareness.
2. It does so by inhibiting higher-order cognitive processes related to the encoding of information in terms of its self-relevance.
3. By inhibiting these encoding processes and thus decreasing the individual's sensitivity to self-relevant information, alcohol consumption has the opposite affective and behavioral consequences of manipulations that increase self-awareness. It therefore: (a) decreases the correspondence of behavior with external and internal standards of appropriate conduct, and (b) decreases self-evaluation based on past performances.
4. The fact that alcohol decreases negative self-evaluation following failure [proposition 3(b)] is a sufficient condition to induce and sustain alcohol consumption.

Evidence for each of these propositions will be considered in turn.

## The Effects of Alcohol on Measures of Self-Awareness

What is self-awareness? How could one measure the effects of alcohol on self-awareness? According to one model (Hull & Levy, 1979), self-awareness involves the organization of information according to its self-relevance. Hofstadter and Dennett (1981) provide a vignette that nicely illustrates the difference between processing information as self-relevant and processing information as non-self-relevant:

> Pete is waiting in line to pay for an item in a department store, and he notices that there is a closed-circuit television monitor over the counter— one of the store's measures against shoplifting. As he watches the jostling crowd of people on the monitor, he realizes that the person over on the left side of the screen in the overcoat carrying the large paper bag is having his pocket picked by the person behind him. Then, as he raises his hand to his mouth in astonishment, he notices that the victim's hand is moving to his mouth in just the same way. Pete suddenly realizes that *he* is the person whose pocket is being picked (pp. 20–21).

As Hofstadter and Dennett point out, this dramatic shift in perspective is not so much a difference in the *information* that is being processed as it is a difference in the *way* the information is being processed. Certainly, Pete was processing information prior to his "discovery," and furthermore this information had to do with a man being robbed in a department store. Since the person being robbed is in fact himself, he was actually thinking about himself prior to his discovery. But as Hofstadter and Dennett conclude, "he wasn't thinking about himself *as himself*; he wasn't thinking about himself in the right way." In terms of the model presented by Hull and Levy (1979), Pete was not self-aware prior to his discovery. Furthermore, self-awareness in this sense specifically involves the processing of the information as self-relevant. The difference in the way Pete thinks and acts before and after his discovery depends on a shift in the way the information on the television screen is being organized or encoded. He shifts from encoding information as non-self-relevant to self-relevant. As a consequence, he has become self-aware.

According to the self-awareness model of alcohol, Pete would have been less likely to become self-aware had he been intoxicated, by virtue of the effect of alcohol on the use of higher-order encoding schemes. Hull, Levenson, Young, and Sher (1983) conducted a series of experiments to examine the effects of alcohol on self-awareness. The first two studies involved general measures of self-awareness, while the third study measured the effects of alcohol on self-relevant encoding processes. Previous studies have assessed general levels of self-awareness using two measures: (1) the relative frequency of first person pronouns in response to specific questions (Davis & Brock, 1975) and (2) the frequency of self-focused responses on the Exner (1973) sentence completion questionnaire (Carver & Scheier, 1978). The first two studies by Hull *et al.* (1983) combined these methods in an open-ended free-response format. Subjects gave short speeches that were then coded for relative frequency of (1) first person pronouns, and (2) self-focused statements according to the Exner scheme. The speeches themselves concerned subjects' perceptions of their physical appearance and took place after subjects had consumed either an alcoholic or placebo beverage. The alcohol dose was sufficient to attain a blood alcohol level of 0.07% just prior to the speech phase of the experiment (1 g ethanol/kg of subject body weight). Regardless of condition, the total amount of liquid consumed was in the same proportion to body weight (e.g., approximately 35 ounces of liquid for a 145-pound subject, 7 ounces of which were 80 proof vodka if the subject actually consumed alcohol). In the first study, all subjects were led to believe that the beverage they were consuming contained alcohol. Alcohol consumption was expected to decrease the relative frequency of both self-focused statements and first person pronouns.

Subjects' speeches were transcribed verbatim. Individual statements were then coded using the scheme devised by Exner (1973) for use with his self-focused sentence completion questionnaire. According to this scheme, statements can be coded into one of four major categories: self-focus, external focus, ambiguous focus, or other (nonfocus). Exner (1973) provided both instructions and examples of this coding scheme. In addition to coding speech statements, the total number of words and self-relevant pronouns (I, me, my, myself, mine) was determined.

Relative frequencies of statement categories were analyzed as proportions of total number of statements. In order to avoid overdetermining the data set, ambiguous-focus responses were not analyzed. All effects are illustrated in Table 8.1. In accord with predictions, there was a significant effect of alcohol on relative frequency of self-focused statements such that alcohol reduced self-focus. In addition, there was a significant effect of alcohol on relative frequency of responses coded "other" such that alcohol increased the relative frequency of these statements. There were no effects for externally focused statements.

Alcohol did not affect the total number of words in subjects' speeches. An analysis of the ratio of self-relevant pronouns to total words revealed a marginally significant effect of alcohol such that alcohol reduced the relative frequency of these pronouns.

The results of this first experiment support the proposition that alcohol reduces self-awareness. Thus, alcohol significantly reduced the relative frequency of self-focused statements and increased the relative frequency of statements coded "other." In addition, alcohol tended to reduce the relative frequency of first person pronouns, although this effect did not achieve conventional levels of significance. Unfortunately, there is an alternative explanation of the results that does not depend on the hypothesis that the drug of alcohol is responsible for the effects. Thus, although efforts were made to equate alcohol and placebo subjects in terms of their expectancies regarding the content of their drinks (all subjects were told they were drinking alcohol), these efforts were unsuccessful. Following the speech phase of the experiment, subjects estimated how many ounces of alcohol they had consumed and how intoxicated they felt during the speech. Subjects in the alcohol condition reported consuming more ounces of alcohol and feeling more intoxicated than subjects in the placebo condition. This was probably due to the relatively

TABLE 8.1. Experiment 1: The Effects of Alcohol on Relative Frequency of Speech Statements and First Person Pronouns

| Beverage content | Proportion of speech statements | | | Word proportions |
|---|---|---|---|---|
| | Self-focus | External focus | Other | Self-relevant pronouns |
| Placebo | 0.437 | 0.030 | 0.505 | 0.145 |
| Alcohol | 0.318 | 0.053 | 0.608 | 0.133 |

Note. Results from Hull, Levenson, Young, and Sher (1983).

high alcoholic content of the experimental beverages (1 g/kg). Nevertheless, it is possible that the cognition that one has consumed alcohol and not consumption per se is responsible for decreased self-focused responses in this study.

In order to eliminate this alternative explanation, a second study was conducted that orthogonally manipulated expectancy and consumption. Once again, subjects gave short speeches that were coded for relative frequency of self-focused statements and first person pronouns. These speeches took place under one of four experimental conditions corresponding to a 2 (consume alcohol–consume tonic water) × 2 (expect alcohol–expect tonic water) design. To the extent that the expectancy manipulation is successful, such a design allows for an independent assessment of the effects of expectancy on self-focused responses.

Once again, alcohol was predicted to decrease the relative frequency of both self-focused statements and first person pronouns. Such an effect would replicate the results of the first experiment. In addition, this effect was predicted to be independent of expectancy. Although the expectancy manipulation was predicted to be successful in affecting subjects' cognitions regarding having consumed alcohol, no explicit predictions were made concerning the effect of expectancy on speech and pronoun measures.

Procedures were similar to those employed in the first experiment. All effects are illustrated in Table 8.2. Once again, there was a significant main effect of alcohol on relative frequency of self-focused statements such that consuming alcohol reduced self-focus. Neither the main effect for expectancy nor the interaction of expectancy and consumption was significant.

Both alcohol and expectancy had significant main effects on relative frequency of statements coded "other." As can be seen in Table 8.2, alcohol increased the relative frequency of "other" responses, while the cognition that one had consumed alcohol had the opposite effect. The interaction of

TABLE 8.2. Experiment 2: The Effect of Alcohol and Expectancy on Relative Frequency of Speech Statements and First Person Pronouns

| Experimental design | | Proportion of speech statements | | | Word proportions |
|---|---|---|---|---|---|
| Consume | Expect | Self-focus | External focus | Other | Self-relevant pronouns |
| Tonic | Tonic | 0.496 | 0.010 | 0.483 | 0.148 |
| Tonic | Alcohol | 0.568 | 0.011 | 0.401 | 0.144 |
| Alcohol | Tonic | 0.331 | 0.018 | 0.643 | 0.122 |
| Alcohol | Alcohol | 0.455 | 0.021 | 0.511 | 0.129 |

Note. Results from Hull, Levenson, Young, and Sher (1983).

alcohol and expectancy was not significant. There were no significant effects on externally focused statements.

As in Experiment 1, an analysis of the ratio of self-relevant pronouns to total words revealed a marginally significant main effect of alcohol consumption such that alcohol reduced the relative frequency of these pronouns. Neither the main effect of expectancy nor the interaction of consumption and expectancy approached significance. A meta-analysis was conducted on this measure to statistically combine the results of Experiments 1 and 2. This analysis indicated that the tendency of alcohol to decrease relative frequency of first person pronouns in both Experiments 1 and 2 was significant at conventional levels when these studies were combined.

Analyses were also conducted on subjects' self-reports of their level of intoxication. Once again, subjects who had consumed alcohol rated themselves as being more drunk and having consumed more ounces of liquor than did subjects who consumed tonic. In addition, subjects who were told they were drinking alcohol rated themselves as more drunk and having consumed more ounces of liquor than subjects who were told they were drinking tonic. There were no significant interactions of consumption and expectancy on these measures. Given that subjects' expectancies regarding the content of their drinks were successfully manipulated and this variable had effects on measures of self-awareness that were opposite those of actual alcohol consumption, the alternative explanation of the results of the first experiment as due to subjects' knowledge regarding the content of their drinks is eliminated. In fact, these results suggest that alcohol affects self-aware responses in spite of, rather than because of, subjects' knowledge of being intoxicated.

Taken together, these two experiments provide support for the proposition that alcohol consumption decreases self-awareness. In both experiments alcohol consumption was associated with a decrease in relative frequency of self-focused statements and an increase in other or nonfocused statements. Meta-analysis revealed that alcohol consumption was also associated with a decrease in the relative frequency of first person pronouns. On the basis of these studies, it would appear that alcohol decreases self-awareness. Furthermore, it would appear to do so by virtue of the pharmacologic effects of the drug independent of subjects' expectancies concerning their intoxicated state. We now turn to a consideration of a possible mechanism for these effects.

### The Effects of Alcohol on Self-Relevant Encoding Processes

Although these experiments support the proposition that alcohol decreases self-awareness, they do not provide evidence of how this occurs. The model proposed by Hull (1981) specifies that alcohol reduces self-awareness by interfering with the processing of information in terms of its self-relevance. In order to test this notion, Hull *et al.* (1983) conducted a third experiment designed to investigate the effects of alcohol on self-relevant encoding processes among individuals high and low in dispositional self-awareness.

The experimental procedures were adapted from those used in previous research that contrasted self-relevant with other forms of encoding (Rogers *et al.*, 1977; Hull & Levy, 1979). Briefly, subjects were read a series of 30 adjectives, 1 at a time. Following the presentation of each adjective, subjects consulted a rating sheet. This sheet specified that that particular adjective was to be rated according to one of three different schemes: either the word was to be evaluated according to its structural characteristics (is this word long or short?), semantic characteristics (is this word meaningful?), or self-relevant characteristics (does this word describe you?). Following the rating of all adjectives, subjects were asked to write down as many of the words as they could recall. Since this recall task was unanticipated and since the words had been presented orally, number of words recalled constituted a measure of incidental memory. Furthermore, differences in recall as a function of type of evaluation scheme (structural, semantic, or self-relevant) can be attributed to differences in the organization of the information at acquisition. Research using this technique has found that self-relevant encoding results in better memory than either semantic or structural encoding (Rogers *et al.*, 1977). Furthermore, dispositionally high-self-aware individuals show this effect, while the memory of dispositionally low-self-aware individuals does not vary as a function of evaluation scheme (Hull & Levy, 1979). On the basis of the latter results, Hull and Levy (1979) proposed that self-awareness involves the process of encoding information according to its self-relevance.

Prior to the start of the experiment, subjects completed the Fenigstein, Scheier, and Buss (1975) self-consciousness[1] inventory in order that they could later be classified into dispositionally high- and low-self-aware groups. The private self-consciousness scale was used since this scale had predicted differences in self-relevant encoding in the experiment by Hull and Levy (1979). (The Fenigstein *et al.* questionnaire had not been included in the first two experiments on alcohol and self-awareness.) Following completion of the questionnaire, subjects consumed either an alcoholic or placebo beverage.

---

[1] The terms *self-consciousness* and *self-awareness* will be used throughout the present discussion. Both terms refer to the same cognitive state. The term self-awareness refers to situationally manipulated differences in this state. Since alcohol is a situational manipulation, it will be referred to as altering an individual's level of self-awareness. The term self-consciousness refers to dispositional differences in this state. Since the cognitive state proposed to vary between individuals as a function of their dispositional levels of self-consciousness is the same as the state proposed to vary as a function of situational manipulations of self-awareness, the terms self-consciousness and self-awareness are generally treated as interchangeable.

The alcohol dose was slightly less than in the first two studies by Hull *et al.* (1983) (0.8 g/kg of body weight; mean blood alcohol content = 0.55% just prior to the word task). All subjects were told that they were consuming alcohol. Following beverage consumption and absorption, subjects participated in the incidental memory paradigm detailed above. General instructions for this task were presented both before and after beverage consumption in order to insure that there was no misunderstanding of the procedures due to the level of intoxication.

Hull and Levy (1979) found that individuals high in dispositional private self-consciousness encoded self-relevant words at a deeper cognitive level than non-self-relevant words. Individuals low in private self-consciousness did not distinguish self-relevant and non-self-relevant words and recalled significantly fewer self-relevant words than did high-self-conscious individuals. If alcohol decreases self-awareness by inhibiting self-relevant encoding processes, then it should have a greater impact on recall of self-relevant words for high-private-self-conscious than low-self-conscious individuals. This effect should take the form of an interaction in which (1) high-self-conscious subjects recall more self-relevant words than low-self-conscious subjects under placebo conditions (thus replicating the findings of Hull & Levy, 1979), (2) alcohol reduces recall of self-relevant words for high-self-conscious subjects, and (3) alcohol has less of an effect on recall of self-relevant words for low-self-conscious than for high-self-conscious subjects.

Recall of words encoded according to their self-relevance constituted the primary dependent measure. The results are presented in Table 8.3. In accordance with predictions, alcohol interacted with self-consciousness. Neither

TABLE 8.3. Experiment 3: The Effect of Alcohol and Self-Consciousness on Recall of Words Encoded as Self-Relevant

| Self-consciousness | Beverage content | |
|---|---|---|
| | Placebo | Alcohol |
| High | | |
| M | 2.81 | 1.75 |
| SD | 1.64 | 1.24 |
| N | 16 | 16 |
| Low | | |
| M | 2.06 | 2.31 |
| SD | 1.00 | 1.01 |
| N | 16 | 16 |

*Note.* Subjects could recall a total of ten possible self-relevant words. Results from Hull, Levenson, Young, and Sher (1983).

the alcohol nor the self-consciousness main effects were significant. Individual comparisons revealed that high-self-conscious subjects recalled more self-relevant words than low self-conscious subjects under placebo conditions, thus replicating the findings of Hull and Levy (1979). Alcohol significantly reduced recall of self-relevant words for high-self-conscious subjects, rendering this group equivalent to both low-self-conscious groups. Alcohol did not affect recall of self-relevant words among low-self-conscious subjects. These analyses were repeated on non-self-relevant words. There were no significant effects.

This experiment supports the proposition that alcohol reduces self-awareness by interfering with the process of encoding information in terms of its self-relevance. Thus, high-self-conscious individuals recalled more self-relevant words than did low-self-conscious individuals under placebo conditions, and alcohol eliminated this difference. Stated somewhat differently, alcohol eliminated the self-consciousness contribution to the processing of self-relevant information.

### Alcohol, Self-Awareness, and Affective Reactivity

Previous research has shown that self-awareness is associated with increased emotional responsivity to affect arousing situations (Scheier & Carver, 1977). Hull and Levy (1979) proposed that these effects are due to the self-aware individual's sensitivity to the self-relevance of the affect arousing cues. By inhibiting self-relevant encoding processes and thus decreasing an individual's sensitivity to self-relevant information, Hull (1981) proposed that alcohol consumption should have the opposite affective consequences of variables that increase self-awareness. Hull et al. (1981) designed an experiment to test this hypothesis. As in the two experiments by Hull et al. (1983), subjects gave short speeches about themselves. All subjects were told that the speeches would be videotaped and evaluated by observers for openness, defensiveness, and other psychological variables. To the extent that one is sensitive to the self-evaluative character of the speech act, the speech should become a somewhat stressful instance of self-disclosure. It was therefore hypothesized that high-private-self-conscious individuals should be more affectively stressed in response to giving such a speech than low-self-conscious individuals by virtue of perceiving the situation in terms of its self-relevance (Archer, Hormuth, & Berg, 1982). Alcohol should reduce the affective reactions of high-self-conscious individuals and equate them with those of low-self-conscious individuals.

In addition to the general character of the speech task, certain cues exist within the task of giving a speech that are self-relevant in the sense that they define a specific relationship between self and the act. Thus, given that one's task is to give a speech, cues that indicate one should begin preparing one's thoughts for the upcoming speech and cues that instruct one to begin the speech are self-relevant. High-self-conscious individuals should be more reactive to the onset of such cues than low-self-conscious individuals. Once again, alcohol should reduce the reactivity of high-self-conscious individuals and equate their reactions with those of low-self-conscious individuals.

The experiment conducted by Hull *et al.* (1981) involved a repeated measures design. Subjects gave speeches about themselves on two separate occasions. On the first occasion, subjects were sober. On the second occasion, they were intoxicated (mean blood alcohol content = 0.07% just prior to the speech). On each occasion, subjects were wired for physiologic measurement (galvanic skin response, finger pulse transit time, finger pulse amplitude, ear pulse transit time, and heart rate). In addition, subjects reported their ongoing level of anxiety continuously throughout the experiment on an "anxiety dial." Rather than having subjects give identical speeches on both occasions, they were instructed to talk about acquaintances' reactions to the subject's body and physical appearance in the first experimental session and their own reactions to their body and physical appearance in the second experimental session.

Measurement of all dependent measures was continuous over a given session but was divided into 92 measurement intervals for the purposes of analysis. The procedures of the experiment grouped these measurement intervals into six distinct periods: (1) a preliminary baseline period during which subjects knew they would give a speech but did not know the topic, (2) a countdown initiation cue, (3) a countdown period in which subjects were to read their speech topic from a clipboard and prepare their thoughts for the speech itself, (4) a speech initiation cue, (5) a speech period during which subjects gave their speeches, and (6) a postspeech baseline period. It was predicted that within sober sessions, high-private-self-conscious subjects would show greater arousal than low-self-conscious subjects across measurement periods due to a heightened sensitivity to the self-evaluative character of the speech act, that within sober sessions high-self-conscious subjects would be more reactive to the countdown initiation cue and the speech initiation cue than low-self-conscious subjects, and that alcohol would effectively inhibit self-awareness and would therefore equate the responses of high- and low-self-conscious subjects with regard to both overall levels of arousal and reactivity to the onset of the self-relevant cues (countdown initiation cue and speech initiation cue).

There were significant effects involving private self-consciousness on four of the six dependent measures, and these effects supported the predictions. In general, within no-alcohol sessions subjects high in private self-consciousness showed higher levels of arousal overall and greater reactivity to the countdown and speech initiation cues relative to their initial baselines than did subjects low in private self-consciousness. These differences did not exist in the alcohol session.

Analysis of galvanic skin response revealed a typical pattern. These results are illustrated in Figure 8.1. There was a significant interaction of private self-consciousness and measurement period such that relative to their initial baseline high-private-self-conscious subjects registered greater skin conductance in reaction to the countdown and speech initiation cues than did low private self-conscious subjects. In addition, there was a significant interaction of private self-consciousness and alcohol session such that high-self-conscious subjects were more aroused than low-self-conscious subjects across measurement periods in the no-alcohol session, and these differences were nonexistent in the alcohol sessions.

Analysis of ear pulse transit time revealed similar effects. Once again, there was a significant interaction of private self-consciousness and measure-

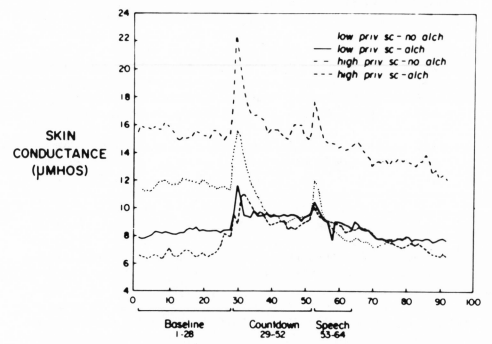

FIGURE 8.1. The effects of private self-consciousness, alcohol, and social stress on galvanic skin response. From Hull, Levenson, and Young (1981).

ment period such that high-self-conscious subjects were more reactive to the initiation of the countdown and speech periods relative to their initial baselines than were low-self-conscious subjects. In addition, there was a significant triple interaction of private self-consciousness, measurement period, and alcohol consumption, indicating that this effect was more marked in the no-alcohol session. Analysis of finger pulse amplitude revealed a similar interaction of private self-consciousness, measurement period, and alcohol session. There were no significant effects involving private self-consciousness for either heart rate or finger pulse transit time.

In summary, high-private-self-conscious subjects showed what might be termed a "reactive" physiologic response pattern under no-alcohol conditions. Thus, relative to their baselines, high-self-conscious subjects showed greater arousal in response to the countdown and speech initiation phases of the experiment than did low-self-conscious subjects. They also showed greater arousal across measurement periods than did low-self-conscious subjects, presumably in reaction to the self-evaluative character of the speech act. Alcohol would appear to have eliminated physiologic differences between high- and low-self-conscious subjects.

These results are consistent with the hypothesis that alcohol consumption inhibits self-awareness: It would appear to have eliminated differences in affective reactions of individuals high as opposed to low in dispositional self-consciousness. Furthermore, alcohol would appear to have this effect by decreasing the individual's reactivity to self-relevant information. Thus, high-self-conscious subjects were more physiologically reactive to situationally self-relevant cues than low-self-conscious subjects during sober but not during intoxicated sessions. Despite this interpretation, it should be pointed out that conclusions regarding these results must be regarded as tenuous. First, for economic and logistic reasons the experiment involved a within subjects design in which all subjects participated in both no-alcohol and alcohol sessions in that order. It is always possible, then, that some aspect of the session other than the content of subjects' drinks was responsible for these effects. Although we feel that this is unlikely, future research should eliminate this design weakness by treating intoxication as a between-subjects factor. Second, it is possible that alcohol had its effects in this study by virtue of directly reducing physiologic responsivity, as opposed to indirectly reducing physiologic arousal by virtue of its effects on self-conscious cognition (Levenson, Sher, Grossman, Newman, & Newlin, 1980). Nevertheless, confidence in the present interpretation of these effects is somewhat bolstered by the fact that they do not exist as isolated findings but rather fit a consistent pattern of results from multiple experiments that suggest that alcohol reduces self-awareness. Given that alcohol has the *effect* of reducing self-awareness, is it also the case that self-awareness can function as a *cause* of alcohol consumption?

## Alcohol and the Strategic Avoidance of Self-Awareness

The results of these experiments support the proposition that alcohol decreases self-awareness. Given that this is true, it follows that some individuals may consume alcohol in order to avoid self-awareness. Previous research has shown that self-awareness is associated with increased sensitivity to information about past performances (Fenigstein, 1979) and heightened negative affect and a desire to avoid the self-aware state following personal failure (Steenbarger & Aderman, 1979). According to Hull and Levy (1979), such reactions are a consequence of the self-aware individual's tendency to encode information about past performances according to its self-relevance. Thus, when a person receives feedback about job performance, he or she is only affected by the feedback to the extent that it is regarded as self-relevant. The more self-relevant the feedback, the greater its capacity to make the individual feel good or bad. As a consequence of the tendency to encode information according to its self-relevance, the self-aware individual is more affected by the positive–negative quality of the feedback and more motivated to maintain or avoid the self-aware state. If alcohol functions to decrease self-awareness, individuals who are experiencing personal failure should be especially likely to resort to alcohol consumption in order to avoid the negative implications of failure. On the other hand, self-aware individuals who are experiencing personal success should be likely not to consume alcohol in order to remain sensitive to the positive implications of success.

In order to test this analysis, it is necessary to manipulate success and failure in an experimental design and directly assess subsequent consumption by high- and low-self-aware individuals. Such a design also allows for the assessment of intermediary processes hypothesized by the self-awareness model. Thus, high-self-aware individuals should show heightened sensitivity and affective reactivity to success and failure feedback followed by alcohol consumption as a function of the quality of personal performance.

Hull and Young (1983b) conducted an experiment to test this analysis. Subjects worked on intelligence-type tasks and were randomly assigned success or failure feedback. Immediate expressions of pleasure/displeasure at their success or failure were recorded as an indication of reactivity to the manipulation. Subjects were then released to participate in a second, ostensibly unrelated experiment during which they completed a mood measure and then tasted and rated a series of wines. The "wine-tasting" experimental design has been used in several previous experiments to assess alcohol consumption in an *ad lib.* situation (Higgins & Marlatt, 1973, 1975). According to this procedure, subjects are asked to sample three different wines and compare them on a list of adjectives that appear one at a time in the window of a memory drum operated by the subject. Subjects are asked to determine which wine a particular adjective describes best, which wine the same adjective describes least, and to record their responses on the taste-rating forms, repeating this procedure for each adjective presented. *Ad lib.* consumption is encouraged by telling subjects: "You can take as many tastes of the drinks as you need to answer the questions. Just pour them into the glasses as you see fit." Procedures for the study by Hull and Young (1983b) were adapted from Higgins and Marlatt (1975). Subjects were allowed 15 minutes to taste and rate the wines.

Three different measures were used to assess processes hypothesized by the self-awareness model of alcohol consumption. First, notes were taken by the experimenter who conducted the intelligence test phase of the experiment that characterized the subject's overt reactions to the feedback. Verbal and nonverbal displays of pleasure or displeasure to the success–failure manipulation were noted as well as the subject's tendency to attribute responsibility for the outcome. Subjects demonstrating any of these characteristics were labeled "reactive"; subjects showing none of these characteristics were labeled "nonreactive." The experimenter's notes and the subsequent evaluation of the subject's reactivity were both made while blind to the subject's level of self-consciousness. It was predicted that high-self-conscious individuals would be more reactive to both success and failure feedback than low-self-conscious individuals.

A second measure of the hypothesized processes involved the Multiple Affect Adjective Checklist (Zuckerman & Lubin, 1965). This was administered just prior to the wine consumption phase of the experiment. It was expected that high-self-conscious individuals would report more negative moods following failure and more positive moods following success than low-self-conscious individuals. Such a finding would be consistent with an experiment by Fenigstein (1979). The final measure was the amount of wine consumed during the 15-minute tasting session. Consistent with the self-awareness model of alcohol use, it was predicted that high-self-conscious individuals would consume the most wine following failure and the least wine following success. Low-self-conscious individuals were predicted to fall between these extremes and not to vary their consumption according to the quality of their performance.

For purposes of analysis, subjects were divided into high- and low-self-conscious groups using the private self-conscious subscale of the Fenigstein *et al.* (1975) inventory. In addition, subjects were divided into high- and low-self-esteem groups using a scale patterned after Watkins (1978). Brockner (1979) has indicated that high-self-conscious subjects who are also low in self-esteem may be especially affected by situational success and failure. The experiment thus consisted of a 2 (high–low private self-conscious) × 2 (high–low self-esteem) × 2 (success–failure) design. Once again, it was predicted that high-self-conscious subjects would show greater overt reactivity to success and failure than would low-self-conscious subjects and that self-reported mood and wine consumption would vary as a function of success and failure for high-self-conscious but not low-self-conscious subjects. Furthermore, given the findings of Brockner (1979), it was felt that in each case the effects might be qualified by the subject's level of self-esteem with the high-self-conscious low-self-esteem subjects showing the greatest overt reactivity to feedback and the largest mood and consumption differences as a function of success and failure.

A log-linear analysis was conducted on the dichotomous reactive–non-reactive ratings. The only significant result corresponded to a main effect of self-consciousness. As predicted, high-self-conscious subjects were more frequently reactive to performance feedback (regardless of its success–failure quality) than were low-self-conscious subjects. Fifty percent of the high-self-conscious compared to only 28% of the low-self-conscious subjects were overtly reactive to the feedback. The self-consciousness by self-esteem interaction was not significant. Neither were any other effects or interactions.

A multivariate analysis of variance was conducted on the Multiple Affect Adjective Checklist subscale categories. In accord with predictions, there was an interaction of self-consciousness and success–failure and an interaction of self-consciousness, success–failure, and self-esteem. The pattern of results was consistent across subscales. High-self-conscious subjects were more negative following failure and more positive following success than low-self-conscious subjects. In addition, subjects who were high in self-consciousness, low in self-esteem, and received failure feedback reported the most negative moods of any group across all subscales. Such findings are consistent with previous research by Fenigstein (1979) and Brockner (1979).

In addition to these results, the analysis revealed a main effect of self-esteem and an interaction of self-consciousness and self-esteem. In general, low-self-esteem subjects reported more negative moods than high-self-esteem subjects, and this was especially true for subjects who were high in self-consciousness. Both of these latter effects should only be interpreted within the context of the previously reported three-way interaction.

The dependent measure of primary interest was the amount of wine consumed during the wine-tasting phase of the experiment. Amount of wine consumed was analyzed using a 2 (high–low private self-conscious) × 2 (high–low self-esteem) × 2 (success–failure) analysis of variance. Subjects' self-reports of amount of alcohol they usually consumed at a given sitting had been measured prior to the wine tasting phase of the experiment and were used as a covariate. This covariate proved to be highly significant. In addition, there was a significant interaction of self-consciousness and success–failure. As predicted, high-self-conscious subjects given failure feedback drank significantly more wine than high-self-conscious subjects given success feedback. Low-self-conscious subjects' consumption fell between these extremes and did not vary as a function of success–failure feedback. The means for these groups are presented in Table 8.4.

In addition to the predicted self-consciousness by success–failure interaction, there was a significant main effect for self-esteem. Low-self-esteem subjects drank more than did high-self-esteem subjects. This finding is consistent with previous research by Schaeffer, Shuckit, and Morrissey (1976). There were no other significant effects or interactions. The complete experimental design with covariate accounted for 26% of the total variance in wine consumption.

The results support the self-awareness model of alcohol consumption. According to this model, alcohol consumption is a function of success and failure for high-self-conscious but not low-self-conscious individuals because self-consciousness is a necessary precondition for reactivity to the self-relevant implications of success and failure (Hull & Levy, 1979). In accord with this analysis, the alcohol consumption of high-self-conscious but not low-self-conscious subjects varied as a function of success and failure feedback. Furthermore, consistent with the mediating processes hypothesized by the model, high-self-conscious subjects were more overtly reactive to performance feedback than were low-self-conscious subjects. They were also more likely to report moods consistent with the quality of performance feedback, although this was especially the case among high-self-conscious subjects who were also low in self-esteem. These results are consistent with previous studies by Fenigstein (1979) and Steenbarger and Aderman (1979) that demonstrate that self-awareness is associated with an intensified reaction to success and failure and research by Greenberg and Musham (1981) showing that self-aware individuals desire to avoid self-awareness inducing stimuli following failure and approach such stimuli following success.

A final analysis of these data involved the calculation of correlations between subjects' self-reported moods and the amount of alcohol consumed. These analyses revealed that moods were consistently and significantly related

TABLE 8.4. The Effect of Self-Consciousness and Success–Failure Feedback on Number of Ounces of Wine Consumed

| | Feedback | |
|---|---|---|
| Self-consciousness | Success | Failure |
| High | $6.21_a$ | $9.03_b$ |
| Low | $8.33_{ab}$ | $7.02_{ab}$ |

*Note.* Means that do not share subscripts differ at the .05 level according to planned comparisons.

to alcohol consumption among high-self-conscious individuals and consistently unrelated to alcohol consumption among low-self-conscious individuals. Furthermore, these differences were statistically significant: Specific comparisons revealed that high- and low-self-conscious individuals differed in the degree to which alcohol consumption was related to mood. These differences in correlations were not associated with differences in ranges or variances of the measures across groups. These results are consistent with a model that proposes that alcohol consumption exists as an attempt to affect mood states indirectly through self-consciousness reduction. Thus, if alcohol affects moods indirectly by reducing self-consciousness, then alcohol consumption will be correlated with mood among individuals whose mood is contingent on the self-conscious state. Negative moods contingent on self-consciousness will motivate alcohol consumption; positive moods contingent on self-consciousness will decrease motivation to consume alcohol. As a consequence, consumption will be positively correlated with mood among high-self-conscious individuals. On the other hand, although mood may vary among low-self-conscious individuals, to the extent that it is not contingent on the self-conscious state and is relatively unaffected by alcohol consumption, it does not provide differential motivation for alcohol consumption. As a consequence, consumption is relatively uncorrelated with mood among low-self-conscious individuals. Note that this explanation of the behavior of low-self-conscious individuals presumes the invalidity of the tension reduction hypothesis (previous sentence: "mood . . . among low-self-conscious individuals . . . is relatively unaffected by alcohol consumption"). Given the correlational nature of these results, causal conclusions remain tentative. Nevertheless, they may serve both as support for self-awareness model of alcohol consumption and as evidence against the tension reduction model.

While the results of the experiment by Hull and Young (1983b) support the self-awareness model of alcohol consumption, it is also necessary to determine if they can generalize to conditions outside of the laboratory. Hull, Young, and Jouriles (in press) report two studies that apply predictions from the model to alcohol consumption in the "real world." In both studies, the basic prediction was that life events indicative of success and failure would be more strongly related to alcohol consumption among individuals high as opposed to low in dispositional private self-consciousness.

The first experiment by Hull et al. (in press) was concerned with predicting patterns of alcoholic relapse. It was hypothesized that alcoholics who are high in private self-consciousness and who have experienced events predominantly indicative of personal failure should be especially likely to relapse following detoxification. Alcoholics who are highly self-conscious and who have experienced events that are predominantly indicative of personal success should be especially likely not to relapse following detoxification. Finally, alcoholics who are low in private self-consciousness should fall between these two extremes and not vary in their likelihood to relapse as a function of the quality of self-relevant life events. Such a pattern would replicate the pattern of results reported by Hull and Young (1983b) in their laboratory experiment on alcohol consumption following success and failure feedback.

A longitudinal study of alcoholic relapse following detoxification was conducted to test these hypotheses. Subjects were 35 males who were nearing completion of an alcoholic detoxification program. All subjects completed the Fenigstein *et al.* (1975) self-consciousness inventory and the Sarason, Johnson, and Siegel (1978) life events survey. Given the hypothesis regarding self-awareness and success–failure experiences, only those events a priori defined as reflecting the individual's successful or unsuccessful performance of a role were included in the calculation of a self-relevant life events score (e.g., trouble with employer, marital reconciliation, change in number of arguments with spouse, and so on). After discharge from the hospital, subjects were contacted at 3- and 6-month intervals to determine whether or not they had relapsed. Relapse was defined as drinking at a level similar to that reported in the preabstinent period. Nonrelapse was defined as either maintaining complete abstinence or drinking at a substantially reduced level such that alcohol did not have a negative impact on the individual's life.

In support of predictions, the quality of self-relevant life events was a significant predictor of relapse at the 3-month interval for high-self-conscious subjects such that the likelihood of relapse increased as the quality of such events became worse. On the other hand, the relationship between such events and relapse was non-significantly in the opposite direction for low-self-conscious individuals. Similar results were found at the 6-month interval.

While the model can be used to predict alcoholic relapse among individuals experiencing personal success and failure, it should be obvious that not all self-conscious individuals who fail become alcoholics. Individuals can cope with failure through various means; alcohol induced self-awareness reduction is only one such means. For example, self-awareness can be reduced through means other than alcohol consumption. Duval and Wicklund (1973) have suggested that physical activity reduces self-awareness. Becoming involved in a variety of activities may be an efficient way to avoid unwanted self-awareness. Wegner and Schaefer (1978) and Diener (1980) have suggested that the presence of others serves to reduce self-awareness by focusing attention away from self. In a more general sense, any environmental stimulus that serves to focus attention away from the self may serve to reduce self-awareness (e.g., television). In addition to reducing self-awareness, the model suggests that the motive to consume alcohol may be eliminated by rendering negative feedback non-self-relevant. For example, one might attribute responsibility for the performance outward (it was due to the fact that the task was so difficult anyone would have failed; it was due to bad luck) or to internal factors that will change in the future (I will get better; I can try harder). By emphasizing the unimportance of performance vis-à-vis personal goals, the nonpermanent implications of performance, or extenuating circumstances surrounding performance, the feedback should be rendered non-self-relevant and as a consequence the motive to consume alcohol should be reduced.

Despite the validity of such reasoning, a recent analysis by Hull and Young (1983a) suggests that alcohol consumption may be a particularly effective means of providing psychological relief for some individuals. These authors reanalyzed data reported by Hull et al. (1983) on the self-awareness-reducing properties of alcohol intoxication. It was found that social drinkers with high scores on the MacAndrew (1965) scale of alcoholic risk were especially likely to show self-awareness reduction as a consequence of intoxication. It may be that these individuals are prone to alcoholism in part because intoxication serves as a particularly effective means of coping with the self-relevant implications of failure.

In addition to the study on alcoholics, Hull, Young, and Jouriles (in press) also conducted a study to examine drinking patterns among high school adolescents. In this study subjects completed a questionnaire booklet that contained measures of self-consciousness (Fenigstein et al., 1975), academic performance (considered an indicator of self-relevant success or failure at an important role), and quantity and frequency of alcohol consumption. In addition, an attempt was made to assess the independent contribution of the self-awareness model by statistically taking into consideration several other variables previously shown to be predictive of adolescent alcohol use. These variables were selected from a study by Donovan and Jessor (1978) and included measures of (1) parental approval and modeling of alcohol consumption, (2) peer approval, pressure, and modeling of alcohol consumption, and (3) general behavioral deviance and conventionality.

In accord with predictions, academic performance was more strongly related to alcohol consumption among individuals high as opposed to low in private self-consciousness. In addition, subjects' general behavioral deviance and their friends' attitudes and behaviors toward alcohol were significant predictors of alcohol use among both high - and low-self-conscious individuals. Parental attitudes and behaviors toward alcohol were significant predictors of alcohol use only among low-self-conscious individuals. Finally, and most importantly, academic performance remained more strongly related to alcohol consumption among high- than low-self-conscious individuals even when the remaining predictors were simultaneously considered within a multiple regression analysis. Put more simply, the self-awareness model proved to be a significant predictor of alcohol use among adolescents; its predictive strength proved to be unique and independent of other known predictors of alcohol use; it did not provide a complete explanation of alcohol use insofar as other variables also proved to be significant and unique predictors of alcohol use.

Together with the experimental study by Hull and Young (1983b), these experiments indicate the generality of the self-awareness model. Alcohol use has been shown to be a joint function of an individual's level of private self-consciousness and personal success–failure. This interaction has been demonstrated across different populations (adolescents, college students, and middle-aged adults), different patterns of alcohol use (social drinkers and alcoholics), different indicators of self-relevant life experiences (experimentally manipulated success–failure, reported academic performance, and reported performance of a significant role), and different measures of alcohol use (situationally measured wine consumption, self-reported alcohol consumption, and measures of alcoholic relapse). Furthermore, the results of the second study by Hull *et al.* (in press) suggest that this relationship is relatively independent of environmental and behavioral factors previously shown to be directly related to alcohol use.

In addition to proposing that alcohol may sometimes be consumed in order to reduce self-awareness, Hull (1981) also proposed that alcohol intoxication has certain behavioral consequences as a function of its self-awareness-reducing properties. Specifically, alcohol was proposed to affect behavior by inhibiting processes related to self-regulation. Since recent research on the self-awareness model has concerned self-regulation, we will briefly consider this topic.

### Alcohol, Self-Awareness, and Self-Regulation

The socially inappropriate consequences of alcohol intoxication are numerous and well-known, ranging from inappropriate conversational styles (Smith, Parker, & Noble, 1975) to inappropriate aggression (Zeichner & Pihl, 1979, 1980) and violent crime (Shupe, 1954). The exact reasons for these behavioral consequences are less clear. While traditional explanations have centered on disinhibition through anxiety or fear reduction (Shuntich & Taylor, 1972), two recent explanations concern the issue of cognitive self-regulation. According to one point of view, alcohol has the pharmacologic effect of disrupting cognitive processes related to self-regulation. The result is disinhibited behavior as a consequence of a drug effect. According to a second point of view, alcohol intoxication provides a socially viable excuse to engage in behavior that is normally sanctioned. The result is that self-regulation occurs, but with respect to a deviant standard as a consequence of the perception that one has consumed alcohol. These two positions are independent, but not mutually exclusive. It is possible that consuming alcohol results in diminished self-regulation with respect to an altered standard.

Much of the early work on the behavioral consequences of alcohol intoxication used designs in which individuals consumed an alcohol or placebo beverage while being told that they were consuming alcohol. This work generally found that alcohol consumption had the effect of increasing socially disapproved behavior. For example, individuals were more aggressive in response to threat when they had consumed alcohol (Taylor, Gammon, & Capasso, 1976).

Research has suggested that these effects may be due in part to the effect of alcohol on the processing of information relevant to the individual's behavior. In one study by Zeichner and Pihl (1979), subjects were instructed to shock their partners in an adjoining room as part of a pain perception experiment. Following each (bogus) shock, participants received feedback from their partners in the form of an aversive tone. The loudness of this tone was either correlated with the severity of the shock or random. The overall duration and intensity of the "shocks" given by the subject constituted the primary dependent measures. Of principal interest is the finding that subjects who had not been given alcohol prior to the experimental task were responsive to the correlated-random manipulation: When increased levels of shock were associated with increasingly obnoxious noise, no-alcohol control subjects decreased their shock severities. In terms of the present analysis, they treated the noise pattern as relevant to their actions. This was not the case for subjects who received an alcohol preload: These subjects gave more severe shocks overall, and this was true regardless of whether the contingencies were shock-correlated or random. In other words, the noise pattern was not treated as self-relevant. Consistent with this analysis of the effects of alcohol, Zeichner and Pihl (1979) conclude: "The findings of the present study suggest that the occurrence of aggressive behavior following the ingestion of alcohol may in part be due to the individual's inability to process information pertinent to the consequences of his behavior" (p. 159). Another study by Zeichner and Pihl (1980) provides additional support for this conclusion.

Hull (1981) proposed that such effects may be mediated by the impact of alcohol consumption on self-awareness and the processing of information according to its self-relevance. As reviewed above, alcohol has been shown to have the effect of reducing self-awareness. In addition, research suggests that alcohol and self-awareness have opposite effects on the appropriateness of behavior: Alcohol decreases and self-awareness increases the probability of appropriate behaviors. Thus, numerous studies indicate that manipulations that increase self-awareness have the effect of increasing self-regulation with regard to internal and external standards of conduct (Carver & Scheier, 1981). Self-aware individuals are less likely to cheat (Diener & Wallbom, 1976) or steal (Beaman, Klentz, Diener, & Svanum, 1979), more likely to help others (Gibbons & Wicklund, 1982), and less likely to aggress when aggression is implicitly proscribed (Scheier, Fenigstein, & Buss, 1974). Furthermore, a distinction has been made between private self-conscious individuals who adhere to internal standards of appropriate conduct and public self-conscious individuals who adhere to external standards of conduct. If alcohol has the general effect of decreasing self-awareness, then it should result in decreased self-regulation with regard to both internal and external standards of conduct.

A recent experiment tested hypotheses related to this aspect of the model (Hull & Young, 1985). The experiment involved a Prisoner's Dilemma Game (a mixed motive game that allows for either cooperative or competitive play). Prior to consuming an alcohol or placebo beverage, subjects read instructions on how to play the game. The instructions included a "strategy section." For half of the subjects, this section emphasized a competitive game playing strategy; for the remaining subjects, this section emphasized a cooperative strategy. Following beverage consumption and absorption, subjects reread the instructions-strategy sheet and played the game. Although subjects thought that they were playing against each other, they actually played against a preprogrammed strategy. For purposes of analysis, subjects were divided according to their dispositional public self-consciousness since the strategy manipulation constituted a manipulation of an external standard of appropriate conduct.

Most interesting for the present discussion, analyses suggested that alcohol had effects on game playing behavior by interfering with self-regulation vis-à-vis the situational standard. Thus, to the extent that subjects self-regulate their behavior with respect to the standard presented on the instruction-strategy sheet, game playing behavior should be a direct function of attention to the sheet: More attention to the cooperative sheet should increase cooperativeness and more attention to the competitive sheet should increase competitiveness. To test such a hypothesis, amount of time subjects spent reading the instruction sheet just prior to playing the game was correlated with amount of competitive play. Consistent with expectations, the two strongest correlations occurred for sober high-public-self-conscious subjects: The longer such subjects attended to competitive instructions, the more competitively they played; the longer they attended to cooperative instructions, the less competitively they played, and these two correlations were significantly different from each other. However, among *intoxicated* high-public-self-conscious subjects these correlations were in the opposite direction and did not differ from each other. By implication, sober public self-conscious individuals regulate their game playing behavior vis-à-vis situational standards of appropriate conduct. Intoxication appears to disrupt such self-regulation: although subjects spent time attending to the material, they were doing so in such a way that it did not affect their subsequent behavior. Interestingly enough, the correlations among intoxicated high-public-self-conscious subjects were virtually identical to those of sober low-self-conscious subjects. Furthermore, none of the correlations for sober or intoxicated low-public-self-conscious individuals were significant, and none were significantly different from each other. Once again, it would appear that alcohol is having effects by virtue of eliminating the self-consciousness contribution to behavior.

By rendering the individual's responses more dependent on the superficial aspects of the situation, decreased self-awareness following alcohol consumption may lead to behavior that appears disinhibited or uncontrolled. According to the self-awareness model, the individual's grosser level of reaction corresponds to a grosser level of understanding. As such, behavior becomes less responsive to existing environmental requirements and often becomes unresponsive to a changing environment.

If one cause of socially inappropriate acts is the intoxicated individual's decreased tendency to encode situational cues of appropriate conduct in terms of their self-relevance, then one possible means of overcoming the inappropriate behavioral consequences of alcohol consumption may be to provide the individual with a cognitive repertoire of self-relevant encoding schemes to employ when he or she has been drinking. For example: What is my behavior saying about the kind of person I am? How would I react if someone was behaving this way toward me? What do I want to say with my behavior? More simply, external cues that heighten self-awareness may have the effect of overcoming such self-regulation deficits. Such a strategy will be effective to the extent that alcohol has its greatest effects on the propensity of the individual to employ self-relevant schemata rather than the ability to benefit from their use (Hull, 1981; Hull & Reilly, 1983). This analysis is consistent with the findings of a recent study by Bailey, Leonard, Cranston, and Taylor (1983). In this study alcohol consumption was shown to increase aggressive responses to threat. At the same time, presence of an external cue to become self-aware had the effect of overcoming this behavioral effect of alcohol. These results have wide-ranging implications for methods of overcoming the negative behavioral consequences of intoxication.

## General Issues and Alternative Models of Alcohol Use

### The Behavioral Effects of Cognitive Expectancies
### Regarding Alcohol Consumption

The self-awareness model attempts to account for some of the pharmacologic effects of alcohol. At the same time, it is recognized that alcohol has effects for reasons other than its pharmacologic properties. For example, the fact that people know they have consumed alcohol is frequently enough to lead them to alter their behavior. In order to study the effects of alcohol expectancies independent of alcohol consumption, it is necessary to employ a "balanced placebo" design. In addition to the traditional experimental conditions (consume alcohol–told alcohol, consume placebo–told alcohol), this design includes a control condition in which the person receives alcohol but is told that they are receiving a placebo, and a control condition in which the person receives a placebo and is told that they are receiving a placebo.

When the balanced placebo design was employed in a self-awareness study by Hull et al. (1983), alcohol consumption was found to decrease self-awareness, while expectancy was found to have weak effects in the opposite direction. The two variables did not interact. In general, research that has employed the balanced placebo design has found that alcohol consumption and expectancy have independent effects on behavior. Some of the effects of alcohol on behavior were reviewed earlier. With regard to expectancy effects, irrespective of the actual beverage content, the expectation that one has consumed alcohol has been shown to increase aggression (e.g., Lang, Goeckner, Adesso, & Marlatt, 1975), to increase sexual arousal in response to deviant stimuli (Wilson & Lawson, 1976), to increase viewing time of erotic stimuli among high-sex-guilt individuals (Lang, Searles, Lauerman, & Adesso, 1980), and to decrease social anxiety (Wilson & Abrams, 1977). These studies support the hypothesis that the belief that one is consuming alcohol can affect self-regulation by providing a socially viable excuse to engage in otherwise disapproved behavior. At the same time, they do not support the hypothesis that the pharmacologic effects of alcohol found in earlier studies are contingent on the cognition that one has consumed alcohol: In none of the above balanced placebo studies was there an interaction of consumption and expectancy such that the effects of having consumed alcohol were dependent on the expectancy of having consumed alcohol. Among all studies that have used the balanced placebo design, the proportion of data analyses that have found significant interactions approaches 1 out of 20. Thus, the socially inappropriate consequences of alcohol consumption found in earlier studies in which all subjects expected alcohol, but some subjects consumed alcohol while others consumed placebo beverages, would appear to be independent of expectancy effects. At the same time, many of the studies that have used the balanced placebo design have only found effects of expectancy (e.g., Abrams & Wilson, 1983), while others have only found effects of alcohol consumption (e.g., Korytnyk & Perkins, 1983). At the present time, it would seem most reasonable to assume that both consumption and expectancy have independent effects. The self-awareness model is specifically addressed to some of the effects of alcohol consumption. Future research should investigate the conditions that are most conducive to expectancy versus consumption effects. In addition, research should attempt to further delineate the self-regulative processes that mediate such effects.

## Models of Alcohol Use

The self-awareness model of alcohol use bears a surface similarity to two other models of alcohol and drug use. The relationship of the model to each of these will now be briefly considered.

### The Self-Handicapping Model of Alcohol and Drug Use

Jones and Berglas (1978; see also Berglas & Jones, 1978) have proposed that performance-debilitating drugs (including alcohol) are sometimes consumed prior to performance in order to create an attributionally ambiguous, no-lose situation. Thus, failure following drug consumption is attributed to the drug itself; success following drug consumption is attributed to personal abilities of sufficient magnitude to overcome the negative effects of the drug. Regardless of the outcome, public and private esteem is maintained. The model is especially applicable when an individual lacks confidence that past successes were due to personal abilities and is required to perform again. Self-handicapping is a means of maintaining esteem gains from past successes perceived to be noncontingent with personal abilities.

A recent study by Tucker, Vuchinich, and Sobel (1981) provides support for this model of alcohol use. In accord with Jones and Berglas (1978), it was hypothesized that subjects who received noncontingent success feedback would desire to avoid having their skills validly reassessed on a second test when compared to subjects given contingent success feedback. In order to avoid valid reassessment, noncontingent success subjects were hypothesized to render their second test performance attributionally ambiguous by consuming alcohol. In accord with this analysis, noncontingent success subjects drank more alcohol than contingent success subjects in two separate experiments. However, the effect was only marginally significant when an alternative strategy was available. If study materials were available such that subjects perceived they could bolster their task-relevant abilities, they were somewhat less likely to adopt the self-handicapping strategy. Tucker et al. (1981) conclude that individuals are most likely to self-handicap when they are denied access to performance enhancing strategies for avoiding anticipated failure.

The self-handicapping model is similar to the self-awareness model of alcohol use in that the individual is proposed to use drugs in order to avoid the negative implications of failure. However, the two analyses postulate different mechanisms whereby this is accomplished. According to Hull (1981), alcohol functions to decrease the individual's sensitivity to the self-relevant implications of the performance by inhibiting higher order encoding processes fundamental to the self-aware state. The individual performs, fails, and then drinks to decrease sensitivity to the performance as a failure. According to Jones and Berglas (1978), alcohol functions to attributionally discount other plausible causes for an individual's performance. The individual drinks and then performs in a no-lose situation: Failure cannot be directly linked to the individual's ineptitude as long as intoxication exists as a plausible cause of the performance. Both accounts would seem to offer valid explanations of different behavior patterns. The results of the experiments on alcohol consumption by Hull and Young (1983b) and Hull *et al.* (in press) would seem to be irrelevant to the Jones and Berglas model.

## The Tension Reduction Model

Conger (1956) has proposed that alcohol is consumed for its tension-reduction properties. According to this analysis, increased tension constitutes a heightened drive state; alcohol consumption has the reinforcing property of lowering drive by reducing tension; and such drive-reducing reinforcement strengthens the alcohol consumption response. Evidence for this model is mixed. There appears to be little support for the proposition that alcohol reduces tension (Brown & Crowell, 1974; Cappell & Herman, 1972). In fact, several studies have found that alcohol increases self-reported anxiety (McNamee, Mello, & Mendelson, 1968; Mendelson, LaDou, & Solomon, 1964; Steffen, Nathan, & Taylor, 1974). More recently, two studies have found that alcohol does decrease physiologic responsiveness to stressful situations (e.g., fear of shock; see Levenson *et al.*, 1980; fear of public evaluation; see Wilson, Abrams, & Lipscomb, 1980), although it is unclear whether this effect is a function of alcohol's impact on tension per se or cognizance of the stressor. At the same time, it is unclear whether or not individuals drink in response to tension. In general, studies have found that individuals drink in response to self-related stress (e.g., anticipated evaluation by others; see Higgins & Marlatt, 1975; Miller, Hersen, Eisler, & Hilsman, 1974) but not in response to non-self-related stress (e.g., threat of shock; see Higgins & Marlatt, 1973).

Despite the lack of empirical support for the tension reduction model, it remains a popular account of the personal causes and effects of alcohol consumption. In addition, it shares with the self-awareness model the notion that consumption is motivated by a negative affective state. According to the tension reduction model, alcohol has the direct effect of reducing this negative physiologic state. According to the self-awareness model, however, alcohol indirectly affects mood states by inhibiting the encoding of information in terms of its self-relevance. Alcohol has the ultimate effect of decreasing negative mood by inhibiting the processing of feedback about past performances in terms of self-relevant failure.

Once again, it is reasonable to hypothesize that both models provide plausible accounts of different alcohol-related effects. Thus, it is almost certainly the case that alcohol has pharmacologic effects independent of those associated with the proposed self-awareness processes. At the same time, the research reviewed in this chapter provides consistent support for the self-awareness-reducing properties of alcohol consumption. In addition, correlational results in the study by Hull and Young (1983b) seem not to support the tension reduction model of alcohol use. Hopefully, future research will be able to clearly define the boundary conditions on the applicability of each model.


## Conclusions

The evidence would appear to support the self-awareness model of alcohol use. First, research suggests that alcohol reduces self-awareness by virtue of interfering with self-relevant encoding processes. Given this self-awareness-reducing property, it follows that alcohol should have the opposite effect of manipulations that increase self-awareness. Research was presented that demonstrates that alcohol reduces the effect of dispositional self-awareness on affective reactions and on behavioral self-regulation with respect to situational standards. Finally, given that alcohol reduces self-awareness, it follows that individuals may drink under conditions in which self-awareness is negative. Previous research has shown that self-awareness is especially negative following personal failure. Research was presented that demonstrates that the motive to consume alcohol in order to escape the negative aspects of self-awareness is both applicable to a wide range of drinking behaviors and independent of other known alcohol consumption motives. One limitation of this research is that it has for the most part been restricted to male subjects. Although it is felt that the model should be equally applicable to males and females, additional work is necessary that tests the model in female populations.

In conclusion, research would appear to support the self-awareness model of alcohol consumption. This is not to say that alcohol consumption is always motivated by a desire to reduce self-awareness or that intoxication only affects behavior by reducing self-awareness. As stated earlier, alcohol is consumed and has effects for a variety of social and personal reasons. It may be stated that the self-awareness model provides a useful framework within which to conceive some of the personal causes and effects of alcohol consumption.

# References

Abrams, D. B., & Wilson, G. T. (1983). Alcohol, sexual arousal, and self-control. *Journal of Pesonality and Social Psychology, 45,* 188–198.

Archer, R. L., Hormuth, S. E., & Berg, J. H. (1982). Avoidance of self-disclosure: an experiment under conditions of self-awareness. *Personality and Social Psychology Bulletin, 8,* 122–128.

Bailey, D. S., Leonard, K. E., Cranston, J. W., & Taylor, S. P. (1983). Effects of alcohol and self-awareness on human physical aggression. *Personality and Social Psychology Bulletin, 9,* 289–295.

Beaman, A. L., Klentz, B., Diener, E., & Svanum, S. (1979). Self-awareness and transgression in children. *Journal of Personality and Social Psychology, 37,* 1835–1846.

Berglas, S., & Jones, E. E. (1978). Drug choice as a self-handicpping strategy in response to non-contingent success. *Journal of Personality and Social Psychology, 36,* 405–417.

Birnbaum, I. M., Johnson, M. K., Hartley, J. T., & Taylor, T. H. (1980). Alcohol and elaborative schemas for sentences. *Journal of Experimental Psychology: Human Learning and Memory, 6,* 293–300.

Birnbaum, I. M., & Parker, E. S. (1977). Acute effects of alcohol on storage and retrieval. In I. M. Birnbaum & E. S. Parker (Eds.), *Alcohol and human memory* (pp. 99–108). Hillsdale, NJ: Lawrence Erlbaum.

Birnbaum, I. M., Parker, E. S., Harltey, J. T., & Noble, E. P. (1978). Alcohol and memory: Retrieval processes. *Journal of Verbal Learning and Verbal Behavior, 17,* 325–335.

Brockner, J. (1979). The effects of self-esteem, success-failure, and self-consciousness on task performance. *Journal of Personality and Social Psychology, 37,* 1732–1741.

Brown, J. S., & Crowell, C. R. (1974). Alcohol and conflict resolution: A theoretical analysis. *Quarterly Journal of Studies on Alcohol, 35,* 66–85.

Cappell, H., & Herman, C. P. (1972). Alcohol and tension reduction: A review. *Quarterly Journal of Studies on Alcohol, 33,* 33–64.

Carver, C. S., & Scheier, M. F. (1978). Self-focusing effects of dispositional self-consciousness, mirror presence, and audience presence. *Journal of Personality and Social Psychology, 36,* 324–332.

Carver, C. S., & Scheier, M. F. (1981). *Attention and self-regulation: A control theory approach to human behavior.* New York: Springer-Verlag.

Cermak, L. S., Butters, N., & Gerrein, J. (1973). The extent of the verbal encoding ability of Korsakoff patients. *Neuropsychologia, 11,* 85–94.

Cermak, L. S., & Reale, L. (1978). Depth of processing and retention of words by alcoholic Korsakoff patients. *Journal of Experimental Psychology: Human Learning and Memory, 4,* 165–174.

Conger, J. J. (1956). Alcoholism: Theory, problem, and challenge. II. Reinforecment theory and the dynamics of alcoholism. *Quarterly Journal of Studies on Alcohol, 17,* 296–305.

Davis, D., & Brock, T. C. (1975). Use of first person pronouns as a function of increased objective self-awareness and performance feedback. *Journal of Experimental Social Psychology, 11,* 381–388.

Diener, E. (1980). Deindividuation: The absence of self-awareness and self-regulation in group members. In P. B. Paulus (Ed.), *The psychology of group influence* (pp. 209–242). Hillsdale, NJ: Lawrence Erlbaum.

Diener, E., & Wallbom, M. (1976). Effects of self-awareness on antinormative behavior. *Journal of Research in Personality, 10,* 107–111.

Donavan, J. E., & Jessor, R. (1978). Adolescent problem drinking: Psychosocial correlates in a national sample. *Journal of Studies on Alcohol, 39,* 1506–1524.

Duval, S., & Wicklund, R. A. (1973). Effects of objective self-awareness on attribution of causality. *Journal of Experimental Social Psychology, 9,* 17–31.

Exner, J. E. (1973). The self-focus sentence completion: A study of egocentricity. *Journal of Personality Assessment, 37,* 437–455.

Fenigstein, A. (1979). Self-consciousness, self-attention, and social interaction. *Journal of Personality and Social Psychology, 37*, 75–86.

Fenigstein, A., Scheier, M. F., & Buss, A. H. (1975). Public and private self-consciousness: Assessment and theory. *Journal of Consulting and Clinical Psychology, 43*, 522–527.

Gibbons, F. X., & Wicklund, R. A. (1982). Self-focused attention and helping behavior. *Journal of Personality and Social Psychology, 43*, 462–474.

Greenberg, J., & Musham, C. (1981). Avoding and seeking self-focused attention. *Journal of Research in Personality, 15*, 191–200.

Hashtroudi, S., Parker, E. S., DeLisi, L. E., & Wyatt, R. I. (1983). On elaboration and alcohol. *Journal of Verbal Learning and Verbal Behavior, 22*, 164–173.

Higgins, R. L., & Marlatt, G. A. (1973). Effects of anxiety arousal on the consumption of alcohol by alcoholics and social drinkers. *Journal of Consulting and Clinical Psychology, 41*, 426–433.

Higgins, R. L., & Marlatt, G. A. (1975). Fear of interpersonal evaluation as a determinant of alcohol consumption in male social drinkers. *Journal of Abnormal Psychology, 84*, 644–651.

Hofstadter, D. R., & Dennett, D. C. (1981). *The mind's I*. New York: Basic Books.

Hull, J. G. (1981). A self-awareness model of the causes and effects of alcohol consumption. *Journal of Abnormal Psychology, 90*, 586–600.

Hull, J. G., Levenson, R. W., & Young, R. D. (1981). *The effects of social anxiety, private self-consciousness, public self-consciousness, and alcohol consumption on response to a social stressor*. Unpublished manuscript, Indiana University, Bloomington.

Hull, J. G., Levenson, R. W., Young, R. D., & Sher, K. J. (1983). Self-awareness reducing effects of alcohol consumption. *Journal of Personality and Social Psychology, 44*, 461–473.

Hull, J. G., & Levy, A. S. (1979). The organizational functions of the self: An alternative to the Duval and Wicklund model of self-awareness. *Journal of Personality and Social Psychology, 37*, 756–768.

Hull, J. G., & Reilly, N. P. (1983). Self-awareness, self-regulation, and alcohol consumption: A reply to Wilson. *Journal of Abnormal Psychology, 92*, 514–519.

Hull, J. G., & Young, R. D. (1983a). The self-awareness reducing effects of alcohol: Evidence and implications. In J. Suls & A. G. Greenwald (Eds.), *Psychological perspectives on the self* (Vol. 2, pp. 159–190). Hillsdale, NJ: Lawrence Erlbaum.

Hull, J. G., & Young, R. D. (1983b). Self-consciousness, self-esteem, and success-failure as determinants of alcohol consumption in male social drinkers. *Journal of Personality and Social Psychology, 44*, 1097–1109.

Hull, J. G., & Young, R. D. (1985). *Alcohol and the self-conscious regulation of public behavior*. Unpublished manuscript.

Hull, J. G., Young, R. D., & Jouriles, E. (in press). Applications of the self-awareness model of alcohol consumption. *Journal of Personality and Social Psychology*.

Jones, B. M. (1973). Memory impairment on the ascending and descending limbs of the blood alcohol curve. *Journal of Abnormal Psychology, 82*, 24–32.

Jones, E. E., & Berglas, S. (1978). Control of attributions about the self through self-handicapping strategies: The appeal of alcohol and the role of underachievement. *Personality and Social Psychology Bulletin, 4*, 200–206.

Korytnyk, N. X., & Perkins, D. V. (1983). Effects of alcohol versus expectancy for alcohol on the incidence of graffiti following an experimental task. *Journal of Abnormal Psychology, 92*, 382–385.

Lang, A. R., Goeckner, D. J., Adeso, V. J., & Marlatt, G. A. (1975). Effects of alcohol on aggression in male social drinkers. *Journal of Abnormal Psychology, 84*, 508–518.

Lang, A. R., Searles, J., Lauerman, R., & Adesso, V. (1980). Expectancy, alcohol, and sex guilt as determinants of interest in and reaction to sexual stimuli. *Journal of Abnormal Psychology, 89*, 644–653.

Levenson, R. W., Sher, K. J., Grossman, L. M., Newman, J., & Newlin, D. B. (1980). Alcohol and stress response dampening: Pharmacological effects, expectancy, and tension reduction. *Journal of Abnormal Psychology, 89*, 528–538.

MacAndrew, C. (1965). The differentiation of male alcoholic outpatients from nonalcoholic psychiatric outpatients by means of the MMPI. *Quarterly Journal of Studies on Alcohol, 26,* 238–246.

McNamee, H. B., Mello, N. K., & Mendelson, J. H. (1968). Experimental analysis of drinking patterns of alcoholics: Concurrent psychiatric observations. *American Journal of Psychiatry, 124,* 1063–1069.

Mendelson, J. H., LaDou, J., & Solomon, P. (1964). Experimentally induced chronic intoxication and withdrawal in alcoholics: Part 3, Psychiatric findings. *Quarterly Journal of Studies on Alcohol* (Suppl. 2), 40–52.

Miller, M. E., Adesso, V. J., Fleming, J. P., Gino, A., & Lauerman, R. (1978). Effects of alcohol on the storage and retrieval processes of heavy social drinkers. *Journal of Experimental Psychology: Human Learning and Memory, 4,* 246–255.

Miller, P. M., Hersen, M., Eisler, R. M., & Hilsman, G. (1974). Effects of social stress on operant drinking of alcoholics and social drinkers. *Behavioral Research Therapy, 12,* 67–72.

Moskowitz, H. (1973). Laboratory studies of the effects of alcohol on some variables related to driving. *Journal of Safety Research, 5,* 185–199.

Parker, E. S., Birnbaum, I. M., & Noble, E. P. (1976). Alcohol and memory: Storage and state dependency. *Journal of Verbal Learning and Verbal Behavior, 15,* 691–702.

Rogers, T. B., Kuiper, N. A., & Kirker, W. S. (1977). Self-reference and the encoding of personal information. *Journal of Personality and Social Psychology, 35,* 677–688.

Ryback, R. S. (1971). The continuum and specificity of the effects of alcohol on memory: A review. *Journal of Studies on Alcohol, 32,* 995–1016.

Sarason, I. C., Johnson, J. H., & Siegel, J. M. (1978). Assessing the impact of life changes: Development of the life experiences survey. *Journal of Consulting and Clinical Psychology, 46,* 932–946.

Schaeffer, G. M., Schuckit, M. A., & Morrissey, E. R. (1976). Correlation between two measures of self-esteem and drug use in a college sample. *Psychological Reports, 39,* 915–919.

Scheier, M. F., & Carver, C. S. (1977). Self-focused attention and the experience of emotion: Attraction, repulsion, elation, and depression. *Journal of Personality and Social Psychology, 35,* 625–636.

Scheier, M. F., Fenigstein, A., & Buss, A. H. (1974). Self-awareness and physical aggression. *Journal of Experimental Social Psychology, 10,* 264–273.

Shuntich, R. J., & Taylor, S. P. (1972). The effects of alcohol on human physical aggression. *Journal of Experimental Research in Personality, 6,* 34–38.

Shupe, L. M. (1954). Alcohol and crime: A study of the urine concentration found in 882 persons arrested during or immediately after the commission of a felony. *Journal of Criminal Law and Criminology, 44,* 661–664.

Smith, R. C., Parker, E. S., & Noble, E. P. (1975). Alcohol's effect on some formal aspects of verbal social communication. *Archives of General Psychiatry, 32,* 1394–1398.

Steenbarger, B. N., & Aderman, D. (1979). Objective self-awareness as a non-aversive state: Effect of anticipating discrepancy reduction. *Journal of Personality, 47,* 330–339.

Steffen, J. J., Nathan, P. E., & Taylor, H. A. (1974). Tension reducing effects of alcohol: Further evidence and some methodological considerations. *Journal of Abnormal Psychology, 83,* 542–547.

Taylor, S. P., Gammon, C. B., & Capasso, D. R. (1976). Aggression as a function of alcohol and threat. *Journal of Personality and Social Psychology, 34,* 938–941.

Tucke, J. A., Vuchinich, R. E., & Sobell, M. B. (1981). Alcohol consumption as a self-handicapping strategy. *Journal of Abnormal Psychology, 90,* 220–230.

Watkins, D. (1978). The development and evaluation of self-esteem measuring instruments. *Journal of Personality Assessment, 42,* 171–182.

Wegner, D. M., & Schaefer, D. (1978). The concentration of responsibility: An objective self-awareness analysis of group effects in helping situations. *Journal of Personality and Social Psychology, 36,* 147–155.

Williams, H. L., & Rundell, O. H. (1984). Effect of alcohol on recall and recognition as functions of processing levels. *Journal of Studies on Alcohol, 45,* 10–15.

Wilson, G. T., & Abrams, D. (1977). Effects of alcohol on social anxiety and physiological arousal: Cognitive versus pharmacological properties. *Cognitive Therapy and Research, 1*, 195–210.

Wilson, G. T., Abrams, D. B., & Lipscomb, T. R. (1980). Effects of increasing levels of intoxication and drinking pattern on social anxiety. *Journal of Studies on Alcohol, 41*, 250–264.

Wilson, G. T., & Lawson, D. M. (1976). Expectancies, alcohol, and sexual arousal in male social drinkers. *Journal of Abnormal Psychology, 85*, 587–594.

Zeichner, A., & Pihl, R. O. (1979). Effects of alcohol and behavior contingencies on human aggression. *Journal of Abnormal Psychology, 88*, 133–160.

Zeichner, A., & Pihl, R. O. (1980). Effects of alcohol and instigator intent on human aggression. *Journal of Studies on Alcohol, 41*, 265–276.

Zuckerman, M., & Lubin, B. (1965). *Manual for the multiple affect adjective check list.* San Diego, CA: Educational and Industrial Testing Service.

# 9 Self-Handicapping Model

STEVEN BERGLAS

> The renown which riches or beauty confer is fleeting and frail; mental
> excellence is a splendid and lasting possession.
> —Sallust 40 B.C.

> We were to do more business after dinner; but after dinner is after
> dinner—an old saying and a true, "much drinking, little thinking."
> —Jonathan Swift (1712)

Since the days when Sallust was an authority on the human condition, it has
been demonstrated that his insightful commentary was slightly in error. Mental excellence *is* splendid, but it is somewhat less stable or lasting than was
once thought to be the case (Anastasi, 1958, 1961; Honzik, 1973). Moreover,
recent research has shown that there is more than one aspect to intelligence,
and that individuals vary in their intellectual capacities across situations (Gardner, 1983). Social psychologists, of course, always knew that mental excellence
was not something that a person could manifest on one or two occasions and
then, for life, reliably manifest on demand. Numerous theories and com-
mentaries on impression management and strategic self-presentation (e.g.,
Goffman, 1959; Jones & Pittman, 1982; Schlenker, 1980) detail the various
techniques that individuals employ to create the impression that they are
intelligent and competent when environmental demands or constraints threaten
their abilities to do so.

Swift's maxim, on the other hand, was absolutely correct. Investigations
of both acute and long-term intoxication have reliably demonstrated that
alcohol consumption has a disruptive effect on intellectual functioning (Levine, Kramer, & Levine, 1975; Miller, Adesso, Fleming, Gino & Lauerman,

STEVEN BERGLAS. Department of Psychiatry, Harvard Medical School/McLean Hospital,
Boston, Massachusetts

1978). Furthermore, alcohol has a widespread and deserved reputation as a performance-inhibitor in realms other than intellectual functioning and is allegedly capable of precipitating a variety of socially undesirable behaviors (MacAndrew & Edgerton, 1969). Clinicians and laymen alike recognize, after Swift, "much drinking, little thinking . . . and probably little else reflective of competence."

The self-handicapping model of alcohol abuse (Berglas & Jones, 1978; Jones & Berglas, 1978) marries the insight of Sallust to that of Swift in order to account for the appeal of alcohol to a significant number of alcohol abusers (see also Berglas, 1985; in press). At the core of this conceptualization is the contention that alcohol's performance-inhibiting reputation can be exploited in social and evaluative interactions by individuals wishing to avoid the negative implications of failure and enhance the positive impact of success. Derived from social psychological principles of attribution (Jones et al., 1971) and impression management theories (Schlenker, 1980), the self-handicapping formulation details a tactic that can enable an individual to protect a favorable competence image by shaping and controlling the attributions drawn from his behavior. The self-handicapping strategist accomplishes this by consuming alcohol in advance of evaluations wherein performances reflective of underlying abilities are known to be disrupted by alcohol. As detailed below, the self-handicapper structures situations within which he chooses to perform by embracing an external causal agent that can serve to reduce his personal responsibility for performance. The self-handicapper's goal in choosing to perform with a self-imposed handicap is straightforward: To protect a positive self-image derived from previous success experiences. In the event of failures enacted under the influence of a handicap, the individual's personal competence is not challenged due to the a priori justification for failure provided by alcohol. In the event of unexpected successes, the self-handicapper's competency image receives a boost since his achievement occurred under less-than-favorable circumstances.

Since its introduction in 1978, the self-handicapping formulation has been replicated and refined (Kolditz & Arkin, 1982; Tucker, Vuchinich, & Sobell, 1981) and extended to areas of clinical psychiatry other than alcohol abuse (Berglas, 1985). Yet despite the fact that this formulation was originally intended to describe an instance of strategic self-presentation designed to protect a *positive* competency image (Baron & Byrne, 1981; Hollander, 1981; Worchel & Cooper, 1979), several authors have employed the term "self-handicapping" to describe tactics that may be initiated by failure (Weidner, 1980) or stem from feelings of *low* self-worth (McHugh, Beckman & Frieze, 1979). Applying the self-handicapping construct in this manner is, at a minimum, quite confusing.

Another source of potential misinterpretation and misapplication derives from the similarities which exist between the self-handicapping model of alcohol abuse and theories of alcoholism which take, as their point of departure, the popular notion that people drink in order to reduce tension (Cappell & Herman, 1972; Higgins, 1976; see also Cappell & Greeley, Chapter 2, this volume). Although the self-handicapping model attempts to restrict its application and predictions to a very specific subtype of alcohol abuser (Berglas, in press-b), its conceptual relatedness to traditional "tension reduction models" is significant enough to risk a blurring of the boundaries between the two perspectives.

As the self-handicapping formulation becomes more widely applied to investigations of actual alcohol consumption (e.g., see Tucker *et al.*, 1981) and the behavior patterns of alcoholics (Wright & Obitz, 1984), the need to understand the model's principles and behavioral implications becomes crucial if it is to retain any heuristic value in clinical contexts (Berglas, 1985). Since the original self-handicapping formulation (Jones & Berglas, 1978) is restricted in its applications to alcohol abusers with some significant history of success which is jeopardized by impending evaluations, it is not applicable to all clinical populations (Berglas, 1985; in press). Yet, if properly understood, a theory such as this with a limited focus and concern is of greater value to the researcher/clinician than one that suffers a loss of predictive power by attempting to account for too many diverse phenomena within a single framework. By retracing the development of the self-handicapping model of alcohol abuse and clarifying its principles and empirical support to date, the benefits of diagnostic, therapeutic, and preventative interventions employing this model should be enhanced materially.

### Theoretical Origins of the Self-Handicapping Formulation

The self-handicapping model of alcohol abuse derives from the premise that people use the principles of attribution theory (Kelley, 1971) in the service of self-image protection (Jones & Berglas, 1978). In a sense, the formulation describes one of several modes of impression management available to people intent upon creating a desired self-image (Schlenker, 1980). Yet the operations of self-handicapping strategies are unique among self-presentational techniques. Specifically, the self-handicapping formulation details the manner in which an individual can structure the contexts of his behavior so as to preserve and protect a favorable self-conception. To do this, the self-handicapper's tactics extend far beyond the verbal claims and disclosures that typify self-presentational behavior. Called "setting the stage for desired attributions" by some (Schlenker, 1980, p. 120), the self-handicapper's behavior is designed to initially lead observers of his actions to question what accounted for observed outcomes, and ultimately control the answers they derive. According to Jones and Berglas, "The self-handicapper . . . reaches out for impediments, exaggerates handicaps, embraces any factor reducing personal responsibility for mediocrity and enhancing personal responsibility for success . . . to shape the implications of performance feedback both in one's own eyes and in the eyes of others" (1978, p. 202).

Research on attributional processes (Heider, 1958; Kelley, 1971), and self-attributions where actors focus on their own behavior and its implications (Bem, 1972), addresses a two-part question: Why a person acted as he did, and why his action took on a particular form (Jones & Davis, 1965, p. 220). At a sharper level of focus, attribution theorists contend that both actors and observers endeavor to determine the extent to which a particular behavior or behavioral sequence is a function of environmental factors (e.g., social pressure, intense physical stimuli to which all people would respond, and so on) or factors inherent in the personal qualities of an actor (e.g., abilities, attitudes, and the like). As Heider (1958) noted, observers of behavior are motivated to determine the underlying causes of an event for a very simple reason: it increases their understanding of their world and renders it more predictable in the future. If, after observing a behavioral sequence, we can confidently derive a situational attribution—that is, determine that some force external to a particular actor accounted for the outcome—we are better able to predict the consequences of entering that context or situation wherein the behavior occurred at some future time. Specifically, we can assume that most everyone will behave as the observed actor did when his actions are determined to be attributable to situational dispositions. When observers derive a personal attribution—that is, conclude that aspects of the actor's unique personal qualities or dispositions accounted for a behavior or behavioral sequence—they are better able to predict how future interactions with this person will unfold. In a word, we know what to expect from him. In the case of self-attributions, when the actor and observer are the same person, the same principle still holds true: following a self-attribution we gain greater confidence in predicting what our own behavior should be like in the future.

Attribution theorists who built upon Heider's (1958) seminal work (Jones & Davis, 1965; Kelley, 1971) formulated an elaborate set of rules that specify how individuals systematically determine the underlying causes of observed behaviors. Jones and Davis's (1965) "correspondent inference theory," for example, focused on how observers account for behaviors in terms of the personal dispositions of actors by specifying the criteria that are used to judge the informational value ("information gain") provided by a sampling of that actor's behavior. One of the more informative principles contained in their analysis of attributional processes argues that to the extent that an actor's behavior deviates from that which would appear to be dictated by his role or contextual constraints placed upon him, observers can be confident that the behavior in question is a reflection of an underlying quality of that particular actor (Jones & Davis, 1965). Stated in other terms, we learn nothing about an individual's personal dispositions when he behaves in a manner identical to all others subjected to comparable situational forces. We learn nothing, for example, about a 15-year-old who declares that he likes Michael Jackson. If the same teenager declared that he likes Stravinsky, then our information gain would be great.

Kelley's (1971) refinement of attributional theorizing concerned the manner in which observers determine an underlying cause for observed behavioral events. Specifically, Kelley addressed himself to the potentially ambiguous situation wherein a behavioral outcome could be the result of a number of possible factors, or, in Kelley's words, "multiple plausible causes" (1971, p. 8). The consequences for an observer who is confronted with several plausible causes for a particular behavioral outcome he would like to understand is detailed in Kelley's "discounting principle" as follows:

> If [an observer] is aware of several plausible causes [for an event], he attributes the [event] less to any of them than if he is aware of only one as a plausible cause. In other words, he makes his attributions according to a discounting principle: the role of a given cause in producing a given [event] is discounted if other plausible causes are also present. (1971, p. 8)

The implications of the ambiguity created by situations where "multiple plausible causes" exist for a particular outcome will be examined further after noting Kelley's consideration of a "reverse" version of the discounting principle, called the "augmentation principle." While it is quite common to find situations in which there are several potential reasons why an event should have occurred, some situations contain obvious reasons why particular behavioral outcomes should not have occurred. Kelley describes the observer's analysis of behavioral outcomes that occur in the presence of "plausible inhibitory causes" as follows:

> If for a given [event], both a plausible inhibitory and a plausible facilitative cause are present, the role of the facilitative cause in producing the [event] will be judged greater than if it alone were present as a plausible cause for the [event]. The central idea here is that the facilitative cause must have been effective, and potently so, if the [event] occurred despite the opposing effect of the inhibitory cause. (1971, p. 12)

A final attributional principle with direct bearing upon the self-handi-capper's use of alcohol as an agent to protect his favorable competence image is the distinction between causality and responsibility. Simply stated, a person need not be held responsible for an outcome in spite of the fact that he or she was the cause of it. More specifically, an actor will only be held responsible for a behavior and its effects to the extent that he was capable of choosing alternative courses of action based upon an unencumbered assessment of their probable effects and was not subject to the influence of constraining forces either prior to or during his performance.

As Ryle (1949) and Heider (1958) noted, assessments of causality proceed from possible causes closest in time and space (proximal) to the event in question backward to more distant (distal) causes. Actors are presumed to be responsible for a behavioral outcome only if they are primary—most distal—in the "causal chain" that leads ultimately to the event. Any plausible causal factor that precedes an individual actor in a causal sequence leading to an event must be judged to assume at least part of the responsibility for the outcome. Unencumbered and acting without constraint, individuals caus-ing an outcome through their behavior will be held responsible for it.

The self-handicapping alcohol abuser, it is argued, is wise to these at-tributional principles and exploits them in order to preserve a positive com-petence image. Consider the following scenario:

> An individual receives much desired and valued accolades pertaining to his competence along a particular behavioral dimension (e.g., verbal or rea-soning abilities). At some point thereafter, he is called upon to once again manifest the ability which was previously praised. He is concerned and anxious regarding the upcoming performance, fearing failure and a loss of his favorable competency image. He consumes an excessive amount of al-cohol and enters the evaluation interaction obviously inebriated.

According to the self-handicapping model of alchol abuse (Berglas, 1985; Jones & Berglas, 1978), the hypothetical actor depicted above has succeeded in structuring himself a truly no-lose situation in terms of the competency image that can be derived following his performance enacted "under the influence." There exists, in the causal chain created by the self-handicapper, a salient impediment to successful performance muddying the attributional waters that will prevent observers from deriving informational gain from the self-handicapper's behaviors. Whatever outcome obtains may be attributable to multiple causes: the actor's ability *or* the performance-inhibiting influence of alcohol.

The self-handicapper is protected against the negative implications of a failed or substandard performance since the cause of the failure may plausibly be attributed to the effects of alcohol. As Kelley's (1971) discounting principle argues, the presence of alcohol as a plausible inhibitory cause for a behavioral outcome external to, and apart from, the actor's ability causes observers to discount the role played by the actor himself in bringing about the poor performance. If the sotted self-handicapper is successful, he has defied expectations of a substandard performance that would be drawn by observers who know the reputation that alcohol has as a performance inhibitor. According to Kelley's (1971) augmentation principle, the self-handicapper's underlying ability (a facilitative causal agent), should be presumed to be greater than would otherwise be the case had he performed without the presence of an inhibitory cause opposing his behavior.

At a minimum, the self-handicapper's alcohol abuse creates a sense of attributional ambiguity regarding the role of his competence in bringing about a particular outcome. While he is undoubtedly a causal agent, the *responsibility* for the quality of the outcome is potentially attributable to a plausible inhibitory causal agent—alcohol. And, as will be discussed at length below, for as long as a self-handicapper is judged to be *unaddicted*—that is, not physically dependent upon alcohol—he can protect his competence image prior to entering threatening evaluative interactions by exploiting alcohol's reputation.

## The Presumed Utility of Self-Handicapping Alcohol Abuse beyond "Setting the Stage for Desired Attributions"

It has been argued that self-handicapping alcohol abuse can serve to control the implications of performance feedback by structuring the context of evaluative interactions in a manner which will protect previously accrued self-esteem gains. Although this formulation maintains that the impetus for engaging in self-handicapping alcohol abuse "lies in the exaggerated importance of one's own private conception of self-competence and the need to protect that conception" (Jones & Berglas, 1978, p. 202), the effect of alcohol consumption for the self-handicapper appears to be quite independent of alcohol's pharmacologic effects on the "self." It is not apparent what unique effects, if any, self-handicapping alcohol abuse has upon an individual's self-system apart from providing transient competence-image protection.

Since it is apparent that self-handicapping's self-protective benefits may be derived by strategists who merely present the *appearance* of being "under the influence" of alcohol, that is, not actually debilitated by alcohol's physiologic effects, questions arise as to what target person or persons the self-handicapper has in mind in advance of his tactical drinking behavior. More specifically, confusion exists about the actual intent of self-handicapping alcohol abuse: Whether it serves only to save an individual from having to alter his self-conception, control the judgements made by observers, or provide the self-handicapper with a viable excuse or explanation for potential failure should one be needed at some future point in time.

Clinical investigations of self-handicappers (Berglas, in press) suggest that for those individuals prone to self-handicap, this particular mode of self-protective behavior serves numerous functions including those mentioned above. Empirical investigations of self-handicapping drug-choice behavior in university psychology department laboratories (Berglas & Jones, 1978; Kolditz & Arkin, 1982) do little to resolve this concern. One set of studies (Berglas & Jones, 1978) concludes that self-handicapping serves a self-protective function, while the other (Kolditz & Arkin, 1982) favors an impression-management interpretation. What will probably emerge once subgroups of self-handicappers are identified within alcoholic and other psychiatric populations is the recognition that the attributional intent of a self-handicapper may be self-directed, other-directed, or both. The critical concern is that self-handicappers maintain an awareness of how judgments of competency become clouded following alcohol consumption, and exploit this awareness when their competency image is threatened by impending evaluations.

As noted above, self-handicapping alcohol abuse is one among a multitude of techniques available to individuals intent upon protecting their self-esteem (Jones & Pittman, 1982). Moreover, alcohol abuse is but one subset of a variety of strategic behaviors capable of effecting self-handicapping strategies. Self-handicappers can protect themselves in two ways: By either finding or creating impediments that will inhibit successful performance, or by withdrawing their effort, thereby inviting probable failure (see Berglas, 1985 for a detailed discussion of the range of self-handicapping disorders).

### The Effects of Self-Handicapping Alcohol Abuse upon Mood

Although it has been argued above that self-handicapping alcohol abuse is one among many tactics available for self-image protection, this should in no way minimize self-handicapping's claim to a unique status within the realm of self-defending maneuvers. Specifically, self-handicapping alcohol abuse is not equivalent to a post hoc rationalization or excuse for poor performance, nor is it a mechanism for denying negative outcomes which have occurred (Berglas, 1985). As an a priori self-protective strategy, self-handicapping is assumed to have both a pragmatic value for esteem-maintenance concerns as well as an important immediate impact upon the mood of the self-handicapper occurring *in advance* of evaluative interactions. And, as noted in the original self-handicapping formulation (Jones & Berglas, 1978), self-handicappers can achieve self-image protection in a variety of ways employing numerous self-handicapping "agents" other than alcohol:

> The high school senior who gets but two hours of sleep before taking his SAT exams may be a self-handicapper. The ingratiator who avoids disclosing his true preferences or opinions protects himself from the ultimate implications of rejection as a person. Even if he gets rejected, this isn't so bad if he was "just trying to be nice," if he held his true self in reserve. . . . Self-handicappers are legion in the sports world, from the tennis player who externalizes a bad shot by adjusting his racket strings, to the avid golfer who systematically avoids taking lessons or even practicing on the driving range. (1978, p. 201)

Although insufficient sleep, ingratiation, poor equipment and lack of practice are adequate agents for enacting self-protection self-handicapping behavior, they all lack alcohol's unique capacity to assume responsibility for impaired performance without implicating the ability of an unaddicted imbiber. The reason for this, quite simply, is the commonly held assumption that alcohol has a uniform impact and effect upon anyone who consumes it. While some people function quite well with minimal rest and can hit a tennis ball with a poor racket or a golf ball with no lessons, it is assumed that no one can perform "up to par" while drunk. Thus, the self-handicapping alcohol abuser is in the enviable position of having a rather foolproof justification for substandard performances: Transient alcohol intoxication that would hamper anyone. Moreover, the effects of alcohol consumption among the unaddicted acts independently of the "wishes" of those who consume it. The assumption here is that golfers are free to choose to take a lesson or not, thereby making "lack of practice" a second-rate self-handicapping strategy. The "social drinker" is provided with a resilient self-handicapping strategy following excessive alcohol consumption since he can plausibly argue that he did not anticipate the extent of debilitation he was about to suffer following consumption of all the alcohol he did; once drunk, however, he was incapable of altering his ability to manifest his competence.

In order to understand the mood-altering effects of self-handicapping strategies it is important to recall the presumed impetus of this tactical behavior: The exaggerated importance of one's own conception of self-competence. When the outcome of performances that have direct bearing on an individual's competence image become excessively important, the anxiety aroused by this situation is both unpleasant and typically self-defeating (Spence & Spence, 1966). Specifically, it is widely acknowledged that the impact of motivation and arousal on cognitive and motoric performance tasks typically follows the Yerkes–Dodson law: As arousal increases above a discernible "optimum" level necessary to sustain goal-directed behaviors, responses irrelevant to efficient task execution become energized and compete with appropriate task execution (Malmo, 1957; Paul & Bernstein, 1973). The so-called "inverted-U" relationship between anxiety and behavioral efficiency has direct bearing on the self-handicapper's affective state and actual performance capabilities prior to entering evaluative interactions. It is assumed that owing to his excessive concern with the outcome of his evaluation, the self-handicapper's anxiety level will be elevated to a point where it *will* actually hamper his performance; that is, unless he consumes alcohol (Berglas, 1977).

In a manner identical to that by which observers of a self-handicapper's performance enacted "under the influence" make allowances for the impact of alcohol upon skilled behaviors, the self-handicapper as self-observer also analyzes the implications of being impaired prior to entering evaluative settings. Recognizing that his capacity to manifest abilities has been reduced, and aware that there exists a plausible explanation for potential failure which will not implicate his abilities directly, it is assumed that the self-handicapper will actually experience less anxiety when he enters evaluative interactions than would be the case if he were sober (Berglas, 1977). Morever, if following the consumption of performance-inhibiting alcohol the self-handicapper's anxiety and evaluation apprehension are actually allayed, the paradoxical possibility of improved performance following intoxication presents itself. Specifically, following the Yerkes–Dodson inverted-U formulation, the individual who is overinvested (aroused) in the outcome of a performance and believes that his failure will be attributed to the actions of an agent external to himself would be predicted to experience a reduction in arousal to a more optimum level and, despite being "under the influence," would outperform comparable aroused individuals who have not elected to self-handicap (Berglas, 1977).

To some, the previous description of paradoxical performance effects predicted following self-handicapping alcohol abuse may be reminiscent of the "negative placebo effect" (Storms & Nisbett, 1970). A negative placebo effect is so-called because it represents the reverse of the direct suggestion placebo effect: The patient feels even worse when the pill that was supposed to make him feel better leaves his symptoms unchanged (Snyder, Schulz, & Jones, 1974). Thus, both the self-handicapping and negative placebo effects are similar in that they involve consequences that reverse alleged effects of drugs and/or placebos. However, careful consideration of the psychological processes presumed to be operating in the negative placebo effect suggests that the two effects may involve rather different processes.

A negative placebo effect is presumed to obtain when a drug with an alleged effect on an individual's subjective state (affective or somatic) fails to act in the suggested manner. The result is that the individual who has ingested the placebo contrasts his unaffected internal state with the expected state "promised" by the reputation of the drug. The consequence of this analysis is that there is an augmentation of the individual's subjective state, in much the same manner as attributional inferences are augmented (Kelley, 1971). Thus, if an anxious person ingests an alleged anxiety-reducing placebo and does not experience relief in spite of the actions of the pill (a plausible inhibitory agent), he is led to infer that he is now, and was, prior to ingesting the pill, experiencing a great deal of anxiety.

On the other hand, the facilitative actions of self-handicapping agents are presumed to obtain when the suggestion of impaired performance relieves an individual's state of performance anxiety or evaluation apprehension by freeing him from the responsibility for failure. In essence, alcohol consumption in the service of self-image protection is initially anxiolytic and then self-protective in its operation. Figure 9.1 illustrates the psychological processes presumed operative in the action of self-handicapping alcohol abuse and negative placebo effects.

## Self-Handicapping and Expectancy Effects

Predictions of how self-handicapping alcohol abuse will affect the performance of individuals who are excessively invested in the outcome of evaluative interactions share many assumptions with other investigations of the role that expectations play in determining a drinker's response to alcohol consumption (see Maisto, Conners, & Sachs, 1981; Marlatt & Rohsenow, 1980; Wilson, 1978 for reviews). Simply stated, numerous methodologically sophisticated research studies have demonstrated that the consumption of alcohol alone is *not* a determinant of many behaviors (e.g., aggressive or sexual behavior) previously thought (Chafetz & Demone, 1962; Kessel & Walton, 1966) to be "released" or "disinhibited" by the physiological effects of alcohol upon the nervous system (Marlatt & Rohsenow, 1980). Rather, it is the belief on the part of individuals—often experimentally manipulated—that they have consumed alcohol, that exerts a "causal" influence over their behavior regardless of the actual content of their drinks. Specifically, for many behaviors (e.g., sexual arousal), the belief that one has consumed alcohol despite not having done so leads to a greater manifestation of the behavior (e.g., sexual arousal in response to a stimulus film) than is seen after actually consuming alcohol under conditions where the cognitive set is that only tonic water is being consumed (see Wilson, 1978 for details).

In commenting on this body of literature, Marlatt and Rohsenow (1980) acount for the phenomenon of "expectancy effects" in a manner comparable to the self-handicapping formulation. They argue, following the reasoning of MacAndrew and Edgerton (1969), that alcohol consumption may serve as a cue or discriminative stimulus for the expression of sexual behavior in part

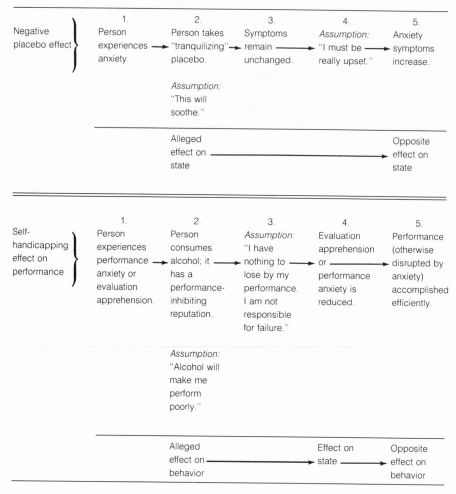

FIGURE 9.1. Psychological processes presumed to operate in the action of self-handicapping alcohol abuse and negative placebo effects.

because "we have come to expect that people will sometimes do things under the influence of alcohol that they would never otherwise do. . . . Later, whatever the actual outcome, the drinker can absolve himself of responsibility for his actions claiming that, 'It wasn't my fault—I was drunk at the time.'" (Marlatt & Rohsenow, 1980, p. 190). The conclusion drawn by Marlatt and Rohsenow (1980) is that the reinforcement for disinhibited or impaired social behavior under the influence of alcohol is the provision to people who drink excessively of temporary immunity for responsibility for their behavior.

Although the Marlatt and Rohsenow (1980) assessment of expectancy effects is, for the most part, entirely compatible with the hypothesis advanced by the self-handicapping formulation (Berglas, 1985; Jones & Berglas, 1978), the two perspectives part company at one crucial juncture. Marlatt and Rohsenow maintain that only certain classes of behaviors will be affected by expectancy effects and reinforced by temporary immunity from responsibility. This group is said to be characterized by behaviors that usually provide immediate gratification followed by delayed social disapproval; certain antisocial behaviors such as rape which combines both aggressive and sexual components in the assaultive act could serve as examples. Marlatt and Rohsenow speculate, "Perhaps alcohol is consumed partly under the belief that it will act as a disinhibitor (to fortify courage, and so on), and partly because it serves as an explanation or excuse for the act" (1980, p. 190).

The logic of this argument concerning which behaviors are effected by expectancy effects continues as follows: "In contrast, memory, motor skills and cognitive abilities are less likely to be performed under similar conditions. Whereas a man who drinks may 'want' to act out his aggression or sexual drives, he probably does not 'want' to impair his cognitive or motor abilities to the same extent," (Marlatt & Rohsenow, 1980, pp. 190–191). The self-handicapping model of alcohol abuse appears to present a limiting condition for Marlatt and Rohsenow's (1980) assertions. Specifically, it describes a circumstance wherein people would prefer to have their cognitive and motor abilities impaired if such transient performance breakdowns could serve to protect dispositional attributions of competence formed in the past. The self-handicapper, it is argued, is willing to temporarily tolerate the label "drunk," and endure impaired cognitive functioning in order to preserve his competency image for future interactions. If successful, that is, if the self-handicapper is confident that his self-protective strategy will be effective, it is assumed that consuming alcohol in the service of self-image protection may actually reduce the self-handicapper's anxiety (see Figure 9.1) enough to counteract the established performance-inhibiting effects of alcohol (Connors & Maisto, 1980; Levine et al., 1975; Miller et al., 1978).

Presumably, empirical support for either the Marlatt and Rohsenow (1980) or self-handicapping (Berglas, 1985) perspectives will be dependent upon the confidence that an individual has in his ability to manifest competency in an upcoming evaluative interaction prior to deciding whether or not to consume alcohol (see also Tucker et al., 1981). The self-handicapping perspective argues, and has demonstrated (Berglas & Jones, 1978; Tucker et al., 1981), that individuals who have achieved a favorable but *fragile* competency image will consume performance-inhibiting drugs or alcohol prior to evaluations that threaten to jeopardize self-esteem gains. This same body of research has also demonstrated, however, that when individuals achieve a favorable competency image under conditions where they are *highly confident* of the factors contributing to their esteem gains, they do not elect to protect themselves by consuming performance inhibitors, a finding that supports the reasoning of Marlatt and Rohsenow (1980). Thus, by gaining a more complete understanding of the confidence that individuals have in their competencies in advance of evaluative interactions, it should be possible to predict the likelihood of their adopting patterns of self-handicapping alcohol abuse.

From the preceding discussion it should now be clear that neither the competency-image protection nor anxiety reduction afforded by self-handicapping alcohol abuse depends, in any apparent manner, upon the pharmacologic effects of alcohol. In fact, an individual need not actually be drunk to enact a self-handicapping strategy; obvious excessive consumption will suffice. What matters most is the *timing* of alcohol consumption-behavior both in terms of contiguity to evaluate interactions and in terms of regularity across time. Obviously, self-handicapping alcohol abuse must occur immediately prior to or in the midst of evaluative interactions for the effects of alcohol to be seen as inhibiting effective performance. Beyond this fact, the most important aspect of the timing of self-handicapping alcohol consumption is that it must appear to be discretionary; that is, not a function of physiologic dependence upon alcohol (Berglas, 1985; in press). Diagnostically, the self-handicapper's alcohol consumption behavior would qualify as substance *abuse* (involving pathologic use causing impairment in social or occupational functioning over a specified time-frame), and not meet criteria established for substance *dependence* (manifesting physiologic dependence evidenced by either tolerance or withdrawal) (American Psychiatric Association, 1980, pp. 163, 165).

This necessary restriction of the self-handicapping formulation to the behavior of alcohol *abusers* derives from the same attributional principles that enable a self-handicapper to exploit the performance-inhibiting reputation of alcohol in self-protective strategies. Specifically, it is argued that self-handicapping alcohol abuse cannot be seen as dispositional due to the fact that dispositional attributions serve to both predict the behavior of individuals across time and assume a causal role in observer's accounts of an actor's behavior (Heider, 1958; Peters, 1958).

One of the primary reasons why self-handicapping alcohol abuse can protect an individual's conception of himself as being a competent, intelligent person, is that since the days when Sallust made his observations about "mental excellence," intellectual competency has been considered to be dispositional; consistent across time and modality in its manifestation (Kelley, 1967). Once observers judge an individual to be intelligent at a particular point in time, they expect that at future observation points his intelligence will not have changed (Heider, 1958). That is, unless a plausible external inhibitory cause exerted a transient influence that impeded the individual's manifestation of intelligence. This is why a self-handicapper's substandard performance enacted following alcohol consumption can be excused: it is assumed that the time-limited effects of alcohol blocked the manifestation of the individual's underlying dispositional competence that had been demonstrated in a previous evaluative interaction.

Should a self-handicapper consistently appear for enough different evaluations in an inebriated state and fail to manifest his competence for a protracted period of time, what was previously judged to be intermittent alcohol abuse would come to assume the permanence of a disposition; observers would label the individual "an alcoholic." Rather than excusing poor performances, the drinking behavior of an individual judged to be dispositionally reliant upon alcohol carries with it two additional features that preclude exploiting alcohol in the service of self-image protection: (1) there is an intercorrelated matrix of traits with negative valences associated with the unfavorable disposition of "alcoholic,"and (2) the disposition "alcoholic" is now judged to be permanent and predictive. Where mental excellence was once expected, disinhibited behavior, poor motor coordination, blackouts, and cirrhosis are now anticipated.

Cronbach (1955) demonstrated the phenomenon of implicit personality theories which, simply stated, are the intuitive judgments people hold regarding how dispositions and attributes cluster within individuals. Someone who is thought to be intelligent, a positive attribute, is likely to be seen as rich and attractive as well. Since "alcoholic" is a negatively toned attribute, self-handicapping strategies cannot be enacted by a person whose drinking behavior would warrant such an attribution. This is due to the likelihood that once he was so labeled he would have difficulty retaining other components of a favorable self-image. While such reasoning is false both in terms of attributional principles (Jones & Nisbett, 1971) and psychiatric assessments of alcoholics (Marlatt, 1983), it is quite powerful and pervasive enough (Mischel, 1968, 1973) to preclude employing an attribute such as "alcoholic" in strategic behavior designed to protect one's competence-image (see Berglas, 1985, for a detailed discussion of this issue).

Although it is difficult to establish empirically how long self-handicappers can engage in patterns of abusive alcohol consumption before being judged "alcoholic," one thing is clear: To retain the positive competency image they are trying to protect, self-handicapping alcohol abusers must periodically manifest competence. Self-handicappers are not losers who drink to improve an undesirable self-conception as some have argued alcoholics are wont to do (e.g., Kinsey, 1966; Vanderpool, 1969). They abuse alcohol in response to excessive evaluation apprehension that is derived from a desire to preserve a favorable but fragile competency image.

## The Impetus to Self-Handicap: Burdensome Expectations and Noncontingent Success

The most commonly held belief about alcohol consumption is that it is motivated by a drinker's desire to alter his mood or emotions (see Freed, 1978; Russell & Mehrabian, 1975 for reviews). Regardless of the fact that following alcohol consumption drinkers commonly report feeling dysphoric (Tamerin, Weiner, & Mendelson, 1970) and manifest, as well as report, more anxiety than prior to drinking (McNamee, Mello, & Mendelson, 1968), abusive alchohol consumption is still typically initiated and maintained by the assumption that it will improve the way the drinker feels. The self-handicapping model of alcohol abuse is consistent with this viewpoint. It posits that abusive drinking is initiated in response to anticipated threats to a favorable competency image, and is sustained by the anxiety reduction and competency-image protection provided by alcohol's performance-inhibiting reputation which can reduce personal responsibility for poor performance and enhance personal responsibility for success.

To better understand the individual who becomes a career self-handicapper (Berglas, 1985), so that prevention programs and therapeutic interventions can be tailored to this alcohol-abusing subtype's needs (Berglas, in press), the impetus to engage in self-handicapping alcohol abuse must be fully understood. While it is recognized that self-handicappers come to invest a disproportionate amount of energy anticipating the outcome of evaluative interactions, the reason why this should be the case has yet to be addressed. More to the point, we must question why evaluative interactions threaten the competency image of self-handicappers and why their self-attributions of competence do not have the resilience and predictive strength that dispositional attributions typically possess (Heider, 1958).

In the original statement of the self-handicapping formulation, Jones and Berglas (1978) argued that something about the learning history of self-handicappers blocked them from determining that their competency-image was entrenched enough to withstand repeated assessments. In an investigation aimed at evaluating this hypothesis, Berglas and Jones (1978) demonstrated that self-handicapping strategies are initiated by noncontingent reinforcement histories.

Noncontingent success refers to positive outcomes not subject to personal control (Abramson, Seligman, & Teasdale, 1978). In terms of the attributional principles discussed above, a lack of contingency between a performer's behavior and an outcome derives when there exists multiple plausible facilitative causal factors that can account for the outcome, thereby discounting the causal significance of any single factor (Kelley, 1971). In everyday terms, the experience of noncontingent success arises when desired outcomes are attributable to extraneous factors such as luck, beauty, personally irrelevant past successes, or the ascribed status of being a member of the "right" family or group. Where these plausible facilitative causal factors exist in conjunction with an actor's instrumental behavior, successes dependent upon a judge's or evaluator's assessments may be clouded with external issues. The result of this state of affairs is that the actor who is successful in the midst of multiple facilitative causal factors must question whether it was who he was, or what he did, that caused success. The rules governing receipt of rewards are unclear to the individual receiving noncontingent success (Abramson *et al.*, 1978; Seligman, 1975).

Conceptually, the lack of contingency referred to is between the actor's subjective uncertainty concerning his control over instrumental behaviors in a given setting and the impression of control conveyed to others by the actor's successful performance outcome. A crucial consequence of experiencing non-contingent success is that the recipient may come to fear that a controlling, effective performance cannot be repeated at will because the degree of control was misjudged in the first place, or that extraneous factors were primarily responsible for prior successes. Consequently, the expectations derived from success experiences are often psychologically "burdensome" in that the only way to avoid the subjective failure of future mediocre performances is to sustain top-level outputs (Berglas, 1985).

It has been argued elsewhere (Berglas, 1985) that self-handicappers can be considered to be *victims* of evaluators who reward them beyond their clearly demonstrated abilities. It is assumed that self-handicappers desire positive feedback from success and want to incorporate it within their self-image. Why else would self-protective strategies following success be necessary? The problem, as noted before, is that competencies are presumed to be the result of dispositions, not transient situational factors such as an evaluator's bias. The actor who internalizes the implications of a noncontingent success experience is thus burdened by the obligation to perform in line with this dispositional attribution; consistently (competent) across time and modality (Kelley, 1967).

Burdensome expectations are typically, although not always, derived ex post facto in evaluative interactions. Yet performance anxiety and evaluation apprehension sufficient to motivate self-handicapping strategies can result from the urgings of others who are invested in a target person's success, provided that these inducements are attributable to external causal loci such as pedigree. Furthermore, "the burden of expectations" is often derived from assertions that an individual will or should be successful in the execution of a particular role or task, if the consequences of successful performance threaten to expose that individual to greater and less "controllable" demands in the future. Considering the fact that some people are rewarded, given social privileges, and expected to perform in a highly competent fashion solely on the basis of who their parents are (e.g., sons of statemen or athletes), it is understandable why so many children of "noble birth" fail to derive an entrenched sense of positive self-regard that would render them resistant to burdensome expectations (Berglas, 1985; in press) and suffer a variety of negative life-styles.

The range of situations that can impose burdensome expectations is virtually limitless. Although these situations all must contain some evaluative component that will convey information pertaining to an individual's competence along a particular dimension, assessments of ability are derived from interactions ranging from tests to cocktail parties. Even discussions with significant others can serve to impose burdensome expectations if the content of these discussions has bearing on an ability dimension that is relevant or important to an individual.

Regardless of the context in which burdensome expectations are imposed, it is critical to remember that they are actually stressful for individuals excessively invested in their performance outcome (Folkman, Schaefer, & Lazarus, 1979; Lazarus, 1981). An individual's involvement in the outcome of a social interaction and his fear that he cannot willingly manifest the competency demanded of him by that situation, result in the affective components of stress (e.g., anxiety and evaluation apprehension) which serve as an impetus to self-handicapping strategies. Although alcohol abuse in the service of self-image protection is not an ideal coping strategy, it is somewhat adaptive when viewed from the perspective of the self-handicapper who is more invested in sustaining an image of competence than in manifesting competence (Kolditz & Arkin, 1982).

### The Role of Noncontingent Success in Self-Handicapping Behavior

Berglas and Jones (1978) conducted two experiments designed to test the hypothesis that individuals would be motivated to subject themselves to the performance-inhibiting effects of drugs such as alcohol when their concerns about protecting a favorable but tenuous competence image were high. The paradigm employed in these experiments involved recruiting subjects for an alleged investigation of the effects of two drugs on intellectual performance, and leading them to expect that they would take two parallel forms of a very challenging intelligence test separated by the ingestion of one of two drugs being evaluated. Subjects were informed that their choice of drug would be between one that allegedly facilitated intellectual performance, and one, modeled after the effects of alcohol, that purportedly exerted a disruptive influence on performance. Through the test/retest protocol, an empirical assessment of the drug's actual effects on intellectual performance would be possible.

To determine if the quality of success experienced by subjects influenced their motivation to self-handicap, conditions of contingent and noncontingent success were established. While all test questions were of the same type [comparable to Scholastic Aptitude Test (SAT) verbal aptitude and analogy questions], one test battery was composed of 80% insoluble questions and 20% soluble, while the other battery was 80% soluble and 20% insoluble. An experimental assistant who administered the intelligence testing gave subjects success feedback following their problem solving attempts regardless of which test battery they received. Success feedback was contingent upon performance only for those subjects receiving the predominantly soluble battery; subjects who were administered test batteries with 80% insoluble problems received noncontingent success. A second experiment reported by Berglas and Jones (1978) added a condition in which subjects received no feedback of any sort following exposure to the intelligence test in order to provide a control condition to assess the effects of mere exposure to the two levels of test solubility.

Drug choice was made immediately following the success feedback manipulation, prior to the promised (actually bogus) posttest. Subject's selection of either the facilitative or the disruptive drug, in anticipation of a reassessment of the ability for which they had just received praise, served as the main dependent measure of their tendency to self-handicap. Subjects' actual confidence in their ability to perform test questions during the pretest—supposedly an indication of how confident they would be of their abilities on a posttest employing comparable questions—was obtained from manipulation checks collected during the posttest.

In both Berglas and Jones (1978) investigations, as well as in two other experimental studies employing an essentially identical paradigm (Kolditz & Arkin, 1982; Tucker et al., 1981), it was revealed that subjects receiving contingent success feedback were more confident in their ability to perform test questions (and, appropriately, felt these questions were less difficult) than subjects receiving noncontingent success. In the Berglas and Jones (1978) studies, subjects receiving soluble questions were overall about 65% certain of the accuracy of their responses to test questions; while subjects receiving insoluble problems reported confidence estimates of only 51%—essentially guessing. Extrapolating from these findings it can be argued that subjects receiving noncontingent success were unaware of how they managed to achieve success and must certainly have doubted their capacity to readily repeat their successful performance. Given their state of subjective uncertainty and ambiguity concerning the factors accounting for their favorable competency image, it is easy to understand why this sense of self-regard would be easily jeopardized by an impending evaluation.

The Berglas and Jones (1978) studies identified the causal role that noncontingent reinforcement and concern about protecting one's competency image play in the initiation of self-handicapping strategies. In line with their predictions, it was found that more than 60% of the males who received noncontingent success feedback elected to receive the performance-inhibiting (alcohol analog) drug, while those males who received contingent success feedback selected this drug less than 20% of the time.

Females did not show a differential pattern of response to either type of success feedback. Indeed, in no study published to date has there been any demonstration of females manifesting the slightest tendency to engage in self-handicapping behavior. Nevertheless, the results of the Berglas and Jones (1978) investigations were conclusive in demonstrating that conditions of contingent success—where subject's confidence about the causes of performance outcomes were high—did *not* reliably motivate subjects to select performance-inhibiting drugs like alcohol for self-protective or any other reasons.

Two experiments conducted by Tucker *et al.* (1981) have replicated and refined the central finding of the Berglas and Jones (1978) investigations. Tucker *et al.* (1981) demonstrated that self-handicapping will occur only when subjects do not have viable performance-enhancing options available to them prior to the pretest. Specifically, these investigations demonstrated, in a study that actually provided subjects with access to an alcoholic beverage, that following noncontingent success and prior to a promised posttest, subjects would study an instructional manual designed to improve posttest performance rather than consume alcohol when both options were presented simultaneously. However, when there was no possibility for subjects to study so as to protect their self-conceptions with a viable performance-enhancing strategy in anticipation of a threatening posttest, those who received noncontingent success consumed significantly greater amounts of alcohol than contingent success subjects. Tucker *et al.* conclude that their data suggest "that seemingly successful persons, who lack obvious financial or interpersonal problems, may be at risk for alcohol problems if they perceive that past successes were due to nonability factors and if they feel that adaptive achievement-oriented strategies to avoid failure are exhausted or inaccessible" (1981, p. 229).

### Self-Handicapping in Response to Burdensome Expectations Generated Outside Intellectual Performance Settings

The preceding discussion and empirical findings published in support of self-handicapping theory (e.g., Berglas & Jones, 1978; Tucker *et al.*, 1981) have focused almost exclusively upon burdensome expectations relating to preserving an image of intellectual competence. Clearly, a wide range of competency attributions other than those pertaining to intellectual skills can be protected by self-handicapping alcohol abuse as documented by clinical studies (see Berglas, in press) and abundant anecdotal evidence.

Although Shakespeare (in *Macbeth*) was not the first to note the phenomenon, he is certainly the most articulate commentator to report the fact that "Drink provokes the desire, but it takes away the performance." Many would-be Casanovas, intent upon, but anxious about, seducing and satisfying a women, report an awareness of the self-protective advantages afforded by consuming excessive quantities of alcohol in advance of the courtship ritual. In an interview study of anxious male alcoholics, 18% of whom met criteria established for a "diagnosis" of self-handicapping alcohol abuse (Berglas, in press), the most commonly reported context for the initiation of self-handicapping alcohol consumption outside of the workplace was the dating bar or the bedroom. It was apparent that these men were aware of the fact that alcohol abuse in the service of "sexual self-handicapping" involved exploiting one reputation in the service of preserving another. These self-handicappers understood that a man who is rendered impotent by excessive "drink," as Shakespeare observed, is only performing as all men "under the influence" would: They'd have the desire, but their "performance" would be taken away . . . presumably, as common knowledge has it, by alcohol.

Here we find an instance wherein alcohol's reputation as a performance inhibitor extends beyond the intellectual realm and, with no loss of efficacy, protects an individual's competency image. With the effects of alcohol serving as an a priori justification for a failure to perform sexually, one particular type of competency image—sexual, manly, or macho—remains intact. In fact, this particular mode of self-handicapping, intended to preserve one's heterosexual reputation, can be initiated well before the sexual strategist enters the bedroom. In countless contexts wherein the display of social skills (charm, wit, charisma, and so on) are necessary, and the ineptitude and/or lack of *savoir-faire* known to derive as a consequence of inebriation can serve as a self-protective explanation for a failure to perform in line with expectations, self-handicapping alcohol abuse is common. The male who is extremely anxious about his ability to perform in bed may elect to self-handicap well in advance of potential amorous involvements by never letting a women relate to him. The drunken boor who is ignored by all eligible females at a party will suffer the torment of social rejection and solitude that he can attribute to alcohol, but will also experience a great deal of psychological relief from being left alone *if* he entered the party with an a priori concern regarding his capacity to perform in bed.

Thus in social activities as in intellectual settings, the self-handicapping alcohol abuser sets himself up to experience the disruptive effects of alcohol consumption with the knowledge that the immediate aversive consequences are far outweighed by the long-term protection afforded his competency-image. Following the arguments raised above regarding the paradoxical possibility of improved performance following self-handicapping alcohol abuse (see Figure 9.1), it is conceivable that socially anxious individuals may also actually succeed as a function of their suffering. Under the influence of alcohol they might become disinhibited and thus more charming than they ever were as tense and inhibited men. Were such a scenario to occur—the individual who drinks in order to self-handicap succeeds remarkably—improved performance would doubtless reinforce drinking behavior which, in turn, would strengthen the motivation to drink; that is, in cases where an individual who was socially anxious and shy had *no* concerns regarding his capacity to perform sexually. It is doubtful, however, that this would occur among men who initiated self-handicapping strategies as a function of *sexual* performance anxiety. Owing to the fact that chronic excessive alcohol consumption does lead to sexual dysfunction, these men, while possibly successful in the short run, would ultimately fall short of their intended goals. What is abundantly clear in all cases is the fact that the range of settings and contexts wherein self-handicapping alcohol abuse will prove to be reinforcing extends far beyond those evaluated to date in experimental investigations.

### Why Don't Women Self-Handicap?

Considering the regularity with which self-handicapping effects have been demonstrated in populations of male subjects (e.g., Berglas & Jones, 1978; Kolditz & Arkin, 1982; Tucker *et al.*, 1981), this is not a trivial question. In fact, finding an answer to this question will both accelerate and help structure alcohol abuse prevention programs for subtypes of alcohol abusers whose maladaptive drinking derives entirely or in part from expectations about the effects of alcohol on mood, social interaction, or self-esteem (Marlatt & Rohsenow, 1980).

Before attempting to answer this question it is instructive to consider that many demonstrated "effects" derived from alcohol consumption either do not hold (Berglas & Jones, 1978) or are actually reversed (Wilson & Lawson, 1978) when findings obtained using male subjects are tested in virtually identical experimental paradigms employing females (Wilson & Lawson, 1976). In the case of Wilson and Lawson, their study of the effects of alcohol administration and expectancy on sexual arousal in males demonstrated that subjects who believed they had consumed alcohol, regardless of the drink's content, showed the greatest levels of arousal in response to erotic films (Wilson & Lawson, 1976). However female subjects participating in this balanced placebo design showed a significantly *reduced* level of sexual arousal in response to an erotic film after consuming alcohol regardless of whether they believed that their drinks contained alcohol or not (Wilson & Lawson, 1978).

While an explanation for the "reversed" outcomes observed by Wilson and Lawson (1976, 1978) can only be obtained through further experimentation, Marlatt and Rohsenow offer an insightful commentary on these investigations that has direct bearing on the self-handicapping formulation as it applies to women:

> At least for the male subjects, the reported expectancy findings are in line with contemporary cultural beliefs and stereotypes about the effects of alcohol: that alcohol will serve to increase aggressive behavior and sexual arousal, while at the same time reducing tension or anxiety. The variable findings obtained with females may reflect the ambivalent attitudes that society has adopted about women who drink and the effects of alcohol upon their behavior. Although society seems to accept the fact that drinking is an acceptable stimulus for "masculine" behaviors (e.g., aggressive and sexual acting out), it is far more critical about acceptable reasons for women to drink. (1980, p. 185)

The applicability of this insightful argument to the question of why women won't self-handicap should be obvious. If society has ambivalent attitudes toward women who drink to excess and is thus likely to not "excuse" poor performance due to alcohol consumption by women, the strategic possibilities of self-handicapping alcohol abuse are denied females! Following the arguments of Marlett and Rohsenow (1980) and a wealth of anecdotal reports, it appears that women who drink—in performance settings and elsewhere—are, a priori, ascribed a deviant label with attendant negatively toned internal dispositional attributions. In exactly the same manner in which the label "alcoholic" denies the recipient any oppotunity to self-handicap via alcohol consumption, women who actively consume alcohol are ascribed a cluster of attributions all of which preclude preserving a favorable competency image.

The preceding sociocultural explanation of why empirical investigations of self-handicapping alcohol abuse have yet to demonstrate that women will drink to protect their self-esteem does not intend to imply that women won't someday engage in this unique mode of strategic behavior. Everyday social interaction reveals that women will regularly self-handicap when agents other than alcohol [e.g., premenstrual syndrome (PMS), psychosocial stressors] are available and exploitable. Morever, as society becomes more tolerant of women assuming roles and behavior patterns previously restricted to men—including excessive alcohol consumption—it is reasonable to assume that women will become more familiar with drinking and increase the quantity and frequency of their consumption in direct proportion to the lifting of social stigmas. As women become more experienced with the effects of alcohol, their awareness of exploiting its reputation in the service of self-image protection should be comparably heightened. Were sex role barriers to continue to fall, it is likely that the Berglas and Jones (1978) studies replicated in 1998 would show comparable results for males and females. If the preceding reasoning is accurate, then alcohol abuse prevention programs must keep pace by both informing potential abusers of the role of expectancy effects in precipitating the untoward effects of alcohol consumption, and training people in methods of responsible drinking capable of preempting the effects of alcohol derived solely from cognitive expectations.

## Self-Handicapping in Perspective

### The Relatedness of the Self-Handicapping Formulation and the Tension Reduction Hypothesis

As noted above, the self-handicapping model of alcohol abuse maintains that consuming alcohol in advance of evaluative interactions that threaten an individual's favorable but fragile competency image serves both a self-protective and anxiolytic effect. More specifically, it is argued (see also Berglas, 1985; in press) that self-handicapping strategies may be considered to be attributional strategies aimed at allaying performance anxiety and evaluation apprehension via alcohol's reputed performance-inhibiting effect. Since the self-handicapping model of alcohol abuse describes the manner in which alcohol can relieve a particular type of "tension"—that associated with threats to one's favorable competency image—it is appropriately compared to models of alcoholism derived from the tension reduction hypothesis (TRH) (Cappell & Herman, 1972; Conger, 1956; Higgins, 1976; also see Cappell and Greeley, Chapter 2, this volume). More importantly, if the self-handicapping model of alcohol abuse is to have utility for clinicians designing subtype-specific therapeutic interventions for empirically derived subgroups of alcohol abusers, the self-handicapping formulation, which focuses on a restricted form of intrapsychic "tension," must also be *contrasted* with comparable yet distinct formulations derived from the TRH focusing upon different forms of tension or stress (see Berglas, in press, for a detailed discussion of this issue).

Conger's (1956) original formulation of the TRH was stated in the most simplistic behavioral terms: Alcohol is consumed for its tension-reducing capabilities. Since increase in tension beyond a certain level constitutes a heightened drive state and alcohol consumption had physiologic consequences that included lowering an organism's level of tension, such drive-reducing properties would be reinforcing and would in turn strengthen the organism's propensity to engage in alcohol consumptive behaviors. Support for this formulation is equivocal.

A systematic and instructive program of research examining the TRH was conducted by R. L. Higgins and G. A. Marlatt. The origianl study performed by this team (Higgins & Marlatt, 1973) attempted to arouse anxiety and consequently heighten the alcohol consumption of nonabstinent alcoholics and matched social drinkers by threatening them with painful electric shock. The findings from this investigation showed that alcohol consumption (on an unobtrusive taste-rating task) was *not* affected by the threat-of-shock manipulation. However, in a later investigation (Higgins & Marlatt, 1975) that attempted to arouse *social* anxiety in subjects, a pattern of significant results were obtained. Conditions of "high threat" were created by informing the male subjects that their responses to personal questions would be evaluated by a group of female peers. Low threat was established by telling the subjects that they would rate the attractiveness of pictures of females. Following these pretreatments, subjects exposed to the high-threat treatment consumed significantly more alcohol than low-threat subjects.

The results from the preceding investigations provide clear-cut support for the contention that any study of the effects of anxiety on the appeal of alcohol must consider the distinct psychological consequences that result from various sources of anxiety. This argument has not escaped Higgins (1976, p. 59) who reports that those studies that provide support for the TRH have employed social-evaluation components. As noted above, the particular type of social-evaluative concerns that initiate self-handicapping strategies have been shown (Berglas & Jones, 1978; Tucker *et al.*, 1981) to be noncontingent reinforcement histories that generate burdensome performance expectations.

The self-handicapping formulation may be capable of accounting for a phenomenon which has been a major problem for TRH theorists. Specifically, the TRH, emphasizing the drive-reducing properties of alcohol, cannot be reconciled with convincing empirical evidence, which leads to the conclusion that alcohol intoxication is, at times, accompanied by *increases* in aversive consequences such as anxiety (see Mello, 1972, for a review). Moreover, some researchers (Mello & Mendelson, 1978; Mendelson, LaDou, & Solomon, 1964; Mendelson & Mello, 1979; Vannicelli, 1972) contend that the aversive consequences of alcohol consumption, such as anxiety induction, *reinforce* drinking for some alcoholics.

While the self-handicapping formulation is, obviously, an anxiety *reduction* model, it also explains the role of aversive consequences of alcohol intoxication in the perpetuation of problem drinking. Specifically, the self-handicapping formulation maintains that "aversive consequences" of drinking such as the impairment of cognitive functioning, psychomotor skills, and socially desirable interpersonal behavior, are anticipated, primary reinforcing properties of alcohol for a certain type of problem drinker—self-handicappers.

The self-handicapping formulation explicates the manner in which "undesired" consequences of alcohol consumption are potentially reinforcing for the self-handicapper, and argues that alcohol consumption is pragmatic—based on an *anticipation* of "aversive" consequences. This reasoning is supported by findings by Tamerin *et al.* (1970) which indicate that sober alcoholics *predict* that their behavior will be more "irresponsible" when they drink, and by theorists such as Berne (1964) and Carson (1969) who argue that alcohol consumption may be an instance of strategic "negotiation" of role behavior adopted as the best option available to an individual at a particular time.

### Marlatt's and Higgins's Tension Reduction Models

The problems inherent in the TRH have prompted other researchers to examine this intuitively appealing perspective from a variety of unique angles (Higgins, 1976). One of the more compelling of what may be called "new TRH models" has been proposed by Marlatt (1975). His perspective has attempted to synthesize and extend a variety of facts and theories pertaining to the actions of alcohol as both a pharmacologic entity and a drug known to precipitate a variety of mood changes solely on the basis of expectancy effects. For this reason, Marlatt's TRH model is quite compatible with the self-handicapping model of alcohol abuse. Borrowing heavily from Mc-Clelland, Davis, Kalin, and Wanner's (1972) power motivation theory, and Sell's (1970) theory of stress deriving from a loss of personal control, Marlatt proposes the following model:

> The probability of drinking will vary in a particular situation as a function of (a) the degree of perceived stress in the situation, (b) the degree of perceived personal control the individual experiences, (c) the availability of an "adequate" coping response to the stressful situation and the availability of alcohol, and (d) the individual's expectations about the effectiveness of alcohol as an alternative coping response in the situation. If the drinker experiences a loss of personal control in a stressful situation (and has no other adequate coping responses available), the probability of drinking will increase. Alcohol consumption, under these conditions, serves to restore the individual's sense of personal control because of its enhancing effects on arousal and thoughts of "personal power" or control. (1975, pp. 24–25)

In his commentary on Marlatt's (1975) provocative formulation, Higgins contends that, "Quite apart from abandoning notions of tension-reduction, the model proposed by Marlatt appears to make the tension-reducing effects of alcohol secondary to a primary function of enhancing feelings of personal control or 'power' " (1976, p. 62). More to the point, Higgins (1976) contends that models such as Marlatt's, and, presumably, the self-handicapping formulation, create a "problem" for researchers by both inferring the motivations for drinking behavior from the study of its effects, and failing to identify a prescribed set of antecedent conditions for abusive drinking that could not be readily incorporated within existing "direct" tension-reduction models. Leaving aside the validity of this argument for the moment, it is instructive to examine Higgins's own "compromise" tension reduction formulation which can presumably incorporate more limited formulations such as Marlatt's (1975) and the self-handicapping model:

> Alcohol consumption may reduce the stress associated with life circumstances in which an individual experiences a need to act effectively or to exercise control but experiences uncertainty regarding his ability to do so. An inability to exercise control or act effectively might result from either behavioral deficits or constraints (environmental or psychological) on behavior. The reinforcing properties of such stress reduction might lead to increasing alcohol consumption (a) when alcohol is available, (b) when the individual feels a need to act effectively but is uncertain or doubtful about his ability to do so, (c) when the outcome of the individual's behavior or circumstance is highly valued, (d) when the resulting stress is sufficiently arousing, and (e) when there is a basis in the individual's experience to expect that the consumption of alcohol in that specific situation will serve a useful function (i.e., tension reduction). (1976, pp. 64–65)

It is apparent that both Higgins (1976) and Marlatt (1975) have proposed "generic" tension-reduction models of alcohol abuse that share dominant themes with the self-handicapping perspective (Berglas, 1985; Jones & Berglas, 1978). For example, both authors contend that alcohol consumption will occur in response to the burden of expectations, but state this in terms more familiar to researchers who have investigated the consequences of psychological stress: e.g., "when the individual feels a need to act effectively but is uncertain or doubtful about his ability to do so [and] when the outcome of the individual's behavior or circumstance is highly valued" (Higgins); "[in response to] the degree of perceived stress in the situation [and] the degree of perceived personal control the individual experiences" (Marlatt). Significantly, both Marlatt (1975) and Higgins (1976) note, as Tucker et al. (1981) demonstrated, that alcohol abuse in the service of tension reduction occurs when alcohol is the best available option in a situation; implicit in the writings of Higgins (1976) and Marlatt (1975) is the notion that providing an alcohol abuser with more appropriate coping strategies would mitigate the desire for alcohol. Moreover, both Higgins and Marlatt claim that the alcohol abuser intent upon relieving psychological stress recognizes that there is some benefit to be derived from consuming alcohol when either blocked from, or incapable of, exercising action-oriented or instrumental coping strategies (Lazarus & Launier, 1978) which would serve to directly master or manage environmental demands: "[drinking is a function of] the individual's expectations about the effectiveness of alcohol as an alternative coping response" (Marlatt); "[increased alcohol consumption occurs] when there is a basis in the individual's experience to expect that the consumption of alcohol in that specific situation will serve a useful function." (Higgins). An awareness of the functional utility of consuming alcohol is, of course, the cornerstone of the self-handicapping formulation.

One may question, as Higgins (1976) did, what benefits, if any, derive from advancing yet another formulation which demonstrates that alcohol consumption can bring about intrapsychic or palliative coping: the coping behavior that involves cognitive processes which serve to regulate or relieve the dysphoria derived from stressful interactions (Lazarus & Launier 1978; Mechanic, 1972). More specifically, it now seems appropriate to inquire as to what, exactly, differentiates the self-handicapping model of alcohol abuse form these "new" TRH models, and what unique insights it can provide to our understanding of the initiation, maintenance, and treatment of problem drinking.

The importance of this question and its answer can be put into perspective by considering the following footnote to a major review of the literature on the TRH which appeared over a decade ago: "The word 'tension' was selected as the generic construct best summarizing such constructs as fear, anxiety, frustration, etc., all of which share in common that they denote hypothesized aversion states which control behavior" (Cappell & Herman 1972, p. 33). The lessons taught the alcohol research community by the Higgins and Marlatt (1973, 1975) investigations should be proof enough that the failure to differentiate, a priori, hypothesized aversive states thought to control behavior, can markedly alter the course of scientific understanding. It is now widely recognized and extremely well documented (Davidson & Schwartz, 1976) that anxiety states are not a unidimensional phenomenon. Anxiety may be experienced in cognitive terms ("my mind is racing") or purely physical terms ("I'm flushed"; "I have butterflies in my stomach"), and individuals are not equally prone to experiencing both types of anxiety (Duncan & Laird, 1977). Similarly, anxiety-provoking stimuli have decidely different impacts across persons as a function of innumerable idiosyncratic differences, such as learning history, gender, age, or character traits. Stress researchers (e.g., see Lazarus & Launier, 1978) have also made a similar point: the "stressfulness of a demand is truly a perceptual phenomenon, dependent upon the individual's appraisal of that demand based upon an awareness of what resources he posseses to cope with it."

The nature of the antecedent "aversive state" thought to provoke self-handicapping alcohol abuse derives from evaluation interactions which threaten a central component of the drinker's competency image (thereby creating the burden of expectations). Thus, the exact nature of the "tension" which initiates self-handicapping—actually evaluation apprehension—can be understood clearly and differentiated from a variety of other alcohol-abuse-provoking "tensions." If we discover that an academic psychologist gets drunk prior to his wedding reception, despite the stressful aspects of this event and the tension it arouses his drinking would not be "diagnosed" self-handicapping. Were the same psychologist to consume an identical quantity of liquor immediately prior to presenting a colloquium wherein he was discussing his award winning theory of behavior, this instance of alcohol abuse would probably qualify for a "diagnosis" of self-handicapping [Berglas (1985) describes a set of crtiteria developed to define a self-handicapping disorder]. To qualify as self-handicapping, alcohol abuse must be contemporaneous to an evaluation that threatens the drinker's competency in a realm wherein he had previously been successful. This restriction clearly does not apply to TRH models of drinking which do not differentiate the "aversive" states thought to proke "relief" drinking.

The present self-handicapping formulation is restrictive and also somewhat unique in its understanding of the role that perceptions of control or feelings of personal power play in heightening the reinforcing properties of alcohol consumption. According to Berglas and Jones, "As long as people can avoid clearly diagnostic feedback settings, they may maintain the precarious illusion of control. They may, paradoxically, deliberately run the risk of being out of control—through [self-handicapping alcohol abuse]—to protect their belief in ultimately being capable of control when it is really necessary, or when the chips are down" (1978, p. 407). The self-handicapper, it has been argued, seeks to control *attributions* drawn from his behavior in current performance settings, and in so doing, retains control of a *previously* derived positive competency image. After his competency image is protected, he will experience a reduction of performance anxiety or evaluation apprehension which may then impact upon his behavior (see Figure 9.1). This perspective is quite distinct from others which posit a direct pharmacologic like between alcohol consumption and reductions in anxiety (e.g., see Conger, 1956), or alcohol consumption and decreased self-awareness which *in turn* decreases negative self-evaluation following failures (Hull, 1981; Hull & Young, 1983; Hull, Chapter 8, this volume).

In this regard it should be noted that Marlatt's (1975) TRH formulation, in accordance with the theorizing and research of McClelland *et al.* (1972), maintains: "Alcohol consumption . . . serves to restore the individual's sense of personal control because of its enhancing effects on . . . thoughts of 'personal power' or control" (p. 25). The population described in detail by McClelland *et al.* (1972) comprises a distinct population of men who *wish* to be powerful, competent, and the like but are not and have not been so, at least in a manner comparable to the self-handicapper. The difference between the power fantasies of the population described by McClelland *et al.* and self-handicappers (see also Beglas, 1985) is reminiscent of the distinction drawn by psychoanalysts between primary process thinking and secondary process thinking. As noted by Kolb (1977), primary process thinking is highly charged affectively, usually involving visual images and ego defensive operations such as symbolization—not unlike the thinking that dominated the fantasies obtained by McClelland et al. (1972) when they analyzed the Thematic Apperception Test (TAT) stories reported by men, with accentuated needs for personalized power, after they had consumed alcohol. On the other hand, secondary process thinking is characterized by Kolb (1977) as being highly organized and logical, related to abstractions concerned with rules of the external world—in essence, the cognitive style that accounts for the pragmatic understanding of social functioning and inference processes manifest in the strategic maneuvers of self-handicappers (see Figure 9.1, above, and Berglas, in press).

The thinking styles that account for the contrast between the populations described by McClelland et al. (1972) and the present self-handicapping formulation are as different as they are because they are predicated on totally distinct, nonoverlapping antecedent needs. The men studied by McClelland et al. (1972) experienced power deficits that were ameliorated following drinking. Self-handicappers experience threats to existing, albeit vulnerable, positive competency images. The self-handicapper is afraid of losing the type of competency image the McClelland et al. "drinking man" seeks to obtain through alcohol-fueled fantasies. Moreover, McClelland et al. maintain, without qualification, "men do not drink primarily to reduce their anxiety" (1972, p. 333). Self-handicappers are known to drink in response to apprehension centered around evaluations that threaten to jeopardize prior success experiences (Tucker et al., 1981).

The value derived from differentiating and contrasting alcohol abuse typologies that bear some similarity to each other by virtue of their tension-reducing features should now be clear. Given that the impetus for drinking among individuals desirous of protecting favorable but fragile self-conceptions (self-handicapping theory) is quite distinct from generic TRH formulations, the model advanced by McClelland et al. (1972) and, for that matter Hull (1981), who argues that alcohol can decrease negative self-awareness following failure, it follows that remediation for alcohol abusers who are identified by these typologies deserve comparably specialized attention (see Berglas, in press). Clinicians must understand fully the psychological factors that initiate abusive drinking in various subgroups of alcohol abusers in order to plan therapeutic strategies tailored to the disorders or deficits that must be addressed when symptomatic drinking behavior has been brought under control. In a manner identical to that which mandates differential treatment for persons who fear open places (agoraphobics) as opposed to those who fear weight gain (anorexics), it is imperative that alcohol abusers whose drinking is intiated by fears of losing the image derived from prior success experiences (Berglas, 1985; in press; Tucker *et al.*, 1981) be differentiated from one who fears social situations (e.g., Higgins & Marlatt, 1975; Kraft, 1971) or other distinctly threatening interactions.

### Confusion Surrounding the Application of the Self-Handicapping Formulation

A review of the literature that has referenced the original self-handicapping formulation following its publication by Jones and Berglas (1978), reveals that this mode of strategic self-protection behavior is, on occasion, misunderstood. The most critical of these misunderstandings centers around researchers' failing to establish a positive competency image as a prerequisite for defining a self-protective behavior "self-handicapping" (Smith, *et al.*, 1982), or applying the concept to drug-taking behavior that follows the experience of failure (Weidner, 1980). (See Berglas, 1985, for a detailed discussion of this issue.) An obvious example of the tendency to ignore the essence of self-handicapping alcohol abuse—namely, that it is intended to protect a favorable but fragile competency image—appears in a report by McHugh *et al.* (1979). According to these authors, "Jones and Berglas (1978) have proposed a relationship between attributions and alcoholism . . . based on the concept of low self-worth of alcoholics. . . . Jones and Berglas (1978) further suggest that alcoholics . . . are likely to have high expectancies for the future in spite of past failures. . ." (1979, pp. 204–205). Leaving aside the fact that Jones and Berglas (1978) took care to limit their comments to alcohol *abusers*, indicating that the path from abuse to addiction would be beyond the concern of their formulation (p. 202), McHugh *et al.* do a clear disservice to the present formulation when they tie the intiation of self-handicapping alcohol abuse to feelings of "low self worth" and "past failure" and ignore the research (e.g., see Berglas & Jones, 1978) linking self-handicapping behavior with noncontingent *success* experiences.

Without question, a significant proportion of those individuals diagnosed as either alcohol dependent or alcohol abusive suffer, or have suffered, feelings of low self-esteem. Studies comparing alcoholics and nonalcoholics on measures of self-esteem (Vanderpool, 1969) show some qualified support for the contention that alcoholics had lower self-esteem. In a similar vein, Williams's (1965) study of college students categorized as "problem drinkers" revealed that this group manifested more negative self-evaluations than nonproblem drinkers, and had response profiles on the Gough Adjective Check List (Gough, 1955) that were very similar to alcoholic subjects assessed with the same instrument. Yet after examining the results of their investigation of self-esteem in alcoholics and nonalcoholics which lent support to their hyposthesis that alcoholics have significantly lower self-esteem than do nonalcoholics, Charalampous, Ford, and Skinner (1976) concluded: "Examination of the alcoholics' scores separately, however, shows that many alcoholics scored high (in self-esteem)" (pp. 992–993). Despite the existence of equivocal findings such as these, however, researchers cling to the myth that alcohol abuse disorders uniformly afflict individuals who are already disadvantaged, and do so accordingly to a unidimensional pattern of deterioration that involves an intensification or exacerbation of preexistent negative self-conceptions (Berglas, in press).

Laboratory investigations of self-handicapping effects (Berglas & Jones, 1978; Tucker *et al.*, 1981) have demonstrated quite clearly the manner in which *success* experiences serve as the antecedent conditions which can initiate abusive alcohol consumption. By direct implication, moreover, both these studies and clinical observations of alcohol abusers (Berglas, in press) serve to delineate a specific set of conditions within which successful persons with no history of past failures whatsoever are at risk for the development of alcoholism. The goal of self-handicapping is to protect and preserve prior success experiences; it is not a cover-up for failures in the past. While a *fear* of failure will prompt self-handicapping alcohol abuse, alcohol consumed in *response* to failure does not qualify as self-handicapping (Berglas, 1985).

As noted above, there are several formulations that describe alcohol abusers whose disordered behavior can be profitably understood as a response to negative self-conceptions. The most influential of these is the "drinking man" conceptualized by McClelland *et al* (1972). These researchers succeeded in identifying a group of men who have accentuated needs for personalized power and drink excessively in order to activate or disinhibit fantasies of power. The psychological makeup of this type of alcohol abuser may be characterized as being fundamentally weak and/or interpersonally impotent. They want power, specifically dominance over others and the experience of personal glory or influence. Their concern with power is presumed to be compensatory, probably derived from having experienced powerlessness or fearing that they were powerless. Yet, regardless of the origins of their heightened personal power needs, the type of alcohol abuser described by McClelland *et al.* (1972) drinks for the gratification they derive from thoughts of power and fantasies experienced when intoxicated. Thus, alcohol abuse for these men is directly reinforcing: Feelings of weakness are suppressed or forgotten when they experience fantasized strength caused by inebriation.

With this brief comparison we can see that the self-handicapping alcohol abuser and the "drinking man" identified by McClelland *et al.* (1972) are quite distant typologies despite the fact that both groups are exquisitely sensitive to the potentially devastating effects of failure. Since one group endeavors to avoid the implications that authentic failure would have for previously accrued increments to their self-conceptions by consuming alcohol (i.e., self-handicappers), and the other group suppresses feelings of chronic low self-esteem through intoxication ("drinking men"), there exists a need to retain a rigorous distinction between the types. The origin of this need is the understanding that while alcohol abuse may be the final common disordered behavior manifested by various clincial typologies, effective clincial interventions and prevention strategies can only be developed when the alcohol abuser's premorbid life-style and character structure are understood. Typologies of alcohol abusers such as those derived from the self-handicapping model of alcohol abuse (Berglas, 1985; in press) or the work of McClelland *et al.* (1972) serve to facilitate preventive and therapeutic services by identifying the specific conditions most likely to initiate and maintain patterns of abusive drinking in certain restricted samples of drinkers.

## Clinical Implications of the Self-Handicapping Formulation

The preceding attempt to differentiate self-handicapping alcohol abuse from similar, yet distinct, patterns of disordered alcohol consumption, should serve to underscore an awareness that the only way in which alcohol abuse formulations can prove to be heuristic frameworks in clincial settings is to insure that they limit the number and type of persons and settings they try to explain. The self-handicapping model of alcohol abuse (Berglas, 1985; in press; Jones & Berglas, 1978) has a limited, yet significant, "range of convenience"—that portion of the real world wherein a theoretical formulation provides descriptive and predictive power (Kelly, 1955). Recall that self-handicapping alcohol abuse is initiated to serve two distinct functions: (1) reduce performance anxiety derived from evaluative interactions, and (2) provide concomitant esteem-*maintaining* defenses. By serving as a "legitimate" mechanism for avoiding or escaping the threat inherent in one type of behavioral setting— evaluations—self-handicapping alcohol abuse can free an individual from the ruminations and debilitating cognitions that might otherwise heighten anxiety and hamper his performance (Berglas, 1985; in press). It is thus clear that there exists a unique set of antecedent conditions to, and affective instigators of, self-handicapping alcohol abuse that require treatment strategies sensitive to the unique characteristics of self-handicappers (Berglas, 1985; in press).

### Reactions to Success and Failure

As noted above, self-handicapping alcohol abusers exploit alcohol's performance-inhibiting reputation in a strategic attempt to protect a highly favorable self-conception that rests upon an uncertain foundation. Since they are more concerned with preserving their image of social competence than they are in manifesting their abilities (Kolditz & Arkin, 1982), it may be inappropriate to attempt to strengthen the competencies of self-handicapping alcohol abusers during a program of remediation (Berglas, in press). Specifically, any therapeutic intervention that attempted to make self-handicappers *more* skillful at executing tasks expected of them might actually exacerbate the dilemma of these individuals rather than resolve it.

It is widely acknowledged that increases in the power to perform highly skilled behaviors carry increased responsibility to manifest performances and attendant pressures together in one complex package (Berglas, 1985; in press; Schlenker, 1980). Self-handicapping alcohol abusers are subjected to ever-increasing burdensome expectations over time owing to the fact that in order to self-handicap and preserve their competency images, they must achieve intermittent success and demonstrate that they are *not* dependent upon alcohol (Berglas, 1985; in press). Thus, success experiences are a two-edged sword for self-handicappers in that in order to sustain their self-protective career, subsequent performance expectations will, over time, be legitimately more threatening than those previously fulfilled. Therapeutic strategies focusing upon interventions intended to provide the self-handicapping alcohol abuser with competency *enhancement* are likely to have the paradoxical effect of perpetuating the cycle of increased burdensome expectations that lead to intensified performance anxiety (Berglas, in press).

In a similar vein it is instructive to recall that self-handicapping alcohol abusers are arranging to heighten the likelihood of failure a priori by entering performance settings under the influence of an agent with known performance-inhibiting capabilities. In so doing they are both prepared for the occurrence of failure and spared the full force of its implications. In a word, self-handicapping alcohol abusers are unaffected by failure since they have set the stage for its probable occurrence while self-handicapping. This unique responsivity to failure is a discriminating quality of self-handicapping alcohol abusers that sets them apart from a variety of other alcohol abusers (Kinsey, 1966; McClelland *et al.*, 1972; Vanderpool, 1969) thought to drink abusively in an attempt to improve their preexistent negative self-conceptions. For this latter group, it is assumed that the experience of failure would have a high impact and, presumably, would be an instigator of abusive alcohol consumption. Self-handicapping alcohol abusers drink prior to evaluation outcomes and not *in response* to failure, but in advance of failure (Berglas, 1985; in press).

This argument is not intended to imply an endorsement of failure for self-handicapping alcohol abusers. On the contrary, self-handicapping alcohol abusers need to succeed in order to ultimately attain a *stable* and entrenched favorable self-conception. What is needed is a therapeutic program that will assist the self-handicapper in attributing desired performance outcomes to his personal ability or other so-called "internal" factors (e.g., hard work, planning) rather than the "external" factors (e.g., luck, pedigree, evaluator bias) that created the experience of noncontingent success so central to the etiology of all self-handicapping behaviors (Berglas, 1985; in press; Berglas & Jones, 1978).

The work of Beck (1976) and Beck *et al.* (1979) on depressive disorders is particularly applicable to self-handicapping alcohol abusers who need to restructure their cognitions and mental schema pertaining to the causes of successful outcomes. In a nutshell, the thrust of the Beck technique (Beck *et al.*, 1979) is to teach patients to learn to identify, and then alter, the sets of dysfunctional beliefs that predispose them to distort experiences in a particular manner. In the case of the self-handicapping alcohol abuser, the goal of therapy would be to learn to locate multiple sources of confirmation for the abilities he suspects he has based upon his *prior* reinforcement history. Following this, the self-handicapping alcohol abuser would need to develop a new attributional "logic" to account for success experiences. With these attributions about the cause of success appropriately aligned, one factor contributing to the self-handicapper's inordinate evaluation apprehension would be brought within normal ranges of concern.

### Evaluation Apprehension

The task of devising therapeutic interventions for self-handicapping alcohol abusers is made easier by the fact that there exists a limited number of circumstances capable of evoking evaluation apprehension or anticipatory anxiety—which evoke abusive drinking—in this particular typology (Berglas, in press). Since it is known that self-handicapping behavior is initiated in response to threats posed to existing positive competence images, once the exact nature of an individual's positive self-regard is established, it is possible to limit the number of evaluative interactions that have the potential to threaten a central component of the individual's self-esteem. This is not to imply that all evaluative threats to a positive competency image will evoke self-handicapping behavior. Rather, it is possible, once abusive alcohol consumption is observed, to determine if it *is* self-handicapping behavior by assessing the individual's reinforcement history and the timing of his abusive drinking (Berglas, 1985). If the criteria for self-handicapping alcohol abuse are met, treatment can be tailored to address the particular evaluation apprehension experienced by any given self-handicapper.

For example, to qualify as self-handicapping alcohol abuse, an individual's drinking (e.g., binges or "benders") must be contemporaneous with evaluative interactions such as job interviews, school examinations and the like, or shifts in status that heighten an individual's real-world responsibility such as graduation, job promotion, or parenthood (Berglas, 1985). If it is established that an individual has been successful in a particular realm of behavior, and his drinking coincides with a retest of an ability relevant to that behavioral dimension, a "diagnosis" of self-handicapping behavior would be appropriate. The true benefit derived from such a "diagnosis" lies in the identification of the specific type of evaluation apprehension responsible for the self-handicapper's alcohol abuse. Since the success experience is, by definition, limited to some specific ability dimension (e.g., mathematics, English composition, billiards), there are only certain situations that threaten successes achieved on that ability dimension.

Contrast this specificity with the almost limitless range of settings capable of evoking abusive drinking behavior in the typology identified by McClelland *et al.* (1972). For individuals beset by chronic feelings of powerlessness, who drink to suppress these feelings and satisfy their urges for power through intoxication-induced fantasies, any situation that can produce a sense that they are not dominant and powerful is sufficient to initiate abusive drinking.

With an understanding of precisely what types of situations evoke evaluation apprehension in a self-handicapping alcohol abuser, the task of addressing the consequences of this anxiety—self-referential worry and performance-impeding cognitions (Sarason, 1973; Wine, 1971)—is made considerably more manageable. Programs targeted at correcting the "internal dialogue" (Meichenbaum, 1977; Meichenbaum & Butler, 1980) that anxious individuals rehearse in anticipation of situational demands, is easier to correct when it blocks coping behavior for one or two tasks, as opposed to an infinite number of behaviors. For self-handicapping alcohol abusers, irrational cognitions concerning evaluations and their consequences are restricted and thus more vulnerable to challenges posed by the reality of past performances, normative data, and the like. Most importantly, by demonstrating that the number of potentially threatening circumstances is restricted to a manageable few—which the self-handicapping alcohol abuser may actually avoid temporarily by appropriate environmental structuring—the self-handicapper's appraisal of the threat, and subsequent stress that he is confronting, will diminish considerably (Lazarus & Launier, 1978; McGrath, 1970).

*Predicting Long-Term Drinking Patterns*

If the self-handicapping alcohol abuser's reactions to success and failure and his idiosyncratic experience of evaluation apprehension are clearly understood, predicting such an individual's drinking behavior over time becomes academic: Drinking will be in response to burdensome expectations and all relapses will be paradoxical in that they will follow what is commonly construed to be a "favorable" life event such as praise, rewards, and the like. Experiences commonly judged to be aversive by the population at large will not provoke the self-handicapper to abuse alcohol in spite of the fact that they may evoke other stress responses.

Knowing self-handicappers implies knowing that they drink to preserve the image of success. Using the Berglas and Jones (1978) studies as a prototype, it can be said that any conditions that impose a burden of expectations upon an individual desirous of maintaining a favorable competence image are sufficient to initiate self-handicapping. The likelihood of observing self-handicapping behavior is diminished only when an individual gains certainty regarding his capacity to manifest behaviors necessary to bring about successful outcomes on tasks for which he had previously been rewarded. Without performance-enhancing options (Tucker *et al.*, 1981) or a sense of self-efficacy (Bandura, 1977) pertaining to the requirements of a relevent evaluative interaction, self-handicapping alcohol abuse will always remain a viable mechanism for preserving a favorable but fragile self-conception.

## Acknowledgments

The writing of this chapter was supported by Research Career Scientist Development Award #1 K01 AA00050-03 from the National Institute on Alcohol Abuse and Alcoholism. The author would like to thank Richard J. Landau and the editors of the volume, Howard Blane and Ken Leonard, for their helpful comments on a preliminary draft of the manuscript.

## References

Abramson, L. Y., Seligman, M. E. P., & Teasdale, J. D. (1978) Learned helplessness in humans: Critique and reformulation. *Journal of Abnormal Psychology, 87*, 49–74.

American Psychiatric Association. (1980). *Diagnostic and statistical manual of mental disorders* (3rd ed.). Washington, DC: Author.

Anastasi, A. (1958). *Psychological testing* (1st ed.). New York: Macmillan.

Anastasi, A. (1961). *Psychological testing* (2nd ed.). New York: Macmillan.

Bandura, A. (1977). Self-efficacy: Toward a unifying theory of behavioral change. *Psychological Review, 84*, 191–215.

Baron, R. A., & Byrne, D. (1981). *Social psychology: Understanding human interaction* (3rd ed.). Boston: Allyn and Bacon.

Beck, A. T. (1976). *Cognitive therapy and emotionl disorders.* New York: International Universities Press.

Beck, A. T., Rush, A. J., Shaw, B. F., & Emery, G. (1979). *Cognitive therapy of depression.* New York: Guilford Press.

Bem, D. J. (1972). Self-perception theory. In L. Berkowitz (Ed.), *Advances in experimental social psychology* (Vol. 6, pp. 2–62). New York: Academic Press.

Berglas, S. (1976). Strategies of externalization and performance: The facilitative effect of disruptive drugs. Doctoral dissertation, Duke University, Durham, NC.

Berglas, S. (1985). Self-handicapping and self-handicappers: A cognitive/attributional model of interpersonal self-protective behavior. In R. Hogan & W. H. Jones (Eds.), *Perspectives in personality: Theory, measurement and interpersonal dynamics.* Greenwich, CT: JAI Press.

Berglas, S. (in press). Typology of self-handicapping alcohol abusers. In M. Saks & L. Saxe (Eds.), *Advances in applied social psychology* (Vol. 3). Hillsdale, NJ: Lawrence Erlbaum.

Berglas, S., & Jones, E. E. (1978). Drug choice as a self-handicapping strategy in response to noncontingent success. *Journal of Personality and Social Psychology, 36*, 405–417.

Berne, E. (1964). *Games People Play.* New York: Grove Press.

Cappell, H., & Herman, C. P. (1972). Alcohol and tension reduction: A review. *Quarterly Journal of Studies on Alcohol, 33*, 33–64.

Carson, R. C. (1969). *Interaction concepts of personality.* Chicago: Aldine.

Chafetz, M. E., & Demone, H. W. (1962). *Alcoholism and society.* New York: Oxford University Press.

Charalampous, K. D., Ford, B. K., & Skinner, T. J. (1976). Self-esteem in alcoholics and nonalcoholics. *Journal of Studies on Alcohol, 37*, 990–994.

Conger, J. J. (1956). Alcoholism: Theory, problem and challenge. II. Reinforcement theory and the dynamics of alcoholism. *Quarterly Journal of Studies on Alcohol, 17*, 296–305.

Connors, G. J., & Maisto, S. A. (1980). Effects of alcohol, instructions, and consumption rate on motor performance. *Journal of Studies on Alcohol, 41*, 509–517.

Cronbach, L. J. (1955). Processes affecting scores on 'understanding of others' and 'assumed similarity.' *Psychological Bulletin, 52*, 177–193.

Davidson, R. J., & Schwartz, G. E. (1976). The psychobiology of relaxation and related states: A multi-process theory. In D. I. Mostofsky (Ed.), *Behavior control and modification of psychological activity* (pp. 399–442). Englewood Cliffs, NJ: Prentice-Hall.

Duncan, J. W., & Laird, J. D. (1977). Cross-modality consistencies in individual differences in self-attribution. *Journal of Personality, 45*, 191–206.

Folkman, S., Schaefer, C., & Lazarus, R. S. (1979). Cognitive processes as mediators of stress and coping. In V. Hamilton & D. M. Warburton (Eds.), *Human stress and cognition: An information-processing approach* (pp. 265–298). London: John Wiley & Sons.

Freed, E. X. (1978). Alcohol and mood: An updated review. *International Journal of the Addictions, 13*, 173–200.

Gardner, H. (1983). *Frames of mind.* New York: Basic Books.

Goffman, E. (1959). *The presentation of self in everyday life.* Gardent City, NY: Doubleday Anchor.

Gough, H. G. (1950). *Reference handbook for the Gough adjective check list.* Berkeley, CA: University of California Press.

Heider, F. (1958). *The psychology of interpersonal relations.* New York: John Wiley & Sons.

Higgins, R. L. (1976). Experimental investigations of tension reduction models of alcoholism. In G. Goldstein & C. Neuringer (Eds.), *Empirical studies of alcoholism* (pp. 34–37). Cambridge, MA: Ballinger.

Higgins, R. L., & Marlatt, G. A. (1973). Effects of anxiety arousal on the consumption of alcohol by alcoholics and social drinkers. *Journal of Consulting and Clinical Psychology, 41* (3), 426–433.

Higgins, R. L., & Marlatt, G. A. (1975). Fear of interpersonal evaluation as a determinant of alcohol consumption in male social drinkers. *Journal of Abnormal Psychology, 84* (6), 644–651.

Hollander, E. P. (1981). *Principles and methods of social psychology* (4th ed.). New York: Oxford University Press.

Honzik, M. P. (1973). The development of intelligence. In B. B. Wolman (Ed.), *Handbook of general psychology* (pp. 644–655). Englewood Cliffs, NJ: Prentice-Hall.

Hull, J. G. (1981). A self-awareness model of the causes and effects of alcohol consumption. *Journal of Abnormal Psychology*, *90*, 586–600.

Hull, J. G., & Young, R. D. (1983). The self-awareness-reducing effects of alcohol: Evidence and implications. In J. Suls & A. G. Greenwald (Eds.), *Psychological perspectives on the self* (pp. 159–190). Hillsdale, NJ: Lawrence Erlbaum.

Jones, E. E., & Berglas, S. (1978). Control of attributions about the self through self-handicapping strategies: The appeal of alcohol and the role of underachievement. *Personality and Social Psychology Bulletin*, *4*, 200–206.

Jones, E. E., & Davis, K. E. (1965). From acts to dispositions: The attribution process in person perception. In L. Berkowitz (Ed.), *Advances in experimental social psychology* (Vol. 2, pp. 219–266). New York: Academic Press.

Jones, E. E., Kanouse, D. E., Kelley, H. H., Nisbett, R. E., Valins, S., & Weiner, B. (1971). *Attribution: Perceiving the causes of behavior*. Morristown, NJ: General Learning Press.

Jones, E. E., & Nisbett, R. E. (1971). *The actor and the observer: Divergent perceptions of the causes of behavior*. Morristown, NJ: General Learning Press.

Jones, E. E., & Pittman, T. S. (1982). Toward a general theory of strategic self-presentation. In J. Suls (Ed.), *Psychological perspectives on the self* (pp. 231–262). Hillsdale, NJ: Lawrence Erlbaum.

Kelley, H. H. (1967). Attribution theory in social psychology. In D. Levine (Ed.), *Nebraska symposium on motivation*. (pp. 192–238). Lincoln: University of Nebraska Press.

Kelley, H. H. (1971). *Attribution in social interaction*. Morristown, NJ: General Learning Press.

Kelly, G. A. (1955). *A theory of personality: The psychology of personal constructs*. New York: W. W. Norton.

Kessel, N., & Walton, H. (1966). *Alcoholism*. Baltimore: Penguin Books.

Kinsey, B. A. (1966). *The female alcoholic*. Springfield, IL: Charles C Thomas.

Kolb, L. C. (1977). *Modern clinical psychiatry*. Philadelphia: W. B. Saunders.

Kolditz, T. A., & Arkin, R. M. (1982). An impression management interpretation of the "Self-Handicapping Strategy." *Journal of Personality and Social Psychology*, *43*, 492–502.

Kraft, T. (1971). Social anxiety model of alcoholism. *Perceptual and Motor Skills*, *33*, 797–798.

Lazarus, R. S. (1981). The stress and coping paradigm. In C. Eisdorfer, D. Cohen., A. Kleinman, & P. Maxim (Eds.), *Models for clinical psychopathology* (pp. 177–214). New York: Spectrum.

Lazarus, R. S., & Launier, R. (1978). Stress-related transactions between person and environment. In L. A. Pervin & M. Lewis (Eds.), *Perspectives in interactional psychology* (pp. 287–327). New York: Plenum Press.

Levine, J. M., Kramer, G. C., & Levine, E. N. (1975). Effects of alcohol on human performance: An integration of research findings based on an abilities classification. *Journal of Applied Psychology*, *60*, 285–293.

MacAndrew C., & Edgerton, R. B. (1969). *Drunken comportment: A social explanation*. Chicago: Aldine.

Maisto, S. A., Connors, G. J., & Sachs, P. R. (1981). Expectation as a mediator in alcohol intoxication: A reference level model. *Cognitive Therapy and Research*, *5*, 1–18.

Malmo, R. B. (1957). Anxiety and behavioral arousal. *Psychological Review*, *64*, 276–287.

Marlatt, G. A. (1975, June–July). Alcohol, stress, and cognitive control. Paper presented at the NATO-sponsored International Conference on Dimensions of Stress and Anxiety, Oslo.

Marlatt, G. A. (1983). The controlled-drinking controversy: A commentary. *American Psychologist*, *38*, 1097–1110.

Marlatt, G. A., & Rohsenow, D. J. (1980). Cognitive process in alcohol use: Expectancy and the balanced placebo design. In N. K. Mellow (Ed.), *Advances in substance abuse: Behavioral and biological research* (Vol. 1, pp. 159–199). Greenwich, CT: JAI Press.

McClelland, D. C., Davis, W. N., Kalin, R., & Wanner, E. (1972). *The drinking man*. New York: Free Press.

McGrath, J. C. (1970). *Social and psychological factors in stress*. New York: Holt, Rinehart and Winston.

McHugh, M., Beckman, L. J., & Frieze, I. H. (1979). Analyzing alcoholism. In I. H. Frieze, D. Bar-Tal, & J. S. Carrol (Eds.), *New approaches to social problems* (pp. 168–208). San Francisco: Jossey-Bass.

McNamee, B., Mello, N. K., & Mendelson, J. H. (1968). Experimental analysis of drinking patterns of alcoholics: Current psychiatric observations. *American Journal of Psychiatry, 124*, 1063–1069.

Mechanic, D. (1962). *Students under stress.* New York: Free Press.

Meichenbaum, D. (1977). *Cognitive-behavior modification: An integrative approach.* New York, Plenum Press.

Meichenbaum, D., & Butler, L. (1980). Toward a conceptual model for the treatment of test anxiety: Implications for research and treatment. In I. G. Sarason (Ed.), *Test anxiety: Theory, research and applications* (pp. 187–208). Hillsdale, NJ: Lawrence Erlbaum.

Mello, N. K. (1972). Behavioral studies of alcoholism. In B. Kissin & H. Begleiter (Eds.), *The biology of alcoholism: Vol. 2. Physiology and behavior* (pp. 219–291). New York: Plenum Press.

Mello, N. K., & Mendelson, J. H. (1978). Alcohol and human behavior. In L. L. Iversen, S. D. Iversen, & S. H. Snyder (Eds.), *Handbook of psychopharmacology: Vol. 12. Drugs of abuse* (pp. 235–317). New York: Plenum Press.

Mendelson, J. H., & Mello, N. K. (1979). One unanswered question about alcoholism. *British Journal of Addiction, 74*, 11–14.

Mendelson, J. H., Ladou, J., & Solomon, P. (1964). Experimentally induced intoxication and withdrawal in alcoholics. *Quarterly Journal of Studies on Alcoholism,* Supplement 2.

Miller, M. E., Adesso, V. J., Fleming, J. P., (1978). Gino, A., & Lauerman, R. (1978). Effects of alcohol on the storage and retrieval processes of heavy social drinkers. *Journal of Experimental Psychology: Human Learning and Memory, 4*, 246–455.

Mischel, W. (1968). *Personality and assessment.* New York: John Wiley & Sons.

Mischel, W. (1973). Toward a cognitive social-learning reconceptualization of personality. *Psychological Review, 80*, 252–283.

Paul, G. L., & Bernstein, D. A. (1973). *Anxiety and clinical problems: Systematic desensitization and related techniques.* Morristown, NJ: General Learning Press.

Peters, R. S. (1958). *The concept of motivation.* London: Routledge & Kegan Paul.

Russell, J. A., & Mehrabian, A. (1975). The mediating role of emotions in alcohol use. *Journal of Studies on Alcohol, 36*, 1508–1536.

Ryle, G. (1949). *The concept of mind.* New York: Barnes & Noble.

Sarason, I. G. (1973). Test anxiety and cognitive modeling. *Journal of Personality and Social Psychology, 28*, 58–61.

Schlenker, B. R. (1980). *Impression management.* Monterey, CA: Brooks/ Cole.

Seligman, M. E. P. (1975). *Helplessness: On depression, development, and death.* San Francisco: W. H. Freeman.

Sells, S. B. (1970). On the nature of stress. In J. E. McGrath (Ed.), *Social and psychological factors in stress* (pp. 134–139). New York: Holt, Rinehart and Winston.

Smith, T. W., Snyder, C. R., & Handelsman, M. M. (1982). On the self-serving function of an academic wooden leg: Test anxiety as a self-handicapping strategy. *Journal of Personality and Social Psychology, 42*, 314–321.

Snyder, M., Schulz, R., & Jones, E. E. (1974). Expectancy and apparent duration as determinants of fatigue. *Journal of Personality and Social Psychology, 29*, 426–434.

Spence, J. T., & Spence, K. W. (1966). The motivational components of manifest anxiety: Drive and drive stimuli. In C. D. Spielberger (Ed.), *Anxiety and behavior* (pp. 291–326). New York: Academic Press.

Storms, M. D., & Nisbett, R. E. (1970). Insomnia and the attribution process. *Journal of Personality and Social Psychology, 16*, 319–328.

Tamerin, J. S., Weiner, S., & Mendelson, J. H. (1970). Alcoholics' expectancies and recall of experiences during intoxication. *American Journal of Psychiatry, 126*, 1697–1704.

Tucker, J. A., Vuchinich, R. E., & Sobell, M. B. (1981). Alcohol consumption as a self-handicapping strategy. *Journal of Abnormal Psychology, 90*, 220–230.

Vanderpool, J. A. (1969). Alcoholism and the self-concept. *Quarterly Journal of Studies on Alcohol, 30*, 59–77.

Vannicelli, M. (1972). Mood and self-perception of alcoholics when sober and intoxicated. *Quarterly Journal of Studies on Alcohol, 33*, 341–357.

Weidner, G. (1980). Self-handicapping following learned helplessness and the Type A coronary-prone behavior pattern. *Journal of Psychosomatic Research, 24*, 319–325.

Williams, A. F. (1965). Self-concept of college problem drinkers. I. A comparison with alcoholics. *Quarterly Journal of Studies on Alcohol, 26*, 586–594.

Wilson, G. T. (1978). Booze, belief, and behavior: Cognitive processes in alcohol use and abuse. In P. E. Nathan, G. A. Marlatt, & T. Loberg (Eds.), *Alcoholism: New directions in research and treatment* (pp. 315–339). New York: Plenum Press.

Wilson, G. T., & Lawson, D. M. (1976). Expectancies, alcohol, and sexual arousal in male social drinkers. *Journal of Abnormal Psychology, 85*, 587–594.

Wilson, G. T., & Lawson, D. M. (1978). Effects of alcohol on sexual arousal in women. *Journal of Abnormal Psychology, 87*, 358–367.

Wine, J. D. (1971). Test anxiety and direction of attention. *Psychological Bulletin, 76*, 92–104.

Worchel, S., & Cooper, J. *Understanding social psychology.* Homewood, IL: Dorsey Press.

Wright, M. H., & Obitz, F. W. (1984). Alcoholics' and nonalcoholics' attributions of control of future life events. *Journal of Studies on Alcohol, 45*, 138–143.

# 10 Opponent Process Theory

THOMAS E. SHIPLEY, JR.

Opponent process theory was developed and first described over a decade ago by Solomon and Corbit (1973, 1974) and Hoffman and Solomon (1974) as a new theory of acquired motivation. Since the first statement it has been applied in theory and research to a broad range of motivational phenomena including imprinting (Starr, 1978), taking of examinations (Craig & Siegel, 1980), the development of polydipsia (Rosellini & Lashley, 1982), and the motivation for habitual blood donations (Piliavin, Callero, & Evans, 1982). The theory was also applied to addictive smoking by Solomon and Corbit (1973), Ternes (1977), and Pomerleau (1979), and other drugs including alcohol by Solomon (1977, 1980), and by Solomon and Corbit (1974).

In this chapter, following an introductory overview, I present a detailed description of opponent process theory as well as two other formulations that have been proposed to help account (1) for the conditioning of opponent processes (Schull, 1979) and (2) for the effect of chronic opponent processes (Shipley, 1984). Following an explication of the theory I describe research that has confirmed some of the basic propositions of the theory and can help us understand the development and treatment of alcoholism. I conclude the chapter with a discussion of implications for treatment after a brief analysis of opposing positions.

Clearly, one of the advantages of opponent process theory is its breadth of applicability. Another advantage lies in the ease with which, as a psychological theory, it can be integrated with psychological approaches such as learning and attribution theory, or physiologic approaches including hormonal analyses. Thus, it was designed to account for a range of phenomena in acquired motivation and addictive behavior, and it is compatible with other theoretical approaches. I will examine alcohol addiction in this context.

THOMAS E. SHIPLEY, JR. Department of Psychology, Temple University, Philadelphia, Pennsylvania

As a theory of acquired motivation it differs significantly from prior theories of acquired motivation (e.g., see Miller, 1951) which emphasized the effect of hedonic stimulation on prior stimuli. In those formulations the acquisition of motives was said to come about through an associative process. Through Pavlovian conditioning stimuli could acquire either motivational or reward properties and then come as a consequence to drive or reinforce behavior. These were called "derived motives" (D'Amato, 1974), but they did not, according to Solomon (1980), easily account for the properties of addiction which do not appear to rely upon conditioning. Thus, opponent process theory is nonassociative and accounts for the acquisition of motives in terms of the repeated effect of a reinforcer, hedonic stimulus, or unconditioned stimulus upon an organism. Solomon (1980) has stated the basic assumption in his more recent general formulation of the theory:

> The theory assumes that for some reason the brains of all mammals are organized to oppose or suppress many types of emotional arousals or hedonic processes, whether they are pleasurable or aversive, whether they have been generated by positive or by negative reinforcers. The opposing affective or hedonic processes are automatically set in motion by those stimulus patterns that psychologists or ethologists have shown through defining experiments, to function as Pavlovian UCSs, operant reinforcers, or innate releasers. (p. 698)

Briefly, as applied to alcohol, the theory would consider alcohol to be an unconditioned stimulus (UCS) that when drunk elicits an unconditioned response (UCR) that is labeled an $a$ process and is identified with a positive affect (A state). The $a$ process sets in motion an opponent process ($b$ process) identified with a B state which is opposite in affective tone to the A state, and, in the case of alcohol, is typically characterized as a hangover. Finally, the theory assumes that the $b$ process becomes stronger with repetition. In the habitual drinker, the strengthened $b$ process is typically characterized by the dysphoria and other symptoms of withdrawal. These elements of the theory are depicted in Figure 10.1 and will be discussed in detail in Opponent Process Theories, below.

The theory has given systematic status to an affective rebound process. This formulation is different from most homeostatic theories in that it calls for the homeostatic forces to overshoot the point of equilibrium. This failure of equilibrium according to the theory becomes more pronounced with repetition.

Prior motivational formulations which foreshadow the present theory can be found in Pavlov's excitatory and inhibitory opponent processes in the brain. Soltysik (1975) has most recently used Pavlov's formulation to explain certain rebound operant behavior following the cessation of consummatory behavior.

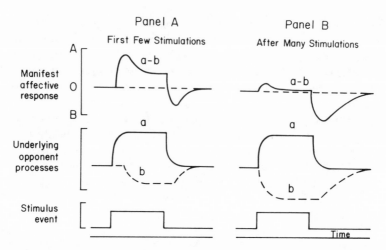

FIGURE 10.1.   The comparison of the effects of *b* processes for relatively novel unconditioned stimuli that are familiar and have frequently been repeated. (Note that the strength of the *b* process is assumed to shorten its latency, increase its asymptotic value, and lengthen its decay time.) From "The Opponent-Process Theory of Acquired Motivation: The Costs of Pleasure and the Benefits of Pain" by R. L. Solomon, *American Psychologist, 35,* 1980, p. 700. Copyright 1980 by the American Psychological Association. Reprinted by permission.

The other important analogy to the present theory may be found in the opponent process theory of color vision of Hurvich and Jameson (1974). They have used opponent process theory to explain the phenomena of negative after images. This suggests that such compensatory processes may be widespread among physiologic processes.

It is the development and characteristics of the opponent process as well as our reaction to it that are central to my approach to alcohol dependence in this chapter. As I have indicated, the continued use of alcohol can lead to the presumed buildup of the opponent process under certain circumstances and the consequent strengthening of the B state and bad feelings that are manifested in withdrawal. Solomon (e.g., 1977) has emphasized that a critical juncture in the development of addiction to alcohol has occurred when the drinker realizes that he or she can avert the withdrawal symptoms by self-dosing with alcohol. The person has, in effect, acquired a new and powerful motive based upon avoidance of extremely unpleasant symptoms. However, Solomon also emphasizes that this is indeed the model for the acquisition of all new motives, and hence in that sense addiction to alcohol can not be considered pathologic.

As a model for understanding alcoholism, opponent process theory is primarily concerned with understanding the transition from normal to addictive drinking. Consequently much of our concern in this chapter will center upon the concepts and phenomena associated with tolerance and alcohol withdrawal. Although the theory does not have any direct relevance for an understanding of how people come to drink in the first place, it may shed some light on the transition to heavy drinking and in conjunction with learning theory can also provide some testable hypotheses about relapse.

In the course of this discussion I have had occasion to refer to such concepts as dependence, addiction, and alcoholism. Throughout the remainder of the chapter I will occasionally refer to such concepts as craving, loss of control, compulsive use, psychological dependence, and physical addiction. All of these concepts have gained much surplus meaning because of their association with one or another discipline, point of view or faction in the long history of our attempts to understand the complex issues provoked by our use of alcohol. George and Marlatt (1983), for instance, seem to suggest that "craving" and "loss of control" are limited to insights proposed by adherents of the medical model. Or one sometimes gets the impression that authors think that "physical addiction" is more real or profound or more difficult to treat than "psychological addiction" or "dependence." For all of these terms that characterize the degree or quality or cause of motivation it is important to be as explicit as possible when defining the referent of the concept. Ludwig and Wikler (1974), for instance, go to some pains to make the concepts of craving and loss of control clear and precise. For present purposes I plan to rely primarily on the concepts of alcoholism and addiction to describe a strong motive to drink. I assume that such terms as "loss of control" or "craving" also refer to different degrees of motivation to drink which occur in varying circumstances. Opponent process theory is not wedded to any specific term or set of terms to describe the degree of motivation. Clearly, our task is to be able to specify the conditions, both external and internal, under which changes in motivation to drink have occurred. Opponent process theory states what some of these factors are and how they contribute to the development of, maintenance of, and relapse to strong motives to drink. In this framework the concepts of "physical" and "psychological" addiction left undefined are often too vague to be useful.

The next section of this chapter is devoted to a detailed description of the opponent process theory in the papers of Solomon and his colleagues (Solomon & Corbit, 1973, 1974; Hoffman & Solomon, 1974). I will rely primarily on the exposition presented by Solomon (1974, 1980). There are other relevant and related theoretical approaches that rely on the basic assumptions of opponent process theory. Thus, Schull (1979) has developed a conditioned opponent theory that draws on the strengths of opponent process theory and Pavlovian conditioning, and Shipley (1984), has explored the implications of a "chronic" opponent process model for understanding shamanic and modern beliefs and practices of healing.

## Opponent Process Theories

A complete theory of alcoholism would enable us to understand the factors involved in the initiation of drinking and the strengthening of the dependence, as well as the factors involved in relapse. I have indicated that the theory does not have anything very specific to contribute to an understanding of the initiation of drinking. Why people get started drinking or why they get drinking more heavily are complicated questions. There are undoubtedly many more or less independent cultural, psychological, and physiologic factors involved in this process.

Opponent process theory assumes that the alcohol is reinforcing. If it is not reinforcing or rewarding for a person then he or she simply won't drink it and will not become dependent. This does not mean that ambivalence and conflict is not often seen on the occasion of the first drink. Indeed, this is quite often the case with early testing for many substances and activities that we can ultimately come to enjoy and sometimes become dependent upon such as cigarettes (Solomon & Corbit, 1973; Ternes, 1977; Pomerleau, 1979), heroin (Solomon 1977, 1980), sky diving (Epstein, 1967; Solomon, 1980), or donating blood (Piliavin et al., 1982). In any event it is assumed that alcohol is a reinforcer or the equivalent of an UCS and elicits an *a* process which is identified with a pleasant affective state labeled the A state. The *a* process in turn gives rise to a *b* process and its associated B state which is opposite in affective sign to the A state. Solomon calls this *hedonic contrast*, and it is one of three critical phenomena stressed by the theory. Solomon underlines the importance of these: "In every case of acquired motivation, *affective* or *hedonic* processes are involved; whenever one identifies an acquired motive, one can, in every case I have found, describe or measure three affective or hedonic phenomena. These are (a) affective or hedonic *contrast*, (b) affective or hedonic *habituation* (tolerance), and (c) affective or hedonic *withdrawal* (abstinence) syndromes" (1980, p. 692).

Some examples of affective contrast will illustrate what is meant by the concept and its broad applicability. In general, the sequence of affect is characterized by an A state followed by a B state and then an eventual return to the initial baseline level. The A and B states are opposite in affective tone and the A state may be either positive or negative, pleasant or unpleasant. Although a large number of such sequences can be listed, only much additional research will indicate the limits of this phenomenon. Examples of positive A states followed by negative B states would include drinking alcohol as well as the use of other drugs such as heroin, cocaine, and the amphetamines. Imprinting a following response in young ducklings is a good nondrug example of a positive A state followed by a negative B state which is evidenced by the distress calls stimulated by the removal of the mother or maternal figure. Examples of the reverse in which unpleasant A states are followed by pleasant B states would include jogging and marathon running as well as sky diving (Solomon, 1980 cites the work of Epstein, 1967). Sometimes examples of negative reinforcers followed by positive affect amounting to euphoric peaks can be quite spectacular such as reports of people struck by lightning. An example from wartime illustrates the contrast of fear and feelings of safety:

> I crouched in the darkness in a front line trench, which was nothing but a muddy ditch, stinking with unburied corpses, amid a tangle of shell-holes. At dawn my battalion was due to attack. I watched the slow movement of the luminous dial of my wrist watch dreading the moment when I must get up and lead my men forward toward the German lines. And suddenly, with absolute certainty, I knew that I was utterly safe . . . it was a vivid sense of being completely safe physically. When the thunder of the barrage broke I went forward quite unafraid. (F. C. Happold, quoted by Greeley, 1974, pp. 25–26)

One more example of affective contrast will help explain the details of affective contrast as well as habituation or the development of tolerance. Solomon (1980) gives us in some detail the example of changes in heart rate of a dog who has received a frightening 10-second shock to its hind feet while restrained in a harness. This example is based on the study of Church, LoLordo, Overmier, Solomon, and Turner (1966). Summarized briefly, the following changes in heart rate take place:

1. There is a sharp increase in heart rate following onset of the shock.
2. Relatively quickly the increase in heart rate is reduced showing adaptation to the shock.
3. Following termination of the shock the heart rate falls below baseline, thereby giving evidence of the opponent *b* process.
4. Ultimately and rather slowly the heart rate returns again to the baseline.
5. In their study Church *et al.* (1966) used two levels of shock. The changes in heart rate reflected the strength of the shock. The rate was higher during the stronger shock and dipped lower following the termination of the stronger shock. This indicates that *a* and *b* processes are a function of the strength of the unconditioned stimulus.

Finally, Katcher *et al.* (1969) did a similar study that showed changes in heart rate following hundreds of shocks over many days. In this case after many shocks the heart rate showed a very small increase at the time of onset but showed a large decrease in heart rate at the termination of the shock. This indicates according to the theory that the animal will show habituation or tolerance with repetition of the stimulus because the b process becomes stronger as a function of repetition.

Solomon summarizes the generalizations of the theory with respect to habituation: "In general, when a UCS of medium intensity is repeated many times within relatively short periods of time, the affective reaction to that UCS often diminishes. This generalization is meant to apply to either positive or negative reinforcers, to UCSs or releasers of either an exteroceptive or interoceptive (drugs, chemicals) sort" (1980, p. 695).

In these two studies the A state initiated by the shock reflects the painful stimulus. The B state reflects the contrasting affect following termination and may fairly be called relief, possibly a pleasant affective state. After chronic administration of shock the curves suggest that the A state of pain is greatly reduced and the B state is magnified and takes much longer to return to baseline. This effect is called the withdrawal or abstinence syndrome. Withdrawal is usually more noticeable for the unpleasant B state associated with alcohol or other drugs because the symptoms are typically more clearcut and often quite dramatic.

These phenomena that I have been discussing are depicted in Figure 10.1 in schematic form. They occur in a wide variety of situations. Solomon (1980, p. 695) summarizes the affective sequence for an often-repeated UCS: "(a) The affective reaction to the onset and maintenance of the UCS will gradually decline; (b) the affective after-reaction will grow in intensity and duration; and (c) a distinctive affective quality of the after-reaction will often emerge, and it will appear to be hedonically opposite to that quality which was engendered by the onset and maintenance of the UCS during the first few presentations." Solomon (1980, p. 690) further underlines the importance of this sequence for our understanding of acquired motives in general: "Repetition of a reinforcer changes the hedonic or reinforcing potency of that reinforcer and results in the emergence of a new reinforcer, which occurs after the termination of the original reinforcer. The new reinforcer has a hedonic quality opposite to that of the original reinforcer's onset. So new or acquired motives arise from the dynamics of affect."

This formulation is very important for an understanding of the opponent process theory of alcohol addiction. It indicates how the affective contrast, tolerance, and abstinence symptoms can interact to strengthen the motive to drink. In the first place the affective contrast is represented for alcohol by the contrast between the good feelings stimulated by the initial drinks and the bad feelings of the hangover or abstinence syndrome. Athough there are many studies (e.g., Gross et al., 1971) that attest to the bad feelings associated with withdrawal, there are few, if any, that systematically document the biphasic course of the affect for the initial drinks early in the drinker's career. However, biphasic effect for other functions have been noted. Mullin and Luckhardt (1934), for instance, report a decreased sensitivity to pain in human subjects following oral administration of alcohol which was usually followed by "a short-lasting period of increased sensitivity" (p. 77). Likewise Mc-Quarrie and Fingl (1958) found a biphasic reduced excitability followed by a transient hyperexcitability in mice given a single dose of alcohol. Furthermore, they report that the hyperexcitability following chronic administration and withdrawal "developed more slowly, was slightly greater in magnitude and was distinctly longer in duration than that which occurs after a single dose of the drug" (p. 269).

Likewise, there are very few, if any, studies that systematically examine the development of affective tolerance or habituation for alcohol. There are, however, many studies of the acute and chronic development of tolerance for other physiologic and behavioral functions that illustrate how compensatory processes may operate over time to weaken the primary effect of the alcohol and ultimately contribute to the expression of the compensatory or opponent processes.

There are, for instance, several studies of the development of tolerance to the hypothermic reaction to alcohol. For example, Mansfield and Cunningham (1980) show that rats administered alcohol in distinctive environments will demonstrate tolerance to the alcohol only in the distinctive environment whereas these same rats give evidence of a hyperthermic reaction when administered a placebo injection in the same distinctive environment. Many other instances of tolerance, both physiologic and behavioral, have been demonstrated (Mello, 1972). Typically, the tolerance does not last very long and will be dissipated within a couple of weeks. However, following chronic administration of alcohol long-lasting changes have been noted (Kissin, 1979).

Finally, consider the third important potential factor in addiction: withdrawal symptoms or the abstinence syndrome. Withdrawal symptoms appear to be highly correlated with tolerance effects and have been implicated by many as an important factor in addiction. Opponent process theory suggests that there is a buildup of the $b$ process with chronic use of alcohol and hence, a strengthening of unpleasant affect which is believed to act as an important negative reinforcer for the addict and also believed to act as an important potential conditioned affective response that stimulates relapse. Such goads for relapse will be discussed in greater detail later in the chapter.

Although depression, anxiety, and other negative emotions have often been observed to accompany the withdrawal from alcohol, there are also many other unpleasant and frightening symptoms including tremor, nausea, cramps, sleeplessness, disorientation, hallucinations, and seizures. A careful study of the symptomatology accompanying detoxication has been made by Hershon (1977). I believe that for the purpose of studying the influence of withdrawal symptoms on the motivation for continued or renewed drinking it will be important to study which symptoms are most likely to occur on specific occasions. For instance, some withdrawal symptoms will occur even before all of the alcohol in the system has been metabolized. It may be important to determine how the motive to continue drinking varies as a function of these and other symptoms.

### Formal Characteristics of the Opponent Process Theory

1. The *a* processes are considered to be unconditioned affective processes that "are postulated to correlate closely in magnitude with the stimulus intensity, quality, and duration of the reinforcer" (Solomon, 1980, p. 699). Formally, in this theoretical system, alcohol is considered to be a UCS that elicits the *a* processes and will have a positive affective state (A state) associated with it. Because of the positive affect it will be considered reinforcing and, as a consequence, will be partially responsible for further drinking behavior.

2. The *a* process elicits a *b* process that opposes the *a* process. The *b* process is said to be sluggish: It is slow to reach its maximum and is slow to weaken after termination of the *a* process. An important assumption of the theory states that the *b* process will increase in strength with frequent elicitations of the *a* process and as a consequence will more rapidly and completely oppose the *a* process. It is this assumption of the theory which accounts for the development of affective tolerance to alcohol. The theory asserts that the tolerance to alcohol will increase with the frequency of the drinking and the elicitation of the *a* and *b* processes.

3. There is evidence (e.g., see Starr, 1978) that the strengthening of the *b* process is a function not only of the strength and frequency of elicitation of the *a* process, but is also a function of the interval between occurrences of *a* processes. Starr (1978) terms this the "critical delay duration." This rule states that there will be no strengthening of the *b* process if the delay between occurrences of the *a* process are long enough to permit the *b* process to weaken to zero strength. These assumptions and empirical findings suggest that the development of tolerance will vary at least in part as a function of frequency and rapidity of drinking occasions. However, the development of tolerance is very complex and has been shown to vary also with conditioning.

4. The affective state of the organism at any given moment is a function of the relative strengths of the *a* and *b* processes. If $a > b$ then the organism

is in the A state and if $a < b$ then the organism is in the B state. At the onset of the UCS, a drink of alcohol, the $a$ process is typically stronger than the $b$ process and the organism is in state A. Upon termination of the UCS, ceasing to drink, the $a$ process fades rapidly and the $b$ process fades more slowly. Consequently, the organism is in state B until the $b$ process fades and returns to baseline.

If the $b$ process has grown from many drinking bouts then when abstinence is initiated the painful effects of the B state are manifest. These have been labeled the abstinence syndrome. Although the withdrawal symptoms will be manifest in theory after a few drinks or chronic stimulation, the theory asserts that the symptoms and hence the dysphoric affect will be much more pronounced after chronic stimulation. I will discuss this issue more fully later in this section.

5. It is asserted that the $a$ and $b$ processes can become conditioned to the situation ($CS_A$ and $CS_B$) in which they occur. This characteristic of the opponent processes may be particularly helpful for our understanding of relapse. Solomon (1977) writes that one cause of relapse after treatment is primarily attributable "to the evocation of the conditioned b-process either by exposure to $CS_A$ or $CS_B$ or both" (1977, p. 100). A similar point is made by Hinson and Siegel (1982) for the conditioned withdrawal to morphine or heroin and will be discussed in the section on implications for treatment.

6. Finally, another process may also contribute to relapse. Solomon suggests that "the action of *generalization gradients* across *aversion* b-processes must be considered" (1977, p. 101). This would mean that relapse might come about if the abstinent alcoholic were to confuse the aversive $b$ process associated with alcohol with other aversive conditions such as sickness or some emotional trauma.

We now can summarize the sequence of events that are postulated to account for the growth of alcohol addiction.

People start to drink because it is enjoyable and/or it helps to solve certain problems such as enabling them to feel more comfortable in certain kinds of social situations. Subsequently they start to drink more heavily and more frequently. This strengthens the $b$ process and a tolerance for alcohol develops and along with it will come signs of discomfort associated with withdrawal or abstinence. The critical juncture comes when they learn that they can relieve the discomfort of withdrawal by drinking more alcohol—in effect, self-dosing. At this point one can stop drinking and the $b$ process effects will subside, or one can continue to drink and thereby strengthen the $b$ process and increase the aversive qualities of the withdrawal.

It is important to emphasize here that the drinking, when a person has become tolerant, is probably still motivated in part by the pleasant affect associated with the *a* process, but such a motive has become relatively less important than the avoidance of the terrors of the B state. Opponent process theory does not insist that the dependency or loss of control is absolute. It does emphasize that important, new, and potentially very powerful motives have been acquired, and stopping the process of self-dosing is very difficult.

### Conditioned Opponent Theory

Schull (1979) designed an associative model of opponent process theory. Combining Rescorla and Wagner's (1972) and Wagner and Rescorla's (1972) mathematical model of Pavlovian conditioning with the Solomon and Corbit opponent process theory, Schull presents a relatively simple formulation of the habituation process. He writes: "Thus, while the conditioned opponent theory necessitates only slight modifications in the theories from which it stems, it promises to organize a larger body of data than does either parent theory, to raise new questions, and to suggest a new interpretation of the mechanisms underlying a number of associative and habituative phenomena" (1979, p. 68). Insofar as Solomon (1977) has allowed for the joint action of opponent processes and conditioning phenomena, it is not clear that these two approaches necessarily will make different predictions. However, the conditioned opponent model is relatively simple, and establishes important similarities with other theories. In this discussion I will present only the basic assumptions and some implications of the many relevant studies.

Schull adds two postulates to the assumptions and postulates of the Solomon and Corbit (1974) formulation. They are:

> *Postulate One*: When a conditioned stimulus is paired with an A state, its ability to elicit conditioned opponents and other conditioned responses (CRs) increases.
> *Postulate Two*: When a conditioned stimulus is paired with a B state, its ability to elicit conditioned opponents and other CRs decreases, and/or its ability to inhibit these $CR_s$ increases. (Schull, 1979, p. 62)

In my discussion I will consider briefly the implications and some supporting data for Postulate One. This postulate asserts that Pavlovian conditioning will be an important factor in the development of tolerance to drugs. Thus, while the Solomon and Corbit (1974) formulation postulates that non-associative factors are important for tolerance, Schull's formulation emphasizes the associative mechanisms and calls upon the early research of Siegel (1975, 1977, 1979) for support.

A brief summary of some of the recent research on drug tolerance will indicate how complex the process is. For instance, a recent review of the biology of tolerance by Tabakoff and Rothstein (1983) categorizes tolerance effects into acute and chronic, environment dependent and environment independent, and dispositional (metabolic) and functional (cellular).

Acute tolerance effects may develop while the initial dose of a drug is still in the system and is presumably best explained by nonassociative factors. However, the relationship of acute to chronic tolerance is not known and may be a function of associative and/or nonassociative factors.

The contribution of learning to chronic tolerance is acknowledged by Tabakoff and Rothstein (1983) and included under their category of environment-dependent factors. However, the degree to which learning enters in or is critical to the development of tolerance is in dispute (e.g., Tabakoff, Melchior, & Hoffman, 1984; Wenger & Woods, 1984).

Nevertheless, both instrumental and classical conditioning have been shown to influence the development of tolerance. Thus, Wenger, Tiffany, Bombardier, Nicholls, and Woods (1981) showed that tolerance could be learned in the context of a stock avoidance task. And Siegel typically has studied the phenomenon in the context of Pavlovian conditioning studies. Most recently, for instance, Krank, Hinson, and Siegel (1984) have shown that the development of tolerance to morphine-induced analgesia and weight loss was attenuated when partial reinforcement procedures were used, an effect predicted by a Pavlovian model.

An important study confirming the first postulate of the conditioned opponent theory has been done by Mansfield and Cunningham. This study showed how tolerance to alcohol injected into rats can be conditioned to a distinctive set of environmental cues. In this study distinctive environments differing in visual cues, brightness, noise level, and odor were associated with saline or alcohol injections, and the tolerance of the hypothermic reaction to alcohol injections was measured. "In subsequent tests, the rats were tolerant only in the presence of cues previously paired with ethanol. Moreover, this environmentally specific tolerance was associated with a conditioned hyperthermic response to placebo (saline) injections in the drug environment" (Mansfield & Cunningham, 1980, p. 962). Finally, they were able to demonstrate extinction of the tolerance by injecting the animals with saline in the environment that had been associated with alcohol. The extinction of the tolerance is the theoretical equivalent of the extinction of the b process, and that has implications for treatment that I will discuss more fully in Implications of the Theory for Treatment, below.

The preponderance of studies do indicate, however, that nonassociative factors are also important for the development of tolerance. One particularly relevant and recent study by Kesner and Cook (1983) shows that both habituation and conditioning can enter into the development of tolerance to morphine. Testing for tolerance in a nondistinctive environment leads to the appearance of tolerance which resembles nonassociatve habituation whereas the tolerance tested in a distinctive environment appears to be "mediated by a classicial conditioning process that is superimposed on the habituation process" (Kesner & Cook, 1983). In effect this study suggests that the nonassociative strengthening of the opponent process emphasized by Solomon as well as the associative strengthening of the compensatory process emphasized by Siegel and Schull and others may both be found in the development of tolerance depending upon the relative distinctiveness of the cues in the development and testing situations.

Other nonassociative factors that enter into the development of tolerance would include the particular properties of the drug. One of the first studies of conditioned opponent processes in humans, for instance, examined the development of tolerance to caffeine in two response systems: salivation and alertness. In this study, Rozin, Reff, Mark, and Schull (1984) report that different drug effects of caffeine show different conditioning properties. They report: "In contrast with salivation, the alerting effects of caffeine show little tolerance, and no evidence for conditioning opponent processes" (Rozin et al., 1984, p. 117). And they conclude: "Our data suggest that conditioning in different caffeine-sensitive response systems can proceed according to opposite principles. Furthermore, the drug positive (wakefulness) and drug negative (salivation) systems seem to operate independently even in the same individual" (Rozin et al., 1984, p. 120).

Finally, I call attention here to the recent studies of individual differences in tolerance apparently attributable to genetic factors. These have included research on different drugs such as opiates (e.g., Ternes, Ehrman, & O'Brien, 1983) and alcohol (e.g., Crabbe, Johnson, Gray, Kosobud, & Young, 1982). Although not much is known yet about these genetic factors I will discuss some of the findings and implications in greater detail in the section Some Empirical Generalizations of the Theory, below.

Even though the suggested importance of conditioning factors in the development of tolerance originated with Pavlov (1927/1960) much of the research has been done very recently stimulated by the work of Siegel. Although the research has concentrated on the opiates, many parallel results have been obtained with alcohol. Thus, Wenger et al. (1981) were able to show tolerance to alcohol in rats when measured by a behavioral index (avoidance of shock on a treadmill), and Mansfield and Cunningham (1980) were able to show conditioned tolerance to the hypothermic effect in rats. Finally, Newlin (1984) has reported "conditioned compensatory responses for finger pulse amplitude, finger temperature, and heart rate when he administered a tonic water placebo to human subjects in place of a vodka and tonic on which they had been trained."

It is clear that the development of tolerance to drugs is very complicated depending on many different factors such as the drug, the behavioral or physiologic system measured, and the distinctiveness of the environment in which the tolerance develops. There is evidence that both associative and nonassociative factors may be operating to promote the development of tolerance. However, it is abundantly clear that the opponent process theory and the conditioned opponent theory of habituation may both provide useful formulations for understanding tolerance at the behavioral level. The stakes are high because of the apparent pivotal place of tolerance in the development of drug dependence. A better understanding of tolerance would undoubtedly help in drug education as well as treatment programs.

### Chronic Opponent Processes

I now discuss briefly some potential opponent process effects that may be manifested in the course of a chronic stress process. Although opposing states may be manifest after very few elicitations, they should according to the theory be much stronger and be "more easily detected after chronic exposure to events or substances having affective value" (Donegan, Rodin, O'Brien, & Solomon, 1983). A consideration of the opponent processes involved in chronically stressful situations may help account for a different array of psychological phenomena. In situations of chronic stress, associated sequences of alternating and contrasting emotions may become involved in new motives, and perhaps as important, the emotions might be related to people, or institutions, or situations because of an attributional process. As a consequence, important people in the environment might be "blamed" for the good feelings following a stressful situation which might more appropriately be attributed to the opponent process. For the person experiencing the mood shifts, an inaccurate attribution for the cause of the shift may be readily available in the form of salient environmental factors and the dictates of cultural customs and expectations. For example, good feelings arising at the beginning of therapy because of the rebound from relief of chronic stress may be attributed solely to the power and technique of the therapist, and, as a consequence, play an important role in the subsquent treatment. Attributions such as these may account for some of the transference phenomena occuring early in therapy.

These considerations simply assume that long term stresses also set up long-term opponent-processes that generate opposite mood states. Furthermore, it is assumed, as in the Solomon and Corbit model, that the mood apparent at any given moment will depend on the relative strengths of the $a$ and $b$ processes at that moment. Thus, we might consider chronic stress as an unstable balance of opposing processes, and the participating $a$ and $b$

processes might be strengthened and weakened by many accidental or systematic, physiologic, or environmental factors that, as a consequence, would also have the effect of influencing the dominant mood.

By way of illustration, I will cite examples of three different chronic stresses: hunger, threat of death, and heavy alcohol use. Each of these cases involve a chronic stress with accompanying unstable mood changes. Typically, the attributions for the mood changes are heavily dependent upon the immediate situation as well as the personal experience and cultural background of the actors. Although these mood changes do not typically initiate new motives, they may nevertheless have an important influence on the perception of the situation and future life choices.

The University of Minnesota studies of semistarvation conducted during World War II give us a closely observed example of the effect of chronic hunger stress on humans. During the 6-month period of semistarvation, the volunteers were subjected to a balanced diet designed to reduce the body weight by 24 percent. The observers report: "cumulative effects of the stress were definitely associated with emotional instability . . . unexpected spells of elation, sometimes bordering on ecstasy occurred. Feeling 'high' was sometimes attributed by the men to a 'quickening' effect of starvation or to success in adjusting to the semi-starvation diet. Feelings of well-being and exhilaration lasted from a few hours to several days, but were inevitably followed by ensuing 'low' periods" (Franklin, Schiele, Brozek, & Keys, 1948). They report other symptoms: "Tolerance to heat was greatly increased, e.g., subjects could hold extremely hot plates without discomfort and they required their food, coffee, and tea served unnaturally hot" (Franklin et al., 1948). Such observations suggest important compensatory physiologic processes, possibly involving the endorphins.

My second example of chronic stress calls on Arthur Koestler's accounts (1937/1966, 1954) of his imprisonment as a spy during the Spanish Civil War in which he was kept in solitary confinement for 3 months. "I was neither tortured nor beaten, but a witness to the beating and execution of my fellow prisoners and, except for the last forty-eight hours lived in the expectation of sharing their fate" (1954, p. 345). Koestler's accounts are particularly interesting for illustrative purposes because they clearly describe the extreme swings of mood that occurred throughout the prison stay. Thus, he describes his mood on one such occasion:

> Then I was floating on my back in a river of peace, under bridges of silence. It came from nowhere and flowed nowhere. Then there was no river and no I. . . . It is this process of dissolution and limitless expansion which is viewed as the "oceanic feeling," as the draining of all tension, the absolute catharsis, the peace that passeth all understanding.
> The coming-back to the lower order of reality I found to be gradual

. . . but there was no unpleasant hangover as from other modes of intoxication. On the contrary: there remained a sustained and invigorating, serene
and fear-dispelling after effect that lasted for hours and days. It was as if a
massive dose of vitamins had been injected into the veins. (1954, pp. 351–
352)

Koestler describes these periods of good feeling as occurring initially two
or three times a week and then at longer intervals, but they "could never be
voluntarily induced. After my liberation it recurred at even longer intervals,
perhaps once or twice a year. But by then the groundwork for a change of
personality was completed" (1954, pp. 352–353). Koestler offers one more
summary of his affective life during his imprisonment: "I had hours of acute
despair, but these were hours, and in between were entire days of newly
discovered peace and happiness" (1954, p. 348). This period of chronic stress
in Koestler's life illustrates the alternation of extreme moods, which, I am
suggesting, results from chronic opposing processes. It also illustrates how
extremely important these good feelings were to Koestler who emphasized
their contribution to his religious conversion, an interesting instance of the
attributions for this affective contrast molding a belief system.

My final example points to the emotional instability following alcohol
withdrawal. Withdrawal typically follows many months or years of drinking,
during which the body has developed a tolerance for alcohol, and abstinence
initiates a new process in which the body adapts without alcohol. It seems to
me possible that *either* the stress that occurs with chronic drinking *or* the
stress of withdrawal and readjustment without alcohol could initiate the opponent process. As Gross has pointed out "alcohol behaves as though it were
several different substances, depending upon the blood-alcohol concentration" (Gross, 1977, p. 109). It is at least conceivable that alcohol could serve
as both a positive and negative *a* process depending on the concentration and
chronicity. Again Gross summarizes the research: "Prolonged exposure to
alcohol appears to increase the varieties of toxic effects which may develop
at the intermediate and high blood-alcohol concentrations" (1977, p. 111).
And there is some evidence that positive opponent processes (Shipley, 1982)
or compensatory responses (Barry, 1982) are expressed following severe acute
intoxication as well as prolonged use.

A person's affective life and sequences of mood changes following withdrawal are not altogether clear; although the technical literature has tended
to emphasize the depressive affect, there are many reports in the self-help
literature of Alcoholics Anonymous (AA) of extended periods of euphoria
which they have labeled a "pink cloud." There are also systematic studies of
mood after withdrawal, indicating extended periods of good feeling (Freed,
Riley, & Ornstein, 1972a, 1977b) and earlier reports (Tiebout, 1949; Mads-
den, 1974) calling attention to the periods of euphoria. The reasons called

upon to account for the euphoria range from defensive denial, surrender, and identification with the group, to theistic and inspirational explanations. A remarkable illustration of a positive rebound following an all-out weekend spree in a nonalcoholic is reported by Russell Baker (1982, p. 217). In that anecdote Baker attributed his own newfound experience of power and control in flight training to the aftereffects of the hangover that followed the spree.

Recently, I have called for study of these phenomena in the context of opponent process theory (Shipley, 1982). I suggest that these elevated mood changes are a normal reaction of the organism to the acute and chronic stress of heavy drinking and withdrawal. I have suggested that these good feelings have important implications for treatment, and I will elaborate on those implications later in this chapter.

In this section of the chapter I have outlined opponent process theory as developed by Solomon (Solomon, 1980; Solomon & Corbit, 1974). I have also briefly outlined how Schull (1979) has integrated opponent process theory with Rescorla and Wagner's interpretation of Pavlovian conditioning. Finally, I have suggested how opponent processes may prove important in understanding mood changes and attributions following chronic stress. The implications of these three points of view for understanding some of the factors involved in alcohol addiction have been discussed.

## Some Empirical Generalizations of the Theory

I now present two studies of particular interest that support opponent process theory and provide a possible foundation for an explanation for dependency on drugs in general and alcohol specifically. These studies are well designed and controlled; they test specifically the operation of the opponent processes in a motivational context that is also relevant to alcohol dependency.

The first study reported by Starr (1978) was designed to study the development of imprinting in ducklings. Starr suggested that the distress calling which marks the behavior of ducklings in aversive situations can be taken as an index of the *b* process in the imprinting situation. In this formulation of the imprinting situation, the mother or object to be imprinted elicits a pleasurable *a* process in the duckling which is then promptly replaced by the opponent *b* process and distress signals when the maternal object disappears. Instead of the distress calling arising as a function of externally aroused curiosity or fear or more simply as an expression of increased arousal, the Starr formulation hypothesizes that the distress calling represents an unlearned response to the *a* process. In other words, the distress calling represents a response to a process which is building strength in the presence of the imprinting object and, hence, represents withdrawal pains when the maternal object is removed. Prior research by Hoffman, Eiserer, Ratner, and Pickering (1974) showed that the removal of the mother was a reliable occasion for the distress calling in ducklings. Starr designed his research to study the effect of the schedule of presentation and removal of the object on the strength of the distress calling. The first experiment was designed to determine whether the strengthening of the distress call was a true aftereffect of the present of the object to be imprinted, a result of general arousal, or due to associative factors that might strengthen the distress calling through direct reinforcement ("Scream and mother will appear"). For Experiment 1, Starr adopted four schedules of stimulus presentation of the object to be imprinted: (1) 6 minutes continuous presence, (2) 12 30-second presentations with 1-minute interstimulus interval (ISI), (3) 12 30-second presentations with 2-minute ISI, and (4) 12 30-second presentations with 5-minute ISI. The length of time spent distress calling was the dependent variable.

Figure 10.2 presents the results of the experiment that indicates that "the amount of prior exposure did not totally determine the rate of distress calling following stimulus withdrawal" (1978, p. 342). Starr summarizes the results: "Taken together, the data indicate that (a) separation distress is a consequence of events that transpire during exposure to the stimulus and is thus not easily characterized as an independently controlled fear reaction, and (b) these events appear to be nonassociative to the extent that prior experience with the presentation and withdrawal of the stimulus is not necessary for distress calls to be produced when the stimulus is withdrawn" (1978, p. 343). Of particular interest (also depicted in Figure 10.2) is the fact that the distress calling did not become stronger over time and with additional presentations of the object if the interval between presentations was sufficiently long. Starr (1978) and Solomon (1977, 1980) argue that this results from the decay of the opponent process which will not increase in strength unless the period between presentations is short enough. Starr has labeled this requirement the *critical decay duration* and describes the implications: "Once successive stimulus events fall within the decay period, this mechanism develops the characteristics of a positive feedback system. Stimulation both increases the strength of the *b* process and increases the critical decay duration, thus allowing integration of repeated experiences over progressively longer ISIs" (1978, p. 352).

Solomon (1977, 1980) has placed considerable stress upon this concept as at least one of the important factors contributing to the strength of acquired motives in general, including alcoholic addictive behavior. The thesis states that unless a person takes sufficiently large drinks within the critical period, there will not occur the strengthening of the *b* process and expression of the unpleasant affect associated with the *b* process when a person stops drinking. Thus this position implies that without the buildup of the opponent process

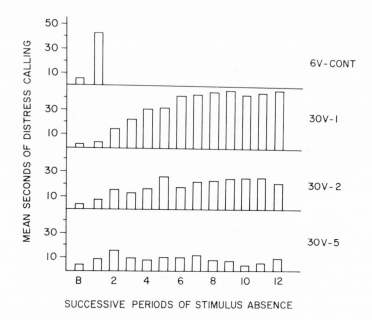

FIGURE 10.2.   Mean number of seconds of distress vocalizing during the preexposure period (B) and during the test period following each successive withdrawal of the stimulus in Experiment 1. (Designations in the right-hand column of the figure represent the experimental groups: 6V-CONT received 6 minutes of uninterrupted stimulus exposure; 30V-1 received 6 minutes of stimulus exposure divided into twelve 30–second presentations at an inter-stimulus interval (ISI) of 1 minute; 30V-2 received the same stimulus presentation as the 30V-1 except that the ISI was 2 minutes; 30V-5 received the same stimulus presentation as 30V-1 except that the ISI was 5 minutes.) From "An Opponent-Process Theory of Motivation: VI. Time and Intensity Variables in the Development of Separation-Induced Distress Calling in Duckings" by M. D. Starr, *Journal of Experimental Psychology: Animal Behavior Processes, 4,* 1978, p. 341. Copyright 1978 by the American Psychological Association. Reprinted by permission of the publisher.

you do not get evidence of the development of tolerance and the withdrawal symptoms associated with sudden abstinence.

   It is also important to point out that Starr was able to show that the buildup had effects on later tests performed after 96 hours. He suggests "a savings in the strength of the opponent, or $b$, process. That is, the structural change or memory function would be interpreted as one that determines the facility and intensity with which the $b$ process is evoked whenever the $a$ process is set in motion" (1978, p. 353).

The second study, performed by Rosellini and Lashley (1982), hypothesizes that the buildup of the opponent process is also in part a function of the size and quality of the hedonic stimulus that initiates the *a* process.

In this study the primary purpose was to extend the opponent process theory to the analysis of adjunctive behavior, that is, the types of behavior that are engaged in shortly after delivery of a reinforcer. Specifically, their research reports the test of the theory with the "schedule-induced polydipsia paradigm" which was originally explored by Falk (1969) and has been conceptualized as a possible model for alcoholic "over-drinking" (Falk & Tang, 1977).

Rosellini and Lashley (1982) describe how polydipsia seems to fit the opponent process paradigm. Typically the animal (a rat), if given an opportunity, will start to drink water shortly after it has eaten some food; the drinking will rise to a maximum shortly thereafter and then decrease during the interpellet interval. They indicate that the time course of the drinking is similar to the presumed time course for the opponent process. There are other similarities, in that deprivation will increase polydipsia and increased food will increase the polydipsia. Finally, they point out that polydipsia will not develop if the interpellet interval is sufficiently long (critical delay duration). In these two experiments the investigators varied the appetitive quality and quantity of the food pellets to see how such variations influence the rate of drinking and amount drunk during the interpellet interval. They assumed that the food pellets stimulate an *a* process which in turn initiates the *b* process which would be aversive in this case. It is presumed that the water that is drunk will have the ability to alleviate the intensity of the underlying aversive motivational state. Thus, the more appetizing the pellet or the larger the pellet the stronger the *a* process, and the stronger the *b* process and the more the animal will drink.

In the first experiment they presented three groups of animals with preferred, less preferred, or least preferred food pellets on a fixed-time 120-second schedule. At the end of the first part of the experiment they presented all three groups with the most preferred food pellets. The results showed that the rats given the preferred food drank the least water until their food was switched to the preferred pellet at which time their water intake increased dramatically.

The second experiment varied appetitive quality and amount factorially. The results also confirm the basic hypothesis: that better quality or greater quantity induced more drinking. In the second study, however, Rosellini and Lashley increased the interpellet interval and found that those rats given the least preferred, small pellets developed no polydipsia. The authors concluded that the lower quality and lower quantity "engender a weaker a-process and consequently a weaker b-process which has a shorter decay duration" (1982,

p. 237), and so drinking behavior is not strengthened. I cite this study because it reinforces the concept of the critical decay duration and illustrates again the relationship of the *a* and *b* process in a study of drinking—albeit non-alcoholic drinking. This underlines how subtle the determination of the stimulus conditions for increases in drinking may be, and also suggests that the tension a person is responding to by drinking may be generated by prior hedonic stimuli or reinforcers, such as peanuts or even tasty cocktails.

I speculate that some people may respond to alcohol with larger *a* and *b* processes, and as a consequence may develop heavy drinking habits early in their drinking careers. At a time when there is no obvious withdrawal pattern early in their career there may still be a significant motivational nudge initiated by a strong *a* or *b* process.

A critical aspect of the present theoretical approach to drug dependency or addiction is the change in motivation that is assumed to take place with the strengthening of the opponent, *b* process. In the case of alcohol dependency the *b* process is presumed to account for the increase in tolerance and the withdrawal symptoms when drinking ceases. Hence, the theory asserts that if tolerance develops there will be withdrawal symptoms, and if tolerance does not develop then there will be no withdrawal symptoms.

Consequently research on this relationship is critical for an understanding of alcohol dependency and also is a critical test for the theory.

In this context the recent report of Ternes, Ehrman, and O'Brien (1983) is of considerable interest. In this study they exposed cynomolgus and rhesus monkeys to hydromorphone (HM) and were unable to obtain either tolerance or withdrawal in the cynomolgus despite their sensitivity to the direct effect of the drug. However, tolerance *was* developed rapidly in the rhesus, who also subsequently showed typical withdrawal symptoms when challenged with naloxone, an opiate antagonist. They summarized their results (p. 327):

> Indeed we found that more than 100 exposures to hydromorphone administered to different monkeys at six different interdose intervals were insufficient to induce measureable tolerance to its sedative effects in this species (cynomolgus). Likewise, no evidence of withdrawal was observed when naloxone, an opiate antagonist, was administered intravenously. By comparison similar procedures with rhesus monkeys produced tolerance and physical dependence after only a few exposures to HM.

The authors concluded that their finding suggested a "genetic mechanism underlying opioid dependence" and also suggested "the unitary nature of tolerance and physical dependence" (1983, p. 329).

There is evidence now (e.g., see Murray, Clifford, & Gurling, 1983) that genetic factors can help account for alcohol dependency. There are many possible ways in which genetic factors can influence alcohol dependency such as through the metabolic process or the reward potency of alcohol. Opponent process theory suggests that the development of tolerance and withdrawal symptoms may be one fruitful area for research, and some recent studies reporting genetic contributions to individual differences in tolerance to alcohol in rats, mice, and humans underlines the importance of this area of research.

For instance, Crabbe *et al.* (1982) report strain differences in mice which indicate that increases and decreases in activity in a field situation as a reaction to alcohol depend on the strain of the mouse. They further conclude that "sensitivity and tolerance to each effect appear to be strain-dependent in mice (i.e., genetically mediated)" (1982, p. 451).

Another clue is supplied in the work reported by Petersen (1983) in which two strains of rats were developed: alcohol tolerant (AT) and alcohol nontolerant (ANT). Petersen reports that "when AT and ANT rats are subjected to the typical two-bottle alcohol preference test, the AT rats will consume twice as much alcohol as the ANT animals" (1983, p. 63).

A comprehensive and systematic series of studies on ethanol-preferring (P) and ethanol-nonpreferring (NP) rats have been reported by Waller, McBride, Gatto, Lumeng, and Li (1984). In summarizing the series they report that the P rats will drink large quantities of 10% ethanol and will work for the ethanol when food and water are available. Furthermore, they report that "when given the opportunity to drink ethanol over long periods P rats develop physical dependence. Studies have also shown that P rats develop tolerance to ethanol's depressant effect more rapidly than do NP rats, that P but not NP rats exhibit an excitatory response to low doses of ethanol" (Waller *et al.*, 1984, p. 78). In this study they were able to show that the preference (and presumably the ethanol rewards) is based upon postabsorptive factors and not merely taste or smell.

Clearly these are interesting and provocative studies, the kind of well-controlled studies that can be done with rats and mice and give promise for additional studies with humans. There are reports in the literature which suggest that the genetic contribution to tolerance in humans would be worth pursuing.

For instance, Wilson, Erwin, and McClearn (1984) were able to demonstrate ethnic effects and effects of prior habits on acute metabolic tolerance. The results on different ethnic groups were complicated, and they concluded that "further studies must be done to determine whether differential AMTE (acute metabolic tolerance to ethanol) scores would be useful for identification of individuals at risk for alcoholism" (1984, p. 231). Clearly the technique is of potential interest as is the work on conditioned tolerance reported by Newlin (1984) who shows that conditioned tolerance to alcohol may be studied in humans.

There has been recognition for some time that different racial and ethnic groups react differently to alcohol; however, there are few if any systematic attempts to relate racial background to differences in the development of tolerance despite some intriguing anecdotal reports. Thus, Heath (1976) citing the work of Levy and Kunitz (1974) reports: "Among the Navaho, another unusual feature is 'negative tolerance,' with long-term heavy drinkers reporting that they require progressively *less* in order to get drunk" (Heath, 1976, p. 43). If patterns of sensitization as well as tolerance could be confirmed for humans it would be of great importance. One would predict that very different kinds of problem drinking would develop for the two kinds of long-term reactions.

At this time the evidence is certainly fragmentary and practically non-existent for humans, nevertheless the theory and some of the animal studies point to potentially important areas of research, important for prevention as well as a causal analysis.

The opponent process theory in conjunction with the studies described earlier in this section suggest that the critical delay duration is an important feature in the etiology of heavy dependence on alcohol. The buildup of the opponent process and thus the postulated buildup of the tolerance is brought about by drinking rapidly enough to stimulate the *a* process within the critical period. The overlap and hence the buildup is more apt to occur when there has been large doses of alcohol; and, if a person has developed a chronic tolerance, then large doses of alcohol are more probable because large doses are needed to achieve the same effect. As a consequence, genetically determined individual differences in the ease of developing tolerance may be one of the important contributions to long-term strengthening of the addictive drinking pattern.

## Evaluation of Recent Criticisms of the Theory

In the past couple of years there have been new points of view emphasized or old points of view revived with both implied and explicit criticisms of Solomon's theoretical position. A most recent example is the positive incentive point of view expressed by Stewart, DeWit, and Eikelboom (1984). In this article they present an incentive theory of drug addiction for cocaine, amphetamines, and heroin although some of their examples are drawn from studies of alcohol. The theory is designed to account for the initiation of drug taking, drug maintenance, and relapse. One of the primary purposes of the article is to bring drugs and drug research into the mainstream of motivational thought, and they devote a considerable part of their analysis to the similarities of drugs to other positive incentives such as food and water.

In this article, Stewart and colleagues "argue that compulsive drug use, even of opiates, is maintained by appetitive motivational processes, that is, by the generation of positively affective motivational states" (1984, p. 252). Furthermore, they state that despite some evidence that these drugs alter the neurochemical properties of the systems that they act on, "it is also true that these drugs are readily self-administered by drug naive animals, and that their long-term use can be maintained in the absence of aversive withdrawal symptoms of physical dependence" (p. 253). And they finally write: "despite repeated demonstrations that physical dependence is not necessary for opiates to be sought and ingested . . . and despite repeated attempts by those reviewing this literature to emphasize this point . . . the prevailing view has been that continued administration of opiates is a function of the need to reduce or avoid concomitant withdrawal symptoms (for a recent example of the revival of this idea, see Solomon and Corbit, 1974)" (1984, p. 253).

Of course, Solomon and Corbit would certainly agree that these drugs contribute an impressive positive incentive (*a* process), and they would also agree that physical dependence is not necessary. Under certain circumstances (small dose with adequate spacing) they would probably agree that these drugs would not induce withdrawal symptoms. However, they do not agree that the positive incentives are sufficient to account for the compulsive/addictive quality of drug use.

An important problem with the theoretical presentation of Stewart *et al.* (1984) is the almost complete lack of attention to the contributions of withdrawal and/or the threat of withdrawal in maintaining these drug habits in humans. There is no discussion, for instance, of the kind of withdrawal symptoms attributed to cocaine or amphetamine, let alone withdrawal pains from heroin. The third edition of the *Diagnostic and Statistical Manual of Mental Disorders* (American Psychiatric Association, 1980), for instance, describes the withdrawal symptoms for cocaine: "One hour or longer after the characteristic behavioral and physical effects have subsided, anxiety, tremulousness, irritability, and feelings of fatigue and depression often ensue. During this period, referred to as 'crashing,' there often is a craving for more cocaine" (p. 146).

More recently, Smith (1984) gives a very similar picture of withdrawal: "following the intense euphoria of high dose cocaine abuse, the withdrawal symptoms are depression, lethargy, insomnia, and irritability. Because there is no well-defined physical dependency syndrome cocaine has been described as nonaddicting" (1984, p. 6).

In addition to a lack of a serious discussion of the human data on withdrawal, Stewart *et al.* call upon priming studies for support of the incentive thesis which could just as readily be explained by opponent process theory. Thus, they explain the increase in self-dosing following an injected priming dose by the increase in the positive affect. They conclude that "the fact that responding is reinstated in the presence of drug in the blood stream and not in its absence during the extinction sessions is the critical finding to be taken from all these experiments" (Stewart *et al.*, 1984, p. 256). But surely one might expect that the opponent *b* process would also be elicited in this procedure, which is formally similar to the sequence of experimental procedures of the work by Starr (1978) and the Rosellini and Lashley (1982) studies.

In elaboration of the priming effect Stewart *et al.* (1984) also call upon the tenets of AA about the dangers of one drink. Specifically, they cite "one experimental demonstration of the phenomenon" (p. 257) by Hodgson, Rankin, and Stockwell (1979). In this study Hodgson *et al.* show that priming leads to an increase in craving but only in the severely dependent alcoholic, and in another study (Hodgson & Rankin, 1976) they are able to show that such an increase in craving is closely paralleled by an increase in fear of withdrawal in accordance with the expectations of opponent process theory.

Finally, I would point out that they use the findings of McAuliffe (1982) to indicate that fewer than a third of those addicts questioned reported signs of conditioned withdrawal sickness during periods of abstinence. And yet this same author and his colleague (McAuliffe & Gordon, 1980) are very careful in describing the broad range of reinforcement effects involved with the addicts that they have studied: "Physical dependence on opiates is neither a necessary nor a sufficient condition for the development of addiction. Physical dependence simply sets the stage for experiencing withdrawal distress, reduction of which consitutes one of the drug's powerful reinforcing effects. Other effects (principally euphoria, but including secondary social gains, and relief of pain, anxiety, and fatigue) can themselves produce or contribute to addiction" (1980, p. 138).

The second recent criticism of opponent process theory considered here was made by Alexander and Hadaway (1982) and is also a critique of most of the active research and theorizing taking place today. In this article on opiate addiction the authors support what they call the *adaptive orientation* which is "the view that opiate addiction is an attempt to adapt to chronic distress of any sort through habitual use of opiate drugs" (1982, p. 367). They oppose the *exposure orientation* which they define as "the view that opiate addiction is a condition that occurs when opiate drug use engenders a powerful tendency toward subsequent, compulsive use" (p. 367). They immediately ward off any temptation for an integrated compromise and assert that these orientations "cannot both be accepted because they are logically incompatible conceptualizations of opiate addiction and have contrary implications for treatment and social policy" (p. 36). Despite this assertion they list the three conditions under which opiate use will develop into addiction: "(a) Opiates are used to adapt to distress, (b) the user perceives no better means of adaptation, and (c) opiate use ultimately leads to an *increase* in the original distress" (p. 376). Finally, they argue that "it is apparent that both tolerance and physical dependence could play a role in the positive feedback loop described above, although neither is essential. Therefore, neither tolerance nor physical dependence can be considered essential causal factors in addiction" (p. 377).

Alexander and Hadaway can adopt this position because they can find little or no evidence for the positive or rewarding function of the opiates (see p. 372), and they find so many exceptions to the role of withdrawal that they reject it altogether: "In sum, the metabolic and conditioning theories have to be stretched and contorted beyond reasonable limits to fit the existing data. It would seem more gracious to allow them a dignified retirement" (p. 374). Such a summary dismissal is in odd contrast to their subsequent apology that one of the main problems "impeding the acceptance of the adaptive orientation is that, because its origin lies primarily in clinical psychology, psychiatry and social work, the main evidence supporting it is anecdotal and retrospective rather than experimental" (p. 377).

However, it is clear that the nature of drug reinforcement, both positive and negative, has been very difficult to explain, and the history of theories of alcoholism is strewn with many different attempts to make sense of the sometimes contradictory hedonic effects attributed to alcohol. The assessment of the tension reduction hypothesis (Cappell & Herman, 1972) is a case in point. I will now discuss briefly some of the studies that bear on this issue following a brief summary of the opponent process theory applied to the development of alcoholism:

1. The theory does not specify the conditions under which drinking is initiated, but the assumption is made that the experience is of a positive affective quality or the person simply will not continue to drink.
2. With sufficient alcohol and with appropriate pacing (relatively short time between drinking sessions) the opponent process will strengthen, tolerance will develop, and withdrawal symptoms will begin to be felt before the next drinking session.
3. When individuals learn that drinking will relieve the withdrawal symptoms, then they will be more likely to drink to self-dose, and they have in effect acquired a new motive.
4. The theory does not specify the onset of alcoholism in terms of any critical point in the development of the withdrawal symptoms, nor does the theory suggest that there is any inevitable progression that has been set in motion. However, it is assumed that the motive will be very strong because of the quality of the withdrawal symptoms and dysphoric affect that can develop.

It is at this point late in the career of the alcoholic that people discuss the compulsive quality of the motivation in terms of craving and loss of control. There has been a great deal of controversy involving these terms. Does their acceptance also mean adoption of the medical model? Or do the terms imply that one drink will be sufficient to initiate a new drinking binge in the abstinent alcoholic? Ludwig and Wikler (1974, p. 122) present a balanced analysis of the concepts:

> From our viewpoint, based on extensive clinical experience with alcoholics, all that loss of control connotes is the relative inability to regulate ethanol consumption. Craving is the cognitive state designating ethanol consumption as a source of relief or pleasure. It need not inevitably lead to drinking. Loss of control is the behavioral state initiated by craving and characterized by activities indicative of a relative inability to modulate ethanol consumption; it need not eventuate in gross intoxication or stupor. It may even take the form of abstinence.

The opponent process theory suggests that dysphoria, the craving, and loss of control will be most evident when an addicted drinker has been drinking large quantities for a period of time. In their early systematic studies of the effect of alcohol on alcoholics, Mendelson, LaDou, and Solomon (1964) reported that anxiety levels tended to increase with a 30-ounce dose per day, when the 40-ounce of whiskey level was reached there was a significant increase in anxiety and "associated with the anxiety was an element of despondency, with overt symptoms of depression" (p. 46). There was also an "increased craving for alcohol: Requests for greater amounts of whiskey and for more frequent drinks were most marked during this time" (p. 47). This report is almost identical to the subsequent study of McNamee, Mello, and Mendelson (1968) in which the subject was able to "control both the amount and rate of his alcohol intake" (p. 1065). During the drinking phase they report (1968, p. 1066):

> There were significant changes in the subjects' affect during this period. A marked increase in anxiety and depression occurred in nine subjects during the second or third day of the drinking phase of the study and grew more intense the longer the subject drank. There appeared to be a correlation between the amount of alcohol consumed and the severity of anxiety and depression. The greater the amount of alcohol consumed, the more severe the degree of anxiety and depression. In no case was drinking stopped voluntarily as a result of these changes in mood.

At the end of the study, "most increased their alcohol consumption during the last 24 hours and some made requests to be allowed to store whiskey to ease the withdrawal" (p. 1067) which is reminiscent of the fear of withdrawal found in the Hodgson and Rankin study (1976).

Nathan and O'Brien (1971) have also systematically measured affect and reported systematic increases in depression for drinking alcoholics in contrast to nonalcoholics. Mello (1978) has reviewed this type of study and concluded "virtually every clinical research program has confirmed and extended these initial observations" (p. 1624). Mello added, "Usually, the severity of the dysphoria and anxiety tends to increase as heavy drinking continues" (p. 1624). She further concluded that "it is possible that a comparable (to heroin) transient perception of well-being accompanies the initiation of each successive episode of intoxication for the alcoholic during a drinking spree" (p. 1624), and that "the transition from sobriety *to* intoxication-related elation *to* intoxicated-related depresssion appears to be related to the amount of alcohol consumed" (p. 1624). This is a very succinct statement of what we would expect from opponent process theory; all of these studies suggest, at least for alcohol, that the positive incentive model of Stewart *et al.* (1984) and the adaptive orientation of Alexander and Hadaway (1982) are not sufficient.

## Implications of the Theory for Treatment

One cannot, it seems to me, derive a goal for the treatment of alcoholism from opponent process theory. There is nothing in the theory which implies that it would be impossible for an alcoholic to return to social or controlled drinking. However, there are clear hazards, some of which are more evident for some people than others. Thus, those who have family members with alcohol problems or those who have developed a noticeable and chronic tolerance are particularly at risk. At least one recent study confirms that risk (Foy, Nunn, & Rychtarik, 1984).

Regardless of the immediate goal, opponent process theory implies that recovery from alcoholism will be difficult. However, the theory also suggests some avenues for exploration for the treatment of alcoholism specifically and for the treatment of other disorders as well. First, I will outline some of the hazards of the recovery process, assuming that the person has developed a tolerance for alcohol and has learned to self-dose to minimize the symptoms of withdrawal.

The critical problem according to the theory is the *b* process. One must have a strong motive to give up the alcohol in the first place because of the withdrawal symptoms. This initial step may be made easier to take if the alcoholic is admitted to a detoxication program which uses drugs to alleviate the withdrawal symptoms. This is one of the first hazards to recovery since the client is presented immediately with a chemical solution that has the unfortunate attribute of reinforcing a therapeutic style of chemical or external curative aid. The alcoholic has become addicted because of reliance on just such a quick fix and further proof of the efficacy of alternative chemicals may not help in the long run. Most detoxication programs are, of course, aware of this but are reluctant to try nonchemical solutions. The chemical solution offers medical and legal protections and is clearly reinforcing to the staff as well as the clients. In my earlier article (Shipley, 1982) I have called for a reevaluation of the use of drugs in the detoxification process.

An additional technical problem lies in the possibility that the drug used for detoxication may be cross-tolerant with alcohol which suggests according to Solomon (1977) that the $b$ process opposing the action of alcohol has properties in common with the $b$ process opposing the action of another drug. The use of a cross-tolerant drug might put off the initiation of the recovery process, and/or may initiate a new drinking spree months later if the drug is still in use or taken for a different purpose entirely.

This suggests additional hazards which await the alcoholic who has returned to the community. These hazards include the many different ways that the $b$ process may be elicited through conditioning or through stimulus generalization.

Solomon (1977) discusses the potential for conditioning in terms of the stimulus ($CS_A$) that regularly preceded the onset of the A state, and the stimulus ($CS_B$) that regularly accompanied the B state. "The $CS_A$ will acquire positive reinforcement properties, but the $CS_B$ should be aversive and will be able to select and energize operants that produce State A and $CS_A$" (1977, pp. 97–98). Since there are innumerable situations in the community that have been associated with drinking and hangovers or withdrawal there are many occasions that will stimulate the $a$ and $b$ processes. Solomon describes the potential sequences: "Although the environmental $CS_A$ events may, at any time, mitigate the severity of craving for the moment, they should also arouse the opponent process and so when $CS_A$ is terminated there should be a short period of intensified b-process. Or, if $CS_B$ stimuli are encountered, a temporary intensification of the b-process will occur, and any intensification of the b-process may then activate behaviors culminating in a redose" (1977, p. 98).

Finally, Solomon speculates about the possible role of generalization gradients other than cross-tolerance that may be responsible for a relapse. Presumably substances or events unrelated to alcohol could initiate either $a$ or $b$ processes with characteristics similar to those qualities associated with alcohol. Given sufficient similarity these unrelated reinforcers or emotional occasions could contribute to a relapse. There is unfortunately little known about the generalization characteristics of opponent processes.

Hinson and Siegel (1982) also stress the possible importance of the conditioned compensatory responses in relapse. They make a distinction between acute withdrawal reactions and drug-compensatory conditioned responses. They write that "it is likely that the acute withdrawal reaction contributes little to relapse use following a long, drug-free period. Drug compensatory CRs may crucially mediate this post-treatment relapse" (Hinson & Siegel, 1982, p. 499). In a relevant study Thompson and Ostland (1965) have shown that readdiction to morphine in rats takes place more rapidly in the environment in which they had been originally addicted.

There certainly is sufficient evidence to suggest that opponent processes (or compensatory CRs) are potential goads for relapse. An important implication for treatment should include the possible extinction of these responses. In addition, for alcoholism treatment, extinction procedures would involve the repeated presentation of placebos or simulated alcoholic drinks and the circumstances of drinking without permitting the drinking of alcohol to take place. Such procedures should reduce the tolerance and hence the opponent *b* processes. Blakey and Baker (1980) report the successful utilization of extinction procedures with several alcoholic clients.

Hodgson and Rankin (1976) reported an early attempt to modify drinking behavior by using extinction procedures. They had assumed that "drinking in the alcoholic, is frequently reinforced through the avoidance of unpleasant consequences (e.g., an escalation in anxiety, frustration or withdrawal symptoms)" (Hodgson & Rankin, 1976, p. 305). Their procedure for one patient involved the administration of alcohol to the alcoholic and then blocking further drinking and the binge which they assumed meant the avoidance of withdrawal for the alcoholic. They report that the procedure led to the loss of the fear of withdrawal and the marked reduction in the desire for a drink within 6 days. They conclude: "We have suggested the possibility that craving and addictive behavior, like fear and avoidance behaviour, is amenable to extinction procedures" (1976, p. 307).

I suggest that this procedure is also interpretable in terms of opponent processes. Thus, their procedure involved the administration of a drink and, as a consequence, they stimulated a fear of withdrawal in the alcoholic and this fear in theory should also stimulate its own positive opponent response. Therefore in this case it may be the positive opponent of the fear response which accounted for the extinction or habituation of the fear of withdrawal. This analysis of the loss of the fear of withdrawal is analogous to our opponent process analysis of exposure therapy with phobic patients (Shipley, Chambless, & DeMarco, 1984).

Opponent process theory also suggests other possible therapeutic strategies and I will consider some of these now.

The theory has led me to consider the strong chronic and acute opponent processes that might be in operation, even if not manifest, at the beginning of the recovery process. One would expect that the more or less continuous stress of heavy alcohol consumption as well as the pain and emotional stress of the withdrawal might stimulate opponent processes with positive, even euphoric, emotion associated with them. These were some of the considerations that prompted a small clinical study (Shipley, 1982). Despite the almost uniform emphasis upon the negative and depressive affect of acute withdrawal in the technical literature there were hints of possible positive affect in classical literature (James, 1902/1958), and follow-up studies (Freed, Riley, & Ornstein, 1977a, 1977b) as well as in the interviews we did with alcoholics who had detoxified without the aid of tranquilizers.

Consider the report of Mr. Smith who tells of his emotional reactions following his last spree (Shipley, 1982):

> "A total out-of-control binge—scotch and water, close to a fifth a day."
> He stopped drinking and after a day, maybe longer, he wound up at home.
> He described a brief period at home of agitated depression with "inner
> shakes," lasting somewhere between 8 to 12 hr. Toward the end of this
> period, a physican was called who, in turn, summoned two members of
> A.A. Mr. Smith described his wait for the A.A. members as one of fearful
> anticipation. When they came he reported that "a great peace descended
> . . . I just jumped onto the pink cloud—not false—a very good feeling—
> a feeling I'd never had before in my life. It was different—a very strange
> peace of mind, very comfortable, very much at ease. Compared to 3 hours
> before it was a goddamned miracle—not euphoria—a peace. I communi-
> cated with my wife for the first time in years. I went to bed, slept for 8 to
> 9 hours without medication with my mind at rest. When I woke up the next
> morning it was 'like a child on Christmas morning'." Finally he reported
> that "I have not had a desire to drink from that morning on." He says that
> his mood was very good that weekend, "very much up, high—the following
> week I was very busy, felt very good—not way up. The good mood lasted
> for 3 years until one day I found myself out of work. I didn't get depressed,
> but just faced reality. The A.A. fellowship was also very supportive during
> that time." (pp. 556–557)

Further surveys of the literature showed that this phenomenon had gained earlier recognition. Most recently Barry (1982) has described some of the possible implications of compensatory responses to the withdrawal illness. Much earlier Tiebout (1949) discussed the change of mood and attributed it to the act of surrender: "I know that the positive phase comes, but not just why. Surrender means cessation of fight and cessation of fight seems logically to be followed by internal peace and quiet. That point seems fairly obvious, but why the whole feeling tone switches from negative to positive, with all the concomitant changes, is not clear" (p. 54). Tiebout further describes some of the changes he observed in his clinical work which he attributes to "the act of surrender": "When that happens the individual is open to reality; he can listen and learn without fighting back. He is receptive to life, not antagonistic. He senses relatedness and an at-oneness which becomes the source of an inner peace and security, the possession of which frees the individual from his compulsion to drink. In other words, an act of surrender is an occasion when the individual no longer fights life but accepts it" (p. 54).

Lindt (1959) discusses the elevated mood after withdrawal and attributed it to a defense against anxiety. And Gibson and Becker (1973) attributed the euphoria to the improved physical condition of the alcoholic. They suggested that it may interfere with therapy because the alcoholic is unrealistically optimistic. And finally Madsen (1974) discussed the mood change which he attributed to the combination of giving up alcohol and the influence of AA:

> As one primary alcoholic individual said: "Every drinking bout was like a game of Russian roulette, but I never really wanted to die or go mad. When I met A.A. and found that one can break away from drinking, I experienced rapture. It was too gorgeous to describe. I was free!" The double elation of a new freedom combined with the satisfaction of the group bonding usually produces a period of euphoria, which A.A. calls a "pink cloud." On his pink cloud, the newcomer is safe from alcoholic temptation. However, the euphoria will eventually dissolve and the "A.A. honeymoon" will end. The newcomer must be indoctrinated with the A.A. principles before this happens or he will slip and be off on another drunken binge. (p. 29)

As indicated by Madsen, it turns out that AA is quite familiar with the phenomenon and in their literature they refer to it as the pink cloud (as did Mr. Smith). The early AA literature tends to give the euphoria a theistic interpretation. More recently they appear to be more ambivalent toward the euphoria and tell the newcomer to "enjoy it while you can, but be prepared for coming off the pink cloud." Today, I think it's fair to say that most of the members of AA do not attempt a causal explanation for the good feeling, but many have said that it may have an important function. In a small interview study Fenley (1984) asked members of AA about the pink cloud. Of the 40 respondents 23 reported a clear euphoric experience of the pink cloud. The rest denied it completely or were uncertain, often because the good feelings alternated rapidly with depressive affect. There was wide variability in the interviews with respect to when it started after the initiation of sobriety (the recollections ranged from almost immediately after detoxication to several months into sobriety), and also wide variability in the length (which ranged from several days to over a year). Although there was considerable ambivalence about the ultimate value of the pink cloud, there was, however, general agreement that it could be of positive value for recovery. As one 34-year-old female respondent with less than 6 months of sobriety evaluated the experience: "It's very positive because if I hadn't had the pink cloud there is a good chance I would have resumed drinking right away. It made me so high without a drink that I told myself that if I can get this high without a drink then I could handle being sober. I needed to start sobriety feeling that way. It acted as a buffer. It gave me a foundation and time to build a foundation in A.A. and get some time under my belt before I had to start dealing with my problems."

I would add that it may well have been important that this high was perceived as arising from her own resources rather than from other chemicals. This, it seems to me, is one of the critically important potential therapeutic effects of the mood change. There is reason to believe that these good feelings will lead to feelings of calm and control, and that these feelings can be attributed to one's own resources. But not necessarily. There are probably strong tendencies to attribute the reasons for the elevated mood, at least in part, to the group, such as AA, or the therapist in a one-to-one therapeutic situation. It may be that Madsen has it backward when he attributes the pink cloud to the bonding. It might be just the reverse such that the bonding or transference comes about because the attribution of the power to bring about the mood is directed to the group or therapeutic agent. Thus, Pisani (1977) ascribes the relationship of patient and therapist to similar attributions: "Patients who are regressed either socially, psychologically or physically are prone to be 'imprinted' to the person who appears to be 'rescuing' them. The persons associated with the termination of the unpleasant experiences that the patient is undergoing in his regressed state will in effect be perceived by him as the benevolent figures who have terminated the unpleasantness, and they will be sought out by the patient" (1977, p. 979).

It may be seen that the opponent processes in this type of situation serve a somewhat different function than those processes which are involved in setting up new acquired motives. In this case it seems unlikely that the pink cloud is involved solely or even primarily in initiating a new motive, but it may critically influence the attitudes toward the self as well as other salient people in the family, community, or therapeutic situation.

Regardless of the theoretical status of the pink cloud, or the $c$ process as I labeled it in the earlier article (Shipley, 1982) it is somewhat surprising that this potentially important emotional phenomenon has not been given greater recognition than it has. Perhaps the lack of a theoretical context has kept it isolated and anomalous.

In any event it is clear that research is needed about the phenomenon itself as well as how it can be systematically integrated into treatment programs.

For instance, the timing and duration of the mood changes has shown great variability both within and between individuals. Such variability may turn out to be a function of definition of mood as well as a function of situational stress, and various physiologic factors. Clearly, the quality of the mood and modifying variables would be important to understand. And, also, we need to know how to handle such mood changes in an ongoing therapeutic program. For instance, how does one tackle the apparently unrealistic nature of the affect? The feelings of supreme confidence that are sometimes expressed may well jeopardize therapeutic progress. Thus, unrealistic feelings of confidence might well be more hazardous when the goal of therapy is a return to controlled drinking than when it is total abstinence.

There are other occasions in AA-oriented recovery groups and other treatment programs which may be understood in terms of opponent processes. Consider Jerome Frank's (1974) emphasis upon the role of emotional arousal in therapy: "Finally, all forms of psychotherapy, when successful, arouse the patient emotionally. The role of emotional arousal in facilitating or causing psychotherapeutic change is unclear. One can only note that it seems to be a prerequisite to all attitudinal and behavioral change. It accompanies all confrontations and success experiences, and production of intense arousal is the central aim of emotional flooding techniques" (1974, p. 330).

It is of course one of the main theses of this paper that such emotional arousal would be accompanied by opponent processes that will gain expression when either the emotional arousal is weakened or the opponents are strengthened.

We have just considered the occasion of withdrawal when important emotions are involved, but there are, of course, many other occasions for strong emotions, both contrived and naturally occurring.

Early in the process of joining AA, for instance, there are several occasions in addition to the withdrawal trauma that elicit strong emotional reactions. Typically a new member is asked to give a talk about their own drinking problems on their 90-day anniversary. Members often report strong fears and feelings of inadequacy before the talk and often report strong feelings of relief or elation after the talk. Several members interviewed by Fenley indicate that the 90-day talk was the event that triggered their pink cloud. One member said that the talk reminded her of an initiation procedure, and reported that it was the first time that she felt herself to be a real member of the group.

Consider also the therapeutic phenomena of catharsis, first described by Breuer and Freud (1893/1955) and, since then, both widely acclaimed and distrusted. Catharsis is specifically elicited in AA by Steps 4 and 5, and typically takes place in other therapeutic situations when a distraught client reports on a personal problem that is charged with emotion. Since the therapeutic context is typically warm and imbued with hope, one would expect according to the theory that there would be a reaction in the fear or unpleasant affect (*a* process) and a consequent opportunity for the expression of the positive opponent affective processes. One of the implications of this formulation is that the resulting affect will be positive, and, consequently, a person is most apt to feel good, worthwhile, and in control following a cathartic experience. Some writers have specifically called attention to the elevated affect. Bindrim (1981), for one, writes: "when these negative energies are allowed discharge by expression, the unpleasant feelings first become neutral and then pleasurable" (1981, p. 41).

The potential impact on the recovering alcoholic is illustrated by an anecdote emphasizing the importance of Step 5, which states: "Admitted to God, to ourselves, and to another human being the exact nature of our wrongs." Of course the requirement of taking this step adds to the stress of the AA member. They write about the difficulty of taking this step: "So intense, though is our fear and reluctance to do this, that many A.A.'s at first try to by-pass Step 5" (Alcoholics Anonymous, 1952, p. 56). However, they emphasize the importance of taking Step 5 and explain what they expect to happen:

> Provided you hold back nothing, your sense of relief will mount from minute to minute. The dammed-up emotions of years will break out of their confinement, and miraculously vanish as soon as they are exposed. As the pain subsides, a healing tranquility takes its place. And when humility and serenity are so combined, something else of great moment is apt to occur. Many in A.A., once agnostic or atheist, tell us that it was during this stage of Step Five that he first actually felt the presence of God. And even those who had faith already often became conscious of God as they never were before. (1952, p. 63)

Without the theistic attributions, this is a fairly clear description of what has come to be expected in a therapeutic situation. Our ambivalence, as therapists, may stem in part from our lack of understanding about the mechanism as well as our distrust of the stability and tenuous realism of the cathartic reaction. The interpretations or attributions for the sudden burst of euphoria are apparently determined by the quality of affect and by one's own life experiences as well as the immediate context including the interpretations of other group members or therapist. However, a strong positive affect will reinforce the interpretation that one gives the experience. The affect and one's interpretation are probably two factors that give such experiences a lasting impact. If, as in the example, a strongly positive emotional experience is interpreted in terms of a religious experience, then this is likely to have a long-term influence.

I also suggest that this is, in principle, similar to the impact of interpretation in modern psychotherapy. In modern practice one would expect that a therapist's interpretations and a client's expression of insight would be couched in terms of the accepted wisdom of the immediately relevant scientific theory and cultural framework. Insight is often an important shared attribution arising at an emotional crisis in therapy, and the conviction that attends the insight as a special and unique solution may hinge on the euphoria following the resolution of the crisis. The long-term effects will depend upon the intensity and quality of the affect on the one hand and also the timing of the interpretation and its associated globality, stability, and internality. I am suggesting that interpretation in psychotherapy is analogous to the role of attributions in the revised helplessness theory that is used to account for the generality and chronicity of depression following bad events (Abramson, Seligman, & Teasdale, 1978; Peterson & Seligman, 1984).

The learned helplessness theorists have argued that internality, globality, and stability of attributions have a long-term influence on depression and self-esteem: "When helplessness theory alone proved unable to account for the generality and chronicity of depressive symptoms or for self-esteem loss in depression, it was revised along attributional lines"(Peterson & Seligman, 1984).

Opponent process theory in conjunction with attribution theory can be a very potent combination and may help us account for the effect and effectiveness of strong emotions in therapy as well as the utility and mechanisms of the causal attributions made by the client and the therapist. Certainly a large number of testable hypotheses may be generated for the treatment of alcoholism specifically and other problems in general. I suggest that the opponent processes in conjunction with the attributions may have important influence on the therapeutic process in at least two ways.

In the first case consider the client in a state of chronic stress which I believe involves two opponent processes in dynamic conflict. An interpretation, or causal attribution, can presumably have the effect of reducing the stress. In the present formulation such a reduction in stress would have the effect of enabling the good feelings associated with the opponents to become manifest. And these good feelings would presumably have an important influence on the self-esteem as well as the client's attitudes toward the therapist.

In the second case consider the effect of the interpretation of the new positive emotion associated with the opponent process. If either the therapist or the client account for these new good feelings in terms that are global, stable, and internal then such attributions would tend to make such feelings more chronic, and would tend to increase the probability of good feelings on future occasions. If either or both of these effects can be found in the therapeutic interaction it would help us explore potentially important affective and cognitive factors in therapy.

In short I am saying that opponent process theory can suggest some very specific interpretations of the therapeutic process with alcoholics which depends upon the particular problems and traumas associated with alcohol. I am stating further that the theory supplies an important interpretation of the typical insight-oriented therapeutic process when strong emotional events are involved. Indeed, I believe that the theory could go far in helping us understand many of the so called nonspecific factors and/or placebo effects (see Wilkins, 1984) that tend to pervade modern treatment practices.

## Summary

This chapter has examined the affective dynamics involved in the acquisition of new motives as postulated by the opponent process theory. The development of an addiction to alcohol has been described in terms of the pleasurable *a* process aroused by the alcohol and the unpleasant *b* process that is initiated by the *a* process and is opposed to it. The strengthening of the *b* process through associative and/or nonassociative means and the consequent development of tolerance and withdrawal symptoms were emphasized as critical factors in the acquisition of the new motives for continued heavy drinking.

As a model for the development of alcoholism several studies were discussed that demonstrated how the new motive associated with the *b* process developed as a function of the strength of the *a* process and the interval between reinforcements (critical delay duration). Also several studies were cited which demonstrated possible genetic factors in the determination of tolerance. The implications of such factors for the development of individual differences in susceptibility to alcoholism were discussed.

Two recent alternative explanations of addiction were described briefly. One emphasized the positive incentive quality of the drugs and the other emphasized the importance of the drugs as adaptive mechanisms for some people. Whereas the opponent process theory does not deny the role of drugs as positive reinforcers and as solutions for certain problems, it does emphasize the critical role played by drugs that are used to alleviate the withdrawal symptoms arising from the use of those same drugs. The development of depression and anxiety by alcoholics in studies of prolonged heavy drinking is consistent with opponent process theory.

Finally, some implications, both hopeful and not so hopeful, for the recovery and treatment of alcoholics were outlined. The dangers as well as the possible therapeutic effect of the strong positive mood experienced by the abstinent alcoholic were discussed in relation to the unique emotional problems of the alcoholic and similar emotional problems of others in treatment.

# References

Abramson, L. Y., Seligman, M. E. P., & Teasdale, J. D. (1978). Learned helplessness in humans: Critique and reformulation. *Journal of Abnormal Psychology, 87,* 49–74.

Alcoholics Anonymous. (1955). *Twelve steps and twelve traditions.* New York: Alcoholics Anonymous World Services.

Alexander, B. K., & Hadaway, P. F. (1982). Opiate addiction: The case for an adaptive orientation. *Psychological Bulletin, 92,* 367–381.

Baker, R. (1982) *Growing Up.* New York: Congden & Weed.

Barry, H. III. (1982). Adaptive behavior of alcohol tolerance and withdrawal. In T. J. Cicero (Ed.). *Ethanol tolerance and dependence: Endocrinological aspects* (National Institute on Alcoholism Research Monograph 13, Department of Health and Human Services Publication No. ADM 83-1258, pp. 16–26) Washington, DC: Government Printing Office.

Bindrim, P. (1981). Aqua energetics. In R. J. Corsini (Ed.), *Handbook of innovative psychotherapies* (pp. 32–50). New York: John Wiley & Sons.

Blakey, R., & Baker, R. (1980). An exposure approach to alcohol abuse. *Behavior Research and Therapy, 18,* 319–325.

Breuer, J., & Freud, S. (1955). Studies on hysteria. In J. Strachey (Ed. and Trans.), *The standard edition of the complete psychological works of Sigmund Freud* (Vol. 2). London: Hogarth Press. (Original work published 1893)

Cappell, H., & Herman, C. P. (1972). Alcoholism and tension reduction: A review. *Quarterly Journal of Studies on Alcohol, 33,* 33–64.

Church, R. M., LoLordo, V., Overmier, J. B., Solomon, R. L., & Turner, L. H. (1966). Cardiac responses to shock in curarized dogs: Effects of shock intensity and duration, warning signal, and prior experience with shock. *Journal of Comparative and Physiological Psychology, 62,* 1–7.

Crabbe, J. C., Jr., Johnson, M. A., Gray, D. K., Kosobud, A., & Young, E. R. (1982). Biphasic effects of ethanol on open-field activity: Sensitivity and tolerance in C57BL/6N and DBA/2N mice. *Journal of Comparative and Physiological Psychology, 96,* 440–451.

Craig, R. L., & Siegel, P. S. (1980). Does negative affect beget positive affect? A test of the opponent-process theory. *Bulletin of the Psychonomic Society, 14,* 404–406.

D'Amato, M. R. (1974). Derived motives. *Annual Review of Psychology, 25,* 83–106.

American Psychiatric Association. (1980). *Diagnostic and statistical manual of mental disorders* (3rd ed.). Washington, DC: Author.

Donegan, N. H., Rodin, J., O'Brien, C. P., & Solomon, R. L. (1983). A learning theory approach to commonalities. In P. K. Levison, D. R. Gerstein, & D. R. Maloff (Eds.), *Commonalities in substance abuse and habitual behavior* (pp. 111–156). Lexington, MA: Lexington Books.

Epstein, S. M. (1967). Toward a unified theory of anxiety. In B.A. Maher (Ed.), *Progress in experimental personality research* (Vol. 4, pp. 2–89). New York: Academic Press.

Falk, J. L. (1969). Conditions producing psychogenic polydipsia in animals. *Annals of the New York Academy of Science, 157,* 569–593.

Falk, J. L., & Tang, M. (1977). Animal model of alcoholism: Critique and progress. In M. M. Gross (Ed.), *Alcohol intoxication and withdrawal: III b: Studies in alcohol dependence* (pp. 465–493). New York: Plenum Press.

Fenley, J. (1984). *A study of affective states following alcohol withdrawal.* Honors dissertation, Temple University, Philadelphia.

Foy, D. W., Nunn, L. B., & Rychtarik, R. G. (1984). Broad-spectrum behavioral treatment for chronic alcoholics: Effects of training controlled drinking skills. *Journal of Consulting and Clinical Psychology, 52,* 218–230.

Frank, J. D. (1974). *Persuasion and healing* (rev. ed.) New York: Schocken.

Franklin, J. C., Schiele, B. C., Brozek, J., & Keys, A. (1948). Observations on human behavior in experimental starvation and rehabilitation. *Journal of Clinical Psychology, 4,* 28–45.

Freed, E. X., Riley, E. P., & Ornstein, P. (1977a). Assessment of alcoholics' mood at the beginning and end of a hospital treatment program. *Journal of Clinical Psychology,* *33,* 887–894.

Freed, E. X., Riley, E. P., & Ornstein, P. (1977b). Self reported mood and drinking patterns following hospital treatment for alcoholism. *British Journal of Addiction, 72,* 231–233.

George, W. H., & Marlatt, G. A. (1983). Alcoholism: The evolution of a behavioral perspective. In M. Galanter (Ed.), *Recent developments in alcoholism:* Vol. 1., pp. 105–138. New York: Plenum Press.

Gibson, S., & Becker, J. (1973). Changes in alcoholics' self-reported depression. *Quarterly Journal of Studies on Alcohol, 34,* 829–836.

Greeley, A. M. (1974). *Ecstasy: A way of knowing.* Englewood Cliffs, NJ: Prentice-Hall.

Gross, M. M. (1977). Psycho-biological contributions to the alcohol dependence syndrome: A selective review of recent research. In G. Edwards, M. Gross, M. Keller, J. Moser, & R. Room (Eds.), *Alcohol related disabilities* (WHO offset Publication, No. 32, pp. 107–131). Genenva, Switzerland: World Health Organization.

Gross, M. M., Rosenblatt, S. M., Chartoff, S., Herman A., Schachter, M., Sheinkin, D., & Browman, M. (1971). Evaluation of acute alcoholic psychoses and related states; the daily clinical course rating scale. *Quarterly Journal of Studies on Alcohol, 32,* 611–619.

Heath, D. B. (1976). Anthropological perspectives on the social biology of alcohol: An introduction to the literature. In B. Kissin & H. Begleiter (Eds.), *The biology of alcoholism: Vol. 4., Social aspects of alcoholism* (pp. 37–76.). New York: Plenum Press.

Hershon, H. I. (1977). Alcohol withdrawal symptoms and drinking behavior. *Journal of Studies on Alcohol, 38,* 953–971.

Hinson, R. E., & Siegel, S. (1982). Nonpharmacological bases of drug tolerance and dependence. *Journal of Psychosomatic Research, 26,* 495–503.

Hinson, R. E., & Siegel, S. (1983). Anticipatory hyperexcitability and tolerance to the narcotizing effect of morphine in the rat. *Behavioral Neuroscience, 97,* 759–767.

Hodgson, R. J., & Rankin, H. J. (1976). Modification of excessive drinking by cue exposure. *Behavior Research and Therapy, 14,* 305–307.

Hodgson, R., Rankin, H., & Stockwell, T. (1979). Alcohol dependence and the priming effect. *Behavior Research and Therapy, 17,* 379–387.

Hoffman, H. S., Eiserer, L. A., Ratner, A. M., & Pickering, V. L. (1974). The development of distress vocalization during withdrawal of an imprinting stimulus. *Journal of Comparative and Physiological Psychology, 86,* 563–568.

Hoffman, H. S., & Solomon, R. L. (1974). An opponent-process theory of motivation: III. Some affective dynamics in imprinting. *Learning and Motivation, 5,* 149–164.

Hurvich, L. M., & Jameson, D. (1974). Opponent process as a model of neural organization. *American Psychologist, 29,* 88–102.

James, W. (1958). *The varieties of religious experience.* New York: New American Library. (Original work published 1902)

Katcher, A. H., Solomon, R. L., Tuner, L. H., LoLordo, V. M., Overmier, J. B., & Rescorla, R. A., (1969). Heart-rate and blood pressure responses to signaled and unsignaled shocks: Effects of cardiac sympathectomy. *Journal of Comparative and Physiological Psychology, 68,* 163–174.

Kesner, R. P., & Cook, D. G. (1983). Role of habituation and classical conditioning in the development of morphine tolerance. *Behavioral Neuroscience, 97,* 4–12.

Kissin, B. (1979). Biological investigations in alcohol research. *Journal of Studies on Alcohol* (Suppl. 8), 146–181.

Koestler, A. (1954). *The invisible writing.* New York: Macmillan.

Koestler, A. (1966). *Dialogue with death.* London: Hutchinson. (Original work published 1937)

Krank, M. D., Hinson, R. E., & Siegel, S. (1984). Effects of partial reinforcement on tolerance to morphine-induced analgesia and weight loss in the rat. *Behavioral Neuroscience, 98,* 72–78.

Levy, J. E., & Kunitz, S. J. (1974). *Indian drinking: Navajo practices and Anglo-American theories.* New York: John Wiley & Sons.

Lindt, H. (1959). The "rescue fantasy" in group treatment of alcoholics. *International Journal of Group Psychotherapy, 9,* 43–51.

Ludwig, A. M., & Wikler, A. (1974). "Craving" and relapse to drink. *Quarterly Journal of Studies on Alcohol, 35,* 108–130.

Madsen, W. (1974). Alcoholics Anonymous as a crisis cult. *Alcohol, Health, and Research World,* 27–30.

Mansfield, J. G., & Cunningham, C. L. (1980). Conditioning and extinction of tolerance to the hypothermic effect of ethanol in rats. *Journal of Comparative and Physiological Psychology, 94,* 962–969.

McAuliffe, W. E. (1982). A test of Wikler's theory of relapse: The frequency of relapse due to conditioned withdrawal sickness. *International Journal of the Addictions, 17,* 19–33.

McAuliffe, W. E., & Gordon, R. A. (1974). A test of Lindesmith's theory of addiction: The frequency of euphoria among long term addicts. *American Journal of Sociology, 79,* 795–840.

McAuliffe, W. E., & Gordon, R. A. (1980). Reinforcement and the combination of effects: Summary of a theory of opiate addiction. In D. J. Lettieri, M. Sayers, & H. W. Pearson (Eds.), *Theories on drug abuse* (National Institute of Drug Abuse Research Monograph 30, Department of Health and Human Services Publication No. ADM 80-967, pp. 137–141). Washington, DC: Government Printing Office.

McNamee, H. B., Mello, N. K., & Mendelson, J. H. (1968). Experimental analysis of drinking patterns of alcoholics: Concurrent psychiatric observations. *American Journal of Psychiatry, 124,* 81–87.

McQuarrie, D. G., & Fingl, E. (1958). Effects of single doses and chronic administration of ethanol on experimental seizures in mice. *Journal of Pharmacology and Experimental Therapeutics, 124,* 264–271.

Mello, N. K. (1972). Behavioral studies of alcoholism. In B. Kissin & H. Begleiter (Eds.), *The Biology of Alcoholism: Vol. 2 Physiology and Behavior* (pp. 219–291). New York: Plenum Press.

Mello, N. K. (1978). Alcoholism and the behavioral pharmacology of alcohol: 1967–1977. In M. A. Lipton, A. DiMascio, & K. F. Killam (Eds.), *Psychopharmacology: A generation of progress* (pp. 1619–1637). New York: Raven Press.

Mendelson, J. H., LaDou, J., & Solomon, P. (1964). Experimentally induced chronic intoxication and withdrawal in alcoholics: Part 3, Psychiatric findings. *Quarterly Journal of Studies on Alcohol* (Suppl. 2), 40–52.

Miller, N. E. (1951). Learnable drives and rewards. In S. S. Stevens (Ed.), *Handbook of experimental psychology.* New York: John Wiley & Sons. (pp. 435–472).

Mullin, F. J., & Luckhardt, A. B. (1934). The effect of alcohol on cutaneous tactile and pain sensitivity. *American Journal of Physiology, 109,* 77–78.

Murray, R. M., Clifford, C. A., & Gurling, H. M. D. (1983). Twin adoption studies: How good is the evidence for a genetic role? In M. Galanter (Ed.), *Recent developments in alcoholism:* (Vol. 1. pp. 25–48). New York: Plenum Press.

Nathan, P. E., & O'Brien, J. S. (1971). An experimental analysis of the behavior of alcoholics and nonalcoholics during prolonged experimental drinking: A necessary precursor of behavior therapy? *Behavior Therapy, 2,* 455–476.

Newlin, D. B. (1984, June). *Human conditioned response to alcohol cues.* Abstract of paper presented at the Second Congress of the International Society for Biomedical Research on Alcoholism and the Annual Meeting of the Research Society on Alcoholism. Santa Fe, NM.

Pavlov, I.P. (1960). *Conditioned reflexes.* Oxford: Oxford University Press. (Originally published 1927.)

Petersen, D. R. (1983). Pharmacogenetic approaches to the neuropharmacology of ethanol. In M. Galanter (Ed.), *Recent developments in alcoholism* (Vol. 1, pp. 49–69). New York: Plenum Press.

Peterson, C., & Seligman, M. E. P. (1984). Causal explanations as a risk factor for depression: Theory and evidence. *Psychological Review, 91,* 347–374.

Piliavin, J. A., Callero, P. L., & Evans, D. E. (1982). Addiction to altruism? Opponent-process theory and habitual blood donation. *Journal of Personality and Social Psychology,* *43,* 1200–1213.

Pisani, V. D. (1977). The detoxication of alcoholics—aspects of myth, magic or malpractice. *Journal of Studies on Alcohol, 38,* 972–985.

Pomerleau, O. F. (1979). Why people smoke: Current psychobiological models. In P. Davidson & S. Davidson (Ed.), *Behavioral medicine: Changing health lifestyles* (pp. 94–115). New York: Brunner/Mazel.

Rescorla, R A., & Wagner, A. R. (1972). A theory of Pavlovian conditioning: Variations in the effectivenss of reinforcement and nonreinforcement. In A. H. Black & W. F. Prokasy (Eds.), *Classical conditioning II: Current theory and research* (pp. 64–99). New York: Appleton-Century-Crofts.

Rosellini, R. A., & Lashley, R. L. (1982). The opponent-process theory of motivation: VIII. Quantitative and qualitative manipulations of food both modulate adjunctive behavior. *Learning and Motivation, 13,* 222–239.

Rozin, P., Reff, D., Mark, M., & Schull, J. (1984). Conditioned opponent responses in human tolerance to caffeine. *Bulletin of the Psychonomic Society, 22,* 117–120.

Schull, J. (1979). A conditioned opponent theory of Pavlovian conditioning and habituation. *Psychology of Learning and Motivation, 13,* 57–90.

Shipley, T. E., Jr. (1982). Alcohol withdrawal and its treatment: Some conjectures in the context of the opponent-process theory. *Journal of Studies on Alcohol, 43,* 548–569.

Shipley, T. E., Jr. (1984). *Opponent-processes, stress and attributions: Some implications for shamanism and healing.* Unpublished manuscript.

Shipley, T. E., Jr., Chambless, D. L., & DeMarco, D. M. (1984). *An opponent-process analysis of the exposure treatment of phobis.* Unpublished manuscript.

Siegel, S. (1975). Evidence from rats that morphine tolerance is a learned response. *Journal of Comparative and Physiological Psychology, 89,* 498–506.

Siegel, S. (1977). Morphine tolerance acquisition as an associative process. *Journal of Experimental Psychology: Animal Behavioral Processes, 3,* 1–13.

Siegel, S. (1979). The role of conditioning in drug tolerance and addiction. In J. D. Keehn (Ed.), *Psychopathology in animals: Research and treatment implications* (pp. 143–168). New York: Academic Press.

Smith, D. E. (1984). Diagnostic, treatment, and aftercare approaches to cocaine abuse. *Journal of Substance Abuse Treatment, 1,* 5–9.

Solomon, R. L. (1977). An opponent-process theory of acquired motivation: The affective dynamics of addiction. In J. D. Maser & M. E. P. Seligman (Eds.), *Psychopathology: Experimental Models* (pp. 66–103). San Francisco: W. H. Freeman.

Solomon, R. L. (1980). The opponent-process theory of acquired motivation: The cost of pleasure and the benefits of pain. *American Psychologist, 35,* 691–712.

Solomon, R. L., & Corbit, J. D. (1973). An opponent-process theory of motivation: II. Cigarette addiction. *Journal of Abnormal Psychology, 81,* 158–171.

Solomon, R. L., & Corbit, J. D. (1974). An opponent-process theory of motivation: I. Temporal dynamics of affect. *Psychological Review, 81,* 119–145.

Soltyskik, S. S. (1975). Post consummatory arousal of drive as a mechanism of incentive motivation. In H. E. Rosvold & B. Zernicki (Eds.), *Memorial in honor of Jerzy Konorski* (pp. 447–474). Polish Academy of Sciences. Warsaw, Poland: Polish Scientific Publishers.

Starr, M. D. (1978). An opponent-process theory of motivation: VI. Time and intensity variables in the deveevelopment of separation-induced distress calling in ducklings. *Journal of Experimental Psychology: Animal Behavior Processes, 4,* 338–355.

Stewart, J., DeWitt, H., & Eikelboom, R. (1984). Role of unconditioned and conditioned drug effects in the self-administration of opiates and stimulates *Psychological Review, 91,* 251–268.

Tabakoff, B., & Rothstein, J. D. (1983) Biology of tolerance and dependence. In B. Tabakoff, P. B. Sutker, & C. L. Randall (Eds.), *Medical and social aspects of alcohol abuse* (pp. 187–220). New York: Plenum Press.

Tabakoff, B. Melchior, C. L., & Hoffmn, P. (1984). Factors in ethanol tolerance. *Science, 224*, 52–524.

Ternes, J. W. (1977). An opponent process theory of habitual behavior with special reference to smoking. In M. E. Jarvik, J. W. Cullen, E. R. Gritz, T. M. Vogt, & L. J. West (Eds.), *Research on smoking behavior* (National Institute of Drug Abuse Research, Monograph 17, Department of Health and Human Services Publication No. ADM 78-581, pp. 157–185). Washington, DC: Government Printing Office.

Ternes, J. W., Ehrman, R., & O'Brien, C. P. (1983). Cynomolgus monkeys do not develop tolerance to opioids. *Behavioral Neuroscience, 97*, 327–330.

Thompson, T., & Ostlund, W., Jr. (1965). Susceptibility to readdiction as a function of the addiction and withdrawal environments. *Journal of Comparative and Physiological Psychology, 60*, 388–392.

Tiebout, H. M. (1949). The act of surrender in the therapeutic process: With special reference to alcoholism. *Quarterly Journal of Studies on Alcohol, 10*, 48–58.

Wagner, A. R., & Rescorla, R. A. (1972). Inhibition in Pavlovian conditioning: Application of a theory. In R. A. Boakes, & M. S. Halliday (Eds.), *Inhibition and learning* (pp. 301–336). New York: Academic Press.

Waller, M. B., McBride, W. J., Gatto, G. J., Lumeng, L., & Li, T.-K. (1984). Intragastric self-infusion of ethanol by ethanol-preferring and -non-preferring lines of rats. *Science, 225*, 78–80.

Wenger, J. R., Tiffany, T. M., Bombardier, C., Nicholls, K., & Woods, S. C. (1981). Ethanol tolerance in the rat is learned. *Science, 213*, 575–577.

Wenger, J. R., & Woods, S. C. (1984). Factors in ethanol tolerance. *Science, 224*, 524.

Wilkins, W. (1984). Psychotherapy: The powerful placebo. *Journal of Consulting and Clinical Psychology, 52*, 570–573.

Wilson, J. R., Erwin, V. G., & McClearn, G. E. (1984). Effects of ethanol I: Acute metabolic tolerance and ethnic differences. *Alcoholism: Clinical and Experimental Research, 8*, 226–232.

# 11 Conclusion

KENNETH E. LEONARD
HOWARD T. BLANE

The past 10–15 years have seen tremendous excitement and activity among psychologists interested in drinking and alcoholism. The theoretical approaches described in this book and the impressive empirical efforts that serve as a foundation for them are but one reflection of this. As many of the authors note, these are not fully formalized theories, but rather represent the initial steps in programs of research devoted to delineating the roles of specific psychological processes in the etiology and maintenance of drinking behavior, problem drinking, and alcoholism. The approaches differ among themselves with respect to the scope of phenomena to be explained, the specific phenomena addressed, and the psychological processes employed. Yet, underlying this diversity, several common themes emerge—some implicitly, others explicitly.

Perhaps the most important theme to emerge is the development of a truly psychological focus that nevertheless eschews sole primacy by any one discipline (including psychology) in explaining the multifaceted aspects of alcohol use and alcoholism. This contemporary version of the long-held view that alcoholism is multiply determined is enriched by a growing sophistication in method and concept, with the suggestion that the field is entering an era of inquiry that is not only increasingly multidisciplinary but beginning to be genuinely interdisciplinary. The paradox of simultaneously being more deeply psychological as well as extrapsychological may speak for a yin–yang stage in scientific development in which more intense activity within a discipline sets the groundwork for cross-disciplinary breakthroughs in theory and research. There is ample evidence in this volume of an emphasis upon the part rather than the whole and upon the microscopic rather than the macroscopic, yet both occurring within an intellectual context that respects the complex

KENNETH E. LEONARD and HOWARD T. BLANE. Research Institute on Alcoholism and Department of Psychology, State University of New York at Buffalo, Buffalo, New York.

nature of relationships among the phenomena under study and the immanent possibility of larger interdisciplinary models to explain drinking and alcoholism.

Such a view necessarily questions models that aim to explain wide ranges of alcohol-related behavior or that proceed from relatively invariant positions. While it has become increasingly common among behavioral scientists to excoriate the disease model of alcoholism, most of these critics would be quick to admit that precise identification of this model and its elements is elusive. This is probably because the disease concept is as much a political animal cloaked in biomedical terms as a model designed to guide scientific research. For many years, it has been a force energizing movements to gain adequate treatment facilities for alcoholic persons, to make alcoholism a medically respectable condition, to raise public consciousness concerning alcoholic problems, and, indeed, to provide funding for research.

As an ideological force, its propositions have tended to deal in absolutes instead of probabilities and to generalize clinically sound observations to encompass phenomena considerably removed from the original observation. Among these propositions are the primacy of physiologic dependency, alcoholism as a unitary phenomenon, and alcoholism as a progressive disease. The present volume challenges these propositions, attempting to retain the essential integrity of each, while offering alternative formulations.

One key assumption of the disease model is the motivational potency and primacy of physiologic dependency in the development of alcoholism and the maintenance of drinking among alcoholics. In this view, physiologic dependency overwhelms the individual's control of his or her behavior and explains the paradox of excessive drinking in the face of extremely unpleasant consequences. The focus of this approach is the specific pharmacologic actions of alcohol or the interactions of pharmacology and metabolic processes. The psychological approaches described in this book, by virtue of their focus, imply a reduction in the centrality of physiological dependency as an explanatory concept. This is not to deny that pharmacologic factors may contribute to alcoholism. Several of the approaches, in fact, rely on certain pharmacologic actions of alcohol in their accounting of drinking and alcoholism (stress response dampening, opponent process theory, self-awareness) and other approaches indicate that certain physiologic and pharmacologic factors will probably prove to be involved with drinking and alcoholism on some level. However, unlike a disease model which utilizes such pharmacologic and physiologic factors as exclusive and direct explanatory concepts, the psychological approaches view these factors as interacting with and as being mediated by psychological processes. For example, this deemphasis of physiologic processes is clearly evident in the expectancy and social learning approach. Goldman, Brown, and Christiansen review evidence that suggests that the behavioral phenomena of craving and loss of control which are typically attributed to physical dependence may arise largely from the expectations the individual holds concerning alcohol. Abrams and Niaura, as well, argue that "while recognizing that direct pharmacologic influences are important in the development of tolerance and dependence, it is important to consider how these factors may interact with cognitive and social learning variables to moderate drinking behavior."

Opponent process theory, as presented by Shipley, relies the most heavily of all the approaches on the physiologic impact of alcohol and the body's homeostatic mechanisms to explain tolerance and withdrawal. However, tolerance and withdrawal do not simply arise as a function of the pharmacologic characteristics of alcohol, but rather are a function of a classical conditioning process. Furthermore, the motivational strength of withdrawal in the continuance of drinking rests largely in the person "learning" that further drinking will relieve the withdrawal. Attributions concerning the withdrawal are also potentially important. As Shipley states: "It is the development and characteristics of the opponent process as well as our reaction to it that are central to my approach to alcohol dependence." Recovery from alcohol dependence is also viewed by Shipley as a joint function of physiologic and attributional processes. Even in this model, which stresses the importance of the body's reaction to alcohol in the development of tolerance and withdrawal, the importance of psychological processes such as classical conditioning and attribution in understanding the motivational force of dependence is recognized. Thus, the approaches are in basic agreement that these characteristics of alcoholism are not the direct result of the pharmacology of alcohol, but also involve cognitive and affective processes.

A belief often attributed to disease conceptions of alcohol is the assumption that alcoholism is a unitary phenomenon. While this is not an essential element of the disease model, and many of its supporters might be willing to dispense with it, this assumption has been linked to the model (Pattison, Sobell, & Sobell, 1977; Peele, 1985). It should be noted, however, that this assumption is not specific to the disease model and can be identified among many early psychological models. According to this assumption, alcoholism is a single disorder with a single etiology. Alcoholics are not seen as all the same, but they are seen as very similar in the ways that matter. As noted earlier, the variations are substantially less important than the commonalities.

The psychological approaches found in this book argue very strongly against a unitary view of alcoholism, and do so in several respects. First, they reject the notion of a single etiology implicit in the unitary consequences of alcoholism. The authors frequently observed the possibility of the other psychological approaches as being complementary rather than mutually exclusive. Consistent with this was the call for multiple, multivariate models directed at different aspects of the alcohol problems. The interactional approaches described by Sadava are, of course, explicit attempts to accomplish this. Furthermore, the authors frequently made it clear that such models need to be integrative in nature, incorporating biological, pharmacologic, psychological, and social factors both additively and interactively.

The possibility of different causal pathways to problems with alcohol implies that some alcoholics differ from other alcoholics in a meaningful fashion. Thus, it would seem that the psychological approaches found in this book would view the differences among alcoholics as at least as important, if not more important, than the commonalities. Throughout the chapters, we see an increasing interest in individual differences, and in examining the interaction of these differences with psychological processes. According to Sher, the interest is in stress response dampening among those at high risk for alcoholism. Self-handicapping with alcohol is an issue for individuals with specific characteristics, namely, a high but vulnerable self-esteen. Self-awareness theory identifies individuals with a high proclivity for self-awareness and events in which there is a negative implication for the self as interactive factors in determing alcohol problems. We see this increased interest in individual factors as well in research concerned with the development of typologies of alcoholism. Cox's review of the personality literature identifies at least two types of alcoholics, those with a more sociopathic element and those with a more neurotic element, presumably with different etiologies. Such specification of the individual differences among alcoholics with regard to etiologic processes could potentially lead to differential treatment aimed at specific subpopulations of alcohol abusers.

A final aspect that differentiates the current approaches from the disease model is the treatment of stages or phases of alcoholism. Traditionally, alcoholism was considered a progressive, degenerative disease. That is, if the disease was not arrested, one would pass through a variety of identifiable stages, each more severe than the preceding one. The clearest exposition of this assumption may be found in the phases hypothesized by Jellinek (1952). It must be emphasized that each stage was seen as characteristic of alcoholism, and therefore, the etiology of the different stages was not considered separately from the etiology of alcoholism. They were simply seen as the course of an unarrested disease.

In contrast, the contributors to this book argue that these stages are not necessarily progressive, nor do they have the same underlying etiology. Basically, this is an argument for disaggregating the concept of alcoholism into a number of component parts, some of which may precede others but some of which have no necessary temporal relationship. This argument emerges implicitly in the fact that many of the approaches strictly limit their application to one or two specifically defined phenomena or apply their fundamental processes somewhat differently as a function of the specific phenomena of conern. Thus, the self-awareness approach attempts to explain intoxicated behavior and excessive drinking; opponent process theory focuses on physical addiction, but not on the initiation of drinking; the interaction approaches, while addressing other phenomena, are most relevant to the initiation of drinking and adolescent problem drinking; expectancy theory suggests that different expectancies may influence initiation of drinking rather than excessive drinking. Abrams and Niaura's chapter on social learning theory is the most explicit with regard to the necessity of disaggregation and specification of the alcohol problems and the differential application of theoretical approaches to these problems.

In sum, we believe that the approaches presented in this book argue for a reconceptualization of alcohol use, abuse, and alcoholism. In a variety of ways, there has been a growing recognition that integrative, multivariate models aimed at highly specific aspects of alcohol use will provide a better understanding of the problems associated with such use. The approaches described in this book are on the leading edge of such efforts.

While considerable effort has gone into these theoretical approaches, there is clearly much more to be accomplished. The authors are explicit in this regard, and each has identified areas of necessary expansion with respect to his or her particular approach. Beyond these rather specific recommendations for further research, there are several general issues that require more thought and empirical activity. These include: the extension of these models to, or the development of alternative models for, females; the further exploration of the interaction between pharmacologic and psychological processes; the explicit linkage of antecedent characteristics and early drinking patterns to alcoholic typologies; an increased attention to the integration of motives for excessive alcohol consumption with more positive life-style motivations; and a more careful consideration of the implications of the various approaches for prevention and treatment.

As in many other areas of research, there has been, until recently, insufficient attention to the applicability of psychological models of drinking and alcoholism to women (Wilsnack & Beckman, 1984). Clearly, the processes described by the various approaches appear relevant to excessive alcohol consumption in women. However, in many cases, research documenting this relevance is lacking. More importantly, when the research has been conducted with women, it is not unusual to find theoretical anomalies. Berglas, for instance, notes that women do not appear to engage in drinking as a self-handicapping strategy. The description by Goldman *et al.* of studies of expectancy and sexual arousal in women suggests that, unlike men, women reported subjectively higher levels of sexual arousal under conditions where alcohol was having precisely the opposite physiologic effect. Cappell and Greeley review evidence regarding the tension-reducing effects of alcohol and expectancies and find that, again, females react to the belief that they have consumed alcohol in a manner unlike males in the same situation. Clearly then, some of the factors posited to influence drinking do not seem to apply to females in quite the same way as they apply to males. Consideration of this difference seems to us to be a very important direction for future theory and research.

While the approaches discussed in this book are distinctly psychological, there is an acknowledgment that pharmacologic aspects of alcohol will prove important as main effects, as mediating variables, or as variables that interact with psychological processes. The research by Sher indicating an apparently physiologic dampening of stress reactions among only individuals with certain psychological characteristics (i.e., high scorers on the MacAndrew scale), and that by Hull suggesting an interaction between the self-awareness-reducing effects of alcohol and the motive to avoid unpleasant self-awareness exemplify this research. Other authors point to several avenues of exploration. Several, for example, suggest research to determine how the pharmacologic impact of alcohol may alter vicariously acquired expectancies about alcohol, and how these altered expectancies may interact with the pharmacologic effects of alcohol to influence both drinking behavior as well as behavior while drinking. Additionally, exploring the interrelationships among personality factors, expectancies, pharmacologic influences, and behavior would appear fruitful.

As was noted above, there has been a reemergence of individual differences as critical factors in the study of alcoholism. Differentiating among different types of alcoholics through the use of cluster analytic procedures has become a vital area of research. As part of these clustering studies, characteristics of the individual's early drinking history are sometimes included. Other, more explicit, ties to antecedent characteristics of these alcoholics is an important domain for future research. This would include further cluster analytic studies of alcoholics, utilizing information concerning the individual's early adult personality, social interactions, and drinking patterns; the application of clustering techniques to samples of men who, though not identified as alcoholics, are experiencing difficulties managing their drinking and drinking behavior; and to samples of young men who, because of their current heavy intake, represent an at-risk population for alcoholism and other alcohol problems. Longitudinal studies would be of obvious value, but the cost of following samples large enough to allow clustering techniques would restrict the length of follow-up to a relatively short time frame. However, through the judicious consideration of transitional points, certain short-term longitudinal studies could be of great value. For example, epidemiologic evidence indicates that heavy drinking in males declines in the early twenties and suggests the possibility that this decline may be linked to marriage. Following identified clusters of heavy drinkers over this transition could provide invaluable information concerning which styles of heavy drinking in adolescence should be of concern.

Although the focus of the theories presented in this book has been primarily on excessive alcohol use and alcohol problems, it is clear that these problems do not exist in isolation. For example, alcoholics are known for their prodigious use of coffee and cigarettes. Among adolescent problem drinkers, the use of other drugs is quite common. Other problems of deviance among alcoholics and teenage problem drinkers have been noted. This constellation of features, the apparently strong motivation toward excessive alcohol consumption and the apparently weaker motivations toward more positive and socially approved behaviors, has been implicitly attributed to the reinforcing power of alcohol. That is, for some people, alcohol is so reinforcing, either in inducing a positive affect or relieving a negative one, that other reinforcers pale in comparison. However, there are other perspectives. The pursuit of certain socially approved reinforcers, such as job satisfaction and advancement, and positive family experiences, may exert an inhibitory influence on excessive alcohol consumption. When these socially approved reinforcers are not particularly reinforcing for an individual, there will be fewer constraints on his or her drinking. Thus, it is not that the benefits of heavy drinking are so great, but rather that the costs are relatively less important. Research that addresses this issue, the relationship among motivations to drink and motivations for other reinforcers, strikes us as particularly important.

Finally, there is a critical need for consideration of the prevention and treatment implications following from the psychological theories presented, and for the evaluation of the impact of interventions based on these implications. While some treatments have evolved from social learning theory and the tension reduction theory, most of the theories have yet to yield clear prevention or treatment techniques. However, several of the approaches do offer suggestions as to potential interventions. Goldman *et al.* indicate the possibility of debunking certain positive expectations concerning alcohol, namely, the belief that alcohol may facilitate motor and cognitive performance. This is important not only from the standpoint that this expectancy differentiates problem from nonproblem teenage drinkers, but also from the standpoint that such an expectancy may promote risky and dangerous behavior because of a failure to appreciate the actual impairment as a result of alcohol. Shipley reviews some work concerning cue exposure as a treatment, based on the assumption that drinking cues, through classical conditioning, may come to be able to elicit withdrawal symptoms. Cue exposure is based on the extinction of classically conditioned responses. Sher, Berglas, and Hull all suggest different motives for drinking. Alternative methods of satisfying these motives could serve both as a basis for prevention and treatment. Obviously, more research is necessary to develop potential intervention techniques, to determine the efficacy of these techniques, and to identify the individuals most appropriate to these techniques. We have little doubt that such research is being done, will be done, and will eventually accomplish this.

## References

Jellinek, E. M. (1952). Phases of alcohol addiction. *Quarterly Journal of Studies on Alcohol,* *13,* 637–684.

Pattison, E. M., Sobell, M. B., & Sobell, L. C. (1977). *Emerging concepts of alcohol dependence.* New York: Springer.

Peele, S. (1985). *The meaning of addiction: Compulsive experience and its interpretation.* Lexington, MA: Lexington Books.

Wilsnack, S. C., & Beckman, L. J. (Eds.). (1984). *Alcohol problems in women. Antecedents, consequences, and intervention.* New York: Guilford Press.

# Subject Index